DATE DUE

OCT 2 3 2007		
MAY 0 5 2010		
APR 2 8 2011		

Demco, Inc. 38-293

D1088689

NUTRITION AND ORAL MEDICINE

NUTRITION ◊ AND ◊ HEALTH

Adrianne Bendich, Series Editor

NUTRITION AND ORAL MEDICINE

Edited by

RIVA TOUGER-DECKER, PhD, RD, FADA

Department of Primary Care, School of Health-Related Professions,
Department of Diagnostic Sciences, New Jersey Dental School,
University of Medicine and Dentistry of New Jersey, Newark, NJ

DAVID A. SIROIS, DMD, PhD

Department of Oral Medicine, New York University College of Dentistry,
New York, NY

CONNIE C. MOBLEY, PhD, RD

Department of Professional Studies, University of Nevada Las Vegas School
of Dental Medicine, Las Vegas, NV

Foreword by

DOMINICK P. DEPAOLA, DDS, PhD

The Forsyth Institute, Boston, MA

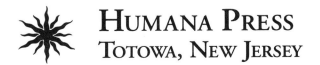

HUMANA PRESS
TOTOWA, NEW JERSEY

© 2005 Humana Press Inc.
999 Riverview Drive, Suite 208
Totowa, New Jersey 07512

www.humanapress.com

Due diligence has been taken by the publishers, editors, and authors of this book to assure the accuracy of the information published and to describe generally accepted practices. The contributors herein have carefully checked to ensure that the drug selections and dosages set forth in this text are accurate and in accord with the standards accepted at the time of publication. Notwithstanding, as new research, changes in government regulations, and knowledge from clinical experience relating to drug therapy and drug reactions constantly occurs, the reader is advised to check the product information provided by the manufacturer of each drug for any change in dosages or for additional warnings and contraindications. This is of utmost importance when the recommended drug herein is a new or infrequently used drug. It is the responsibility of the treating physician to determine dosages and treatment strategies for individual patients. Further it is the responsibility of the health care provider to ascertain the Food and Drug Administration status of each drug or device used in their clinical practice. The publisher, editors, and authors are not responsible for errors or omissions or for any consequences from the application of the information presented in this book and make no warranty, express or implied, with respect to the contents in this publication.

Cover design by Patricia F. Cleary
Production Editor: Robin B. Weisberg

For additional copies, pricing for bulk purchases, and/or information about other Humana titles, contact Humana at the above address or at any of the following numbers: Tel.: 973-256-1699; Fax: 973-256-8341; E-mail: humana@humanapr.com or visit our website at http://humanapress.com

This publication is printed on acid-free paper. ∞
ANSI Z39.48-1984 (American National Standards Institute) Permanence of Paper for Printed Library Materials.

Photocopy Authorization Policy:
Authorization to photocopy items for internal or personal use, or the internal or personal use of specific clients is granted by Humana Press, provided that the base fee of US $25.00 per copy is paid directly to the Copyright Clearance Center (CCC), 222 Rosewood Dr., Danvers MA 01923. For those organizations that have been granted a photocopy license from the CCC, a separate system of payment has been arranged and is acceptable to the Humana Press. The fee code for users of the Transactional Reporting Service is 1-58829-192-8/05 $25.00.

Printed in the United States of America. 10 9 8 7 6 5 4 3 2 1

eISBN 1-59259-831-5

Library of Congress Cataloging-in-Publication Data

Nutrition and oral medicine / edited by Riva Touger-Decker, David A. Sirois, and Connie C. Mobley ;
foreword by Dominick P. DePaola.
    p. ; cm.
    Includes bibliographical references and index.
    ISBN 1-58829-192-8 (alk. paper)
    1. Teeth--Care and hygiene. 2. Dental public health. 3. Mouth--Care and hygiene. I. Touger-Decker, Riva.
II. Sirois, David. III. Mobley, Connie C.
    [DNLM: 1. Oral Health. 2. Diet. 3. Mouth Diseases--etiology. 4. Nutrition Disorders--complications.
5. Nutrition.   WU 113.7 N9757 2004]
    RK61.N88 2004
    617.6'01--dc22

                                                                                    2004001616

Dedication

Former Israeli Prime Minister Golda Meir once said *"I never did anything alone. Whatever was accomplished in this country was accomplished collectively" (1)*. Rarely are accomplishments solo products. They are the result of team work and mutual respect. For the most part, the first person, nominative case plural is the operative pronoun of accomplishment, not the singular. In this regard, our colleagues, students, and fellow practitioners constitute the corporate "we" of accomplishment. We dedicate this work to you with this simple sentence: "We did it!"

Thank you to our parents, who gave us the guidance, inspiration, and encouragement to succeed in anything we do and to our spouses and our children without whose support, patience, and understanding we never would have been able to complete this book.

Thank you to our students, colleagues, faculty, and staff at the University of Medicine and Dentistry of New Jersey, University of Texas Health Sciences Center at San Antonio Dental School, and New York University College of Dentistry for providing insight, support, challenges and opportunities to advance the education, practice, and research surrounding nutrition and oral medicine.

Thank you to the editors and staff at Humana Press, in particular Dr. Adrianne Bendich, for their foresight in seeing the need for this book and their guidance in the technical phases of production and publication.

REFERENCE

1. Meir G. Quote from Remarks to Egyptian President Anwar el-Sadat during his unprecedented visit to Israel, news summaries 21 Nov 77. Bartleby.com. Internet: http://www.bartleby.com/63/31/231.html (Accessed 10 May 2003).

Series Editor's Introduction

The *Nutrition and Health* series of books have an overriding mission to provide health professionals with texts that are considered essential because each includes (1) a synthesis of the state of the science; (2) timely, in-depth reviews by the leading researchers in their respective fields; (3) extensive, up-to-date fully annotated reference lists; (4) a detailed index; (5) relevant tables and figures; (6) identification of paradigm shifts and the consequences; (7) virtually no overlap of information between chapters, but targeted, interchapter referrals; (8) suggestions of areas for future research; and (9) balanced, data-driven answers to patient /health professionals' questions that are based on the totality of evidence rather than the findings of any single study.

The series' volumes are not the outcome of a symposium. Rather, each editor has the potential to examine a chosen area with a broad perspective, both in subject matter as well as in the choice of chapter authors. The international perspective, especially with regard to public health initiatives, is emphasized where appropriate. The editors, whose trainings are both research- and practice-oriented, have the opportunity to develop a primary objective for their book, define the scope and focus, and then invite the leading authorities from around the world to be part of their initiative. The authors are encouraged to provide an overview of the field, discuss their own research, and relate the research findings to potential human health consequences. Because each book is developed *de novo*, the chapters are coordinated so that the resulting volume imparts greater knowledge than the sum of the information contained in the individual chapters.

Nutrition and Oral Medicine, edited by Riva Touger-Decker, David Sirois, and Connie Mobley, clearly exemplifies the goals of the *Nutrition and Health* series. The editors are internationally recognized leaders in the field of dentistry and nutrition. Moreover, they are excellent communicators and have worked tirelessly to develop a book that is destined to be the benchmark in the field because of its extensive, practice-based, in-depth chapters covering the most important aspects of the effects of diet and its nutrient components on the development, growth, maintenance, disease prevention, as well as disease treatment in the oral cavity and pharynx. The editors have chosen 24 of the most well-recognized and respected authors to contribute the 18 informative chapters in the volume. The foreword, contributed by Dominick DePaola, highlights the book's clear, well-organized information about the interactions between nutrition and dentistry that can be used daily by both health professionals and students. Unique appendices, including the latest Dietary Reference Intake charts, oral nutrition risk-assessment tools, a body mass index table, a cranial nerve assessment chart, and diet education tools are provided for the reader, further assuring that this volume will be the key resource for professionals in the fields of nutrition, dietetics, and dentistry. Finally, to fulfill the objectives of the editors to provide clear guidance to readers, where appropriate, chapters include a chart entitled "Guidelines for Practice" that includes columns for oral health professionals and nutrition professionals and examines their roles in both prevention and intervention.

The book chapters are logically organized to provide the reader with all of the basics in both oral health and nutrition. The unique chapters in first section, "Synergistic Relationships Between Nutrition and Health," include a comprehensive discussion of the terms "diet quality" and "nutrition," numerous comprehensive tables that compare the dietary intake recommendations from authoritative sources including the USDA's Dietary Guidelines for Americans; the Dietary Reference Intakes from the National Academy of Sciences; and recommendations from the World Health Organization, the American Heart Association, the American Diabetes Association, and the National Cholesterol Education Program. Tables that describe dietary practices to optimize oral health in infants and young and older children are also included. The process of tooth development and the consequences of tooth loss and caries development; oral health issues in children with special needs; effects of oral surgery and tooth replacement; and the role of culture, ethnicity, religious practices, societal, and technical influences on food choices and feeding practices are also reviewed in the comprehensive chapters in the first section.

There are two ways to look at the interactions between nutrition and oral health: factors that affect the oral cavity and their consequences to nutritional status, and vice versa, nutrient effects—with more emphasis on deficiencies and their effects on oral physiology. The second section contains two complementary, in-depth chapters that examine the "Synergistic Relationships Between Oral and General Health" with an emphasis on nutrition. For example, areas covered in the two chapters include the gingival responses to plaque, pregnancy, menstruation, puberty, diabetes, and other life events. The interactions between diet and caries formation, effects of smoking, orofacial pain, and dysphagia are included as well. Detailed tables that list drugs that can affect nutritional status and oral health, drugs that alter food absorption, and clinical manifestations of vitamin deficiencies that can be detected in the oral cavity provide the reader with clear, easily accessible information.

Cutting-edge discussions of the "Relationship Between Nutrition and Oral Health" are presented in the four chapters in the following section. Areas covered include enamel developmental defects resulting from poor maternal dietary intake; specific discussions of essential nutrients and the oral signs of marginal micronutrient deficiencies; the critical requirement for salivary secretion and an intact oral mucosa; nutritional factors that affect the risk for oral cancers and, additionally, the effects of oral cancers on nutritional status, development of dental plaque and its prevention. Critical issues involved with tooth loss and subsequent loss of alveolar bone; loss of soft tissues in the oral cavity because of congenital defects, accidents, cancer, or other causes are examined in the light of their nutritional consequences. Other topics include oral pain, immune disorders, diminished taste and smell, and the current state of the science with regard to the use of complementary and alternative medicine practices in the oral cavity. Of great importance, the editors and authors have provided chapters that balance the most technical information with discussions of its importance for patients as well as graduate nutrition and dental students, related health professionals and research-based academicians.

The fourth section examines "Selected Diseases/Conditions With Known Nutrition and Oral Health Relationships." Separate in-depth, cutting-edge chapters address the effects of diabetes, oral and pharyngeal cancer, human deficiency virus infection, osteoporosis, and wound healing. Each of the chapters begins with an overall review of the disease and its systemic effects, and then discusses the specific consequences to the oral cavity. Numerous detailed tables and figures assist the reader in comprehending the complexities of each of the disease states and their effects on taste, salivary secretion, mastication, swallowing, and absorption of nutrients. With regard to diabetes, the dental team can be of great service in identifying patients with undiagnosed diabetes as 70% of all adults visit the dentist at least once a year and oral signs of diabetes occur early in disease development. This chapter contains many detailed tables that describe the steps in diabetes surveillance, treatment guidelines for oral infections often seen in diabetics, oral drugs used in diabetes treatment and dosing regimes, another table on the types of insulins used and their dosing schedules, and goals for medical nutrition therapy in diabetics, as well as a list of relevant websites. With regard to oral and pharyngeal cancers, it is critical to note that smoking and alcoholic beverages are linked to 75% of cases. The associations between these cancers and intakes of fruits, vegetables, breads, grains, cereals, meats, dairy, and fiber are shown in detailed tables. Information is also provided concerning dietary supplements and the evidence of their actions in precancerous oral lesions.

The next chapter looks in depth at the effects of HIV infection and treatment in the oral cavity. As with diabetes, the first signs of HIV infection may be seen in the mouth by the oral health team. The clinical signs of immune suppression in the oral cavity may be manifest in viral infections that can include herpes, cytomegalovirus, Epstein-Barr virus, human herpes virus (which can result ultimately in Kaposi's sarcoma) and human papilloma virus—all of which are tabulated. There is also detailed information on the sources of fungal and bacterial infections. Finally, there are in-depth guidelines for the nutritional management of oral HIV and related infections.

Autoimmune diseases, reviewed in the next chapter, are also often diagnosed by evaluating the changes seen in the oral cavity. The example used is pernicious anemia, an autoimmune disease directly related to nutrition as it results in vitamin B_{12} deficiency; its initial symptoms include a red and smooth tongue and general weakness. Other autoimmune diseases discussed include systemic lupus erythematosus, rheumatoid arthritis, and Sjogren's syndrome. The clinical features for each disease that are reviewed include both general diagnosis and treatment, oral complications of the disease, and its clinical management, with separate sections for drugs and nutritional management. The chapter on osteoporosis includes a careful review of the clinical literature on the possible links between loss of systemic and alveolar bone (in the jaw). There appears to be a relationship between osteoporosis in women and periodontal disease. There is a comprehensive review of the current anti-osteoporosis therapies as well as the consistent findings that low intakes of calcium and vitamin D increase the risk of osteoporosis, as well as periodontal disease and alveolar bone loss in the jaw. The final chapter in this section deals with wound healing and reviews the general physiology of wound healing and nutrients that have been found to enhance the process. There are many potential types of injury to the oral cavity including physical, chemical, thermal, and mechanical injuries. Lifestyle choices such as chewing tobacco, and diseases such as kidney disease, and certain medications that impair wound healing are also discussed in depth. Thus, the six chapters in this section provide a wealth of clinical information that focuses on providing detailed data in well-organized tables so that readers have important information at their fingertips.

The last section of the book includes two unique chapters on "Nutrition and Oral Medicine: Education and Practice." The first chapter explores the value of using a novel tool, the "Oral Nutrition Health Risk Assessment" tool in the evaluation of patients. By using the tabulated set of questions, the health care provider can determine the patient's health history, use of drugs and dietary supplements, and eating habits. This tool can be very effective in identifying some of the serious eating disorders such as bulimia and anorexia that can be hidden from family members or never identified early in the disease process by other health providers. The emphasis in this chapter is on the importance of the team approach, including the dietitian, to have a full evaluation of the dental patient. The final chapter provides an integrated plan for the inclusion of nutrition information in the dental education process. Nutrition education should be a core component of both pre- and postdoctoral education and continue to be updated with targeted continuing education courses. Tables are provided that indicate the required areas of focus for both the nutrition and dental professionals in order for the dental education to be optimal. Certainly, this comprehensive volume could easily serve as the text for such education programs.

Hallmarks of all the chapters include complete definitions of terms with the abbreviation fully defined for the reader and consistent use of terms between chapters. There are numerous relevant tables, graphs, and figures, as well as up-to-date references; all chapters include a conclusion section that provides the highlights of major findings. The volume contains a highly annotated index and within chapters, readers are referred to relevant information in other chapters.

This important text provides practical, data-driven resources based on the totality of the evidence to help the reader evaluate the critical role of nutrition, especially in at-risk populations, in optimizing health, and preventing diseases in the oral cavity. The overarching goal of the editors is to provide fully referenced information to health professionals so they may have a balanced perspective on the value of foods and nutrients that are routinely consumed and how these help to maintain oral health.

In conclusion, *Nutrition and Oral Medicine* provides dietitians and dental professionals in many areas of research and practice with the most up-to-date, well-referenced, and easy-to-understand volume on the importance of nutrition in optimizing oral health currently available. Actually, all health professionals can find valuable information about the links between systemic and oral health and nutrition in this benchmark volume. This text will serve the reader as the most authoritative resource in the field to date and is a very welcome addition to the *Nutrition and Health* series.

Adrianne Bendich, PhD, FACN
Series Editor

Foreword

Many of the nation's most significant health problems are linked to poor dietary practices and under- and overnutrition. Most notably, a recent report of the Surgeon General of the United States indicated that a large proportion of the population is overweight with attendant risks for a host of chronic diseases including, among others, cardiovascular disease, diabetes, some forms of cancers, and hypertension. Consequently, there has been a flurry of activity by the food industry, including food manufacturers, the federal government, the academic community, and consumer groups to increase public awareness of the deadly risks of excessive food consumption and the importance of a balanced diet for nutrition and systemic health. The problem, however, is neither simple nor easy to reverse.

It does not help that virtually each day, the public is bombarded with conflicting nutritional messages including the nutrient *du jour* that is associated with cancer, only to be reversed in a few weeks with a confounding study, and the plethora of dietary regimes espoused in best selling books, by charismatic salespeople and seemingly endless infomercials. Even the staid "Food Guide Pyramid" has come under attack because it does not address portion sizes, "good" fats, and on and on. In total, the sum of all these commentaries, whether based on good science or pseudoscience is a confused consumer who does not know what or when to believe. The net result is a public at risk for disease!

So, too, oral health and nutrition! This is a field that has moved forward ever so slowly mainly because of a dearth of investigators and educators adequately trained in nutrition. Additionally, the field of nutrition and oral health has been plagued by a legacy of poor, uncontrolled and flawed nutrition studies; a legacy of oversimplification of research results; a legacy of clinical practitioners who either were true believers that diet and nutrition was critically linked to the diagnosis and treatment of oral disease and disorders, or clinical practitioners who did not believe that nutrition had anything to do with oral disease and disorders, in spite of studies to the contrary. In addition, because of the lack of education and training and paucity of insurance reimbursement for nutrition care, many educators, practitioners and, thus, the consumer are confused and consequently remain at risk for oral disease and disorders. Both the general diet and nutrition dilemma as well as the oral health issue are compounded by the lack of funding of nutrition science by the government and by the small proportion of the health care dollar (less than 5%) that is spent on prevention!

In my considered view, the common denominator between overnutrition, poor dietary practices, and risk of chronic and oral diseases is the lack of an evidence-based approach to nutrition, medicine, and dental medicine. In this text, the editors (Touger-Decker, Mobley, and Sirois) call upon some of the finest investigators, educators, and clinical practitioners to provide the evidence linking (or not) nutrition and dietary practices to oral diseases and disorders. To be sure, in the past decade, nutrition research has seen a major shift in emphasis from epidemiology and food intake studies to outcomes research, clinical studies, molecular biology, genetics and physiology. Thus, the evidence base for linking nutrition causally or as risk factor(s) to specific diseases and disorders, including oral disease, is about to explode.

Indeed, with the vast array of information available about the human genome, it is anticipated that the role of nutrients and, by implication, dietary practices on gene expression, nutrient-relevant metabolomics and proteomics will enable an understanding of the response of whole systems to nutrients (1). The application of these "nutrigenomic" tools will provide a fundamental basis for understanding how, for example, craniofacial defects can be prevented; how oral cancer can be detected early; how periodontal inflammation and metabolic stress are related; and how early molecular biomarkers for individuals can be used to reduce the risk of oral diseases and disorders.

In this same regard, with the growing data that links systemic health and well-being to oral infection, particularly in the areas of low birthweight, cardiovascular disease, stroke, and diabetes, the understanding of gene–nutrient interactions can result in even more profound discoveries. For example, there is growing evidence that the nutrition a fetus receives, as measured by low birthweight, may influence the risk of adult onset diabetes, heart disease, and some cancers. Specific nutrients can create "epigenetic" changes such that the sequence of a specific genome does not change, but, selective nutrients can silence or activate specific genes. If one puts together the growing evidence relating oral infection to low birthweight, it would be easy to speculate how the mother's specific nutrient intake patterns could affect gene expression, and how the combination of oral infections and poor dietary practices can lead to major risk for chronic disease later in life! However, similar to the folate–neural tube relationship, before the clinical practitioner will be able to use this information for the public good, he or she must wait until the preponderance of evidence favors dietary intervention. Unfortunately, that has not always been the case!

Although there is much promise in applying the excitement of nutrigenomics to conditions of oral health and disease, there are also many other relationships that must be explored that have direct implications to the public. Tantamount to these relationships is the understanding that nutrients and dietary intake patterns must be the basis for prevention of diseases and disorders. Indeed, messages to the public must integrate contemporary dietary practice knowledge with scientific nutritional evidence and consumer behavior in order to be effective. In this regard, it is critical that single nutrients are not labeled good or evil, but that there is an understanding that dietary intake patterns themselves can affect specific nutrient absorption, transport, and utilization. Witness the recent publication in *Nature (2)* that demonstrates that although consumption of plain, dark chocolate results in an increased total antioxidant capacity and the (-)epicatechin content of blood plasma, these effects are markedly reduced when the chocolate is consumed with milk. These data are consistent with previous dietary recommendations linking intake of nutrients to dental caries. For it is not only the extent and frequency of the fermentable carbohydrates that contributes to caries risk, but the specific foods ingested and the order in which the foods are consumed.

Because nutrition is one of the truly integrative sciences, where molecules derived from the genome could be traced to use in metabolic pathways, it is likely that data forthcoming from genomics and proteomics will provide confirmatory evidence of the real role of nutrition and dietary practices to diseases and disorders. It is also likely that the forthcoming discoveries will demonstrate that the physiologic system of the human does not discriminate between a tissue found in the liver from one found in the oral cavity. Thus, contemporary nutrition and dietary practices must pay close attention to the evidence derived from these nutrient–genetic metabolic studies in order to provide students, the practitioner, and the consumer with the evidence necessary to prevent, diagnose, and treat human disease. It is also likely that these types of data will enable the public to understand that health and reduced risk of future disease, including oral disease, is what nutrition is all about.

The bottom line is that dietary recommendations and practices must be based on scientific evidence and the scientific community and the education community must not be afraid to change these recommendations if the evidence dictates. In order to get there, we need more education and training practices in nutrition; more linkages between nutrition, medicine, and dentistry; greater involvement of dietetics and clinical nutrition in medical/dental practice; improved funding of nutritional science; informed clinical practitioners and consumers; and a serious evidence-based approach to the science and art of the exciting and dynamic world of nutrition and oral medicine practice! Providing the reader with the evidence to make informed clinical judgments about risk and intervention are what this text is about.

Dominick P. DePaola, DDS, PhD
President and CEO
The Forsyth Institute, Boston, MA

REFERENCES

1. Miller M, Kersten S. Nutrigenomics: goals and strategies. Nature Reviews/Genetics 2003; 4:315–322.
2. Serafini M, Bugianesi R, Maiani G, Valtuena S, DeSantis S, and Crozier A. Plasma antioxidants from chocolate. Nature 2003;424:1013.

Preface

Nutrition and Oral Medicine was written to fill an existing void in the nutrition and dental literature. The primary aims of this book are to target the known complex, multifaceted relationships between diet/nutrition and oral health. The reader will find chapters focusing on oral and dental diseases and disorders, oral manifestations of systemic diseases, and discussions of the synergy between oral tissues and nutrients. Specific topics, such as diet and head, neck, and oral cancers, are examined in the light of nutrition intervention strategies. Oral and systemic diseases and orofacial pain syndromes are addressed via their relationship and impact on nutrition status, the impact of medications and treatments on the oral cavity and nutrition status. Suggested management strategies are paired with selected topics. Cutting-edge research issues regarding the relationship of individual antioxidants, trace elements, polyphenols, and other nutrient substrates and oral health/disease are covered. The links between compromised immunity, oral infections, systemic disease, and nutrient deficiencies in relation to oral diseases and systemic diseases with oral manifestations are included as well as the impact of impaired host defense on oral and nutrition health.

The book is divided into five sections: oral and general health, nutrition and general health, nutrition and oral health, select oral and systemic diseases with known nutrition and oral health interfaces, and nutrition and oral health education and practice. Chapters in each section examine the research and practice relative to the topic as well as address current issues. Several screening and education tools are included for our readers to use for educational purposes. We hope our colleagues in dental, dietetics, allied health, and medical education and practice, as well as students in the fields of nutrition/dietetics, dentistry, and related disciplines whose research, practice, and education includes nutrition and oral medicine find *Nutrition and Oral Medicine* a valuable resource.

Riva Touger-Decker, PhD, RD, FADA
David A. Sirois, DMD, PhD
Connie C. Mobley, PhD, RD, LD

Contents

Contributors

RUTH M. DEBUSK, PhD, RD • *DeBusk Communications, LLC, Tallahassee, FL*

DOMINICK P. DEPAOLA, DDS, PhD • *CEO, Forsyth Institute, Boston, MA*

MICHAEL GLICK, DMD • *Department of Diagnostic Sciences, Division of Oral Medicine, New Jersey Dental School, University of Medicine and Dentistry of New Jersey, Newark, NJ*

MAUREEN HUHMANN, MS, RD • *School of Health Related Professions, University of Medicine and Dentistry of New Jersey, and Cancer Institute of New Jersey, New Brunswick, NJ*

ANGELA R. KAMER, DDS, PhD • *Department of Periodontics, New York University College of Dentistry, New York, NY*

SHELBY KASHKET, PhD • *Forsyth Institute, Boston, MA*

A. ROSS KERR, DDS, MSD •*Department of Oral Medicine, New York University College of Dentistry, New York, NY*

JOANNE KOUBA, MS, RD• *Dietetic Internship, Loyola University Chicago, Chicago, IL*

ELIZABETH A. KRALL, PhD, MPH • *Department of Health Policy & Health Services Research, Boston University Goldman School of Dental Medicine, Boston, MA*

PETER LINGSTRÖM, DDS, PhD • *Department of Cardiology, Goteborg University, Faculty of Odontology,Goteborg, Sweden*

SUZANNE MAKOWSKI, MED, RD, LDN, RDH • *Department of Food and Nutrition, Rhode Island Hospital, Providence, RI*

TERESA MARSHALL, PhD, RD • *Department of Preventive Medicine and Community Dentistry, University of Iowa, Iowa City, IA*

CONNIE C. MOBLEY, PhD, RD • *Department of Professional Studies, University of Nevada Las Vegas School of Dental Medicine, Las Vegas, NV*

DOUGLAS E. MORSE, DDS, PhD • *Department of Epidemiology and Health Promotion, New York University College of Dentistry, New York, NY*

PAULA J. MOYNIHAN, PhD, RD • *School of Dental Medicine, University of Newcastle upon Tyne, Newcastle upon Tyne, UK*

CAROLE A. PALMER, EdD, RD • *Division of Nutrition and Health, Tufts University Dental School, Boston, MA*

ANITA PATEL, DMD • *Department of Diagnostic Sciences, University of Medicine and Dentistry of New Jersey, New Jersey Dental School, Newark, NJ*

ELIZABETH REIFSNIDER, RN, PhD • *Department of Chronic Nursing, School of Nursing, University of Texas Health Science Center at San Antonio, San Antonio, TX*

DIANE RIGASSIO RADLER, MS, RD • *Department of Primary Care, School of Health-Related Professions, Department of Diagnostic Sciences, New Jersey Dental School, University of Medicine and Dentistry of New Jersey, Newark, NJ*

MIRIAM R. ROBBINS, DDS, MS • *Department of Oral Medicine, New York University College of Dentistry, New York, NY*

DAVID A. SIROIS, DMD, PhD • *Department of Oral Medicine, New York University College of Dentistry, New York, NY*

RIVA TOUGER-DECKER, PhD, RD, FADA • *Department of Primary Care, School of Health-Related Professions, and Department of Diagnostic Sciences, New Jersey Dental School, University of Medicine and Dentistry of New Jersey, Newark, NJ*

ANTHONY T. VERNILLO, DDS, PhD • *Department of Oral Pathology, New York University College of Dentistry, New York, NY*

MARION F. WINKLER, MS, RD, LDN, CNSD • *Division of Biology and Medicine, Department of Surgery/Nutritional Support Service, Rhode Island Hospital and Brown University, Providence, RI*

Value-Added eBook/PDA

This book is accompanied by a value-added CD-ROM that contains an Adobe eBook version of the volume you have just purchased. This eBook can be viewed on your computer, and you can synchronize it to your PDA for viewing on your handheld device. The eBook enables you to view this volume on only one computer and PDA. Once the eBook is installed on your computer, you cannot download, install, or e-mail it to another computer; it resides solely with the computer to which it is installed. The license provided is for only one computer. The eBook can only be read using Adobe® Reader® 6.0 software, which is available free from Adobe Systems Incorporated at www.Adobe.com. You may also view the eBook on your PDA using the Adobe® PDA Reader® software that is also available free from Adobe.com.

You must follow a simple procedure when you install the eBook/PDA that will require you to connect to the Humana Press website in order to receive your license. Please read and follow the instructions below:

1. Download and install Adobe® Reader® 6.0 software
   You can obtain a free copy of Adobe® Reader® 6.0 software at www.adobe.com
   Note: If you already have Adobe® Reader® 6.0 software, you do not need to reinstall it.
2. Launch Adobe® Reader® 6.0 software
3. Install eBook: Insert your eBook CD into your CD-ROM drive
   PC: Click on the "Start" button, then click on "Run"
   At the prompt, type "d:\ebookinstall.pdf" and click "OK"
   *Note: If your CD-ROM drive letter is something other than d: change the above command accordingly.
   MAC: Double click on the "eBook CD" that you will see mounted on your desktop. Double click "ebookinstall.pdf"
4. Adobe® Reader® 6.0 software will open and you will receive the message "This document is protected by Adobe DRM" Click "OK"
   Note: If you have not already activated Adobe® Reader® 6.0 software, you will be prompted to do so. Simply follow the directions to activate and continue installation.
   Your web browser will open and you will be taken to the Humana Press eBook registration page. Follow the instructions on that page to complete installation. You will need the serial number located on the sticker sealing the envelope containing the CD-ROM.

If you require assistance during the installation, or you would like more information regarding your eBook and PDA installation, please refer to the eBookManual.pdf located on your CD. If you need further assistance, contact Humana Press eBook Support by e-mail at ebooksupport@humanapr.com or by phone at 973-256-1699.

*Adobe and Reader are either registered trademarks or trademarks of Adobe Systems Incorporated in the United States and/or other countries.

I

SYNERGISTIC RELATIONSHIPS
BETWEEN NUTRITION AND HEALTH

1 Impact of Dietary Quality and Nutrition on General Health Status

Connie C. Mobley and Teresa Marshall

1. INTRODUCTION

Dietary quality and nutrition are important in the promotion and maintenance of health throughout the entire life span and inclusive among the multiple determinants of chronic diseases. They occupy a prominent position in disease prevention and health promotion. When combined with other modifiable risk factors, such as tobacco or physical activity, diet and nutrition may have an additive or multiplier effect for an array of chronic diseases, including cardiovascular disease, diabetes, obesity, cancer, osteoporosis, and dental diseases *(1)*. Furthermore, nutritional status is a primary determinant of responses to medical therapies effective in the treatment of an array of physical and iatrogenic conditions.

This chapter discusses the synergistic relationships of diet and nutrition with other determinants of health and provides a contemporary perspective of related nutrition research. Foundations for practices that include diet and nutrition with respect to both primary and secondary prevention and management of prevalent diseases are reviewed.

2. DEFINTION OF TERMS

Nutrition is the sum of dietary quality and physiological and biological activity necessary to maintain life. The multidimensional impact of nutritional status on health reflects the intricacies of nutrition. *Dietary quality* is often expressed in terms of agricultural or industrial sources of food, nutrient content, organoleptic appeal, variety, and adequacy. Food and foodstuffs are chemical compounds configured by nature or formulated by manmade processes to mimic nature. Beyond human milk for infants, there is no one food that meets all nutritional needs and thus it is a combination of foods and adequacy of the diet that defines quality. Dietary quality to a large extent defines health. Between 20 and 30 biologically distinct types of foods are required for healthy diets in the course of 1 wk *(1)*. Diets evolve over time, are influenced by many factors, and represent complex sociodemographic and political/economic environments associated with availability and accessibility of food. Nutrition is a scientific term that describes how diets meet energy output and balance the needs and demands of cellular activity, growth, and tissue maintenance. An optimum diet, via the nutritional processes, sup-

From: *Nutrition and Oral Medicine*
Edited by: R. Touger-Decker, D. A. Sirois, and C. C. Mobley © Humana Press Inc., Totowa, NJ

ports general health, health promotion, and disease prevention but has yet to be precisely identified for each individual.

Both undernutrition and overnutrition are forms of *malnutrition*. Nutrient inadequacies as well as the malabsorption, utilization, or excretion of a nutrient, can result in undernutrition, whereas excessive intakes of nutrients represent toxicities and overnutrition. Over several million years of human evolution, nutrients and physical activity have influenced gene expression and defined opportunities for both health and susceptibility to disease. Environmental factors determine which individuals among those who are susceptible will develop an illness or chronic condition.

Nutritional status is a measurement of the extent to which an individual's defined physiological need for nutrients are being met by his or her dietary patterns and choices. Thus, these measurements entail review of dietary intake, biochemical markers of nutrient status, and anthropometric changes.

Dietary guidelines are developed based on population-based nutritional status summaries and their associations with indices of disease risk and defined health status. They provide clinicians with markers for both assessing health status and recommending lifestyle behaviors to enhance positive health outcomes.

3. DIET, PHYSICAL ACTIVITY, AND CHRONIC DISEASE

3.1. Dietary Excess and Inadequate Physical Activity

Chronic diseases are largely preventable and associated with lifestyle behaviors—diet, physical activity, and tobacco use. Excessive intakes of energy-dense, highly processed foods and a lack of physical activity contribute to obesity and obesity-related diseases (e.g., insulin resistance, hyperlipidemias, cardiovascular disease, cancer). The prevalence of obesity has increased among all age groups, and obesity-related diseases are observed at increasingly younger ages. Among adults living in the United States, the prevalence of obesity increased by 74% between 1991 and 2001 *(2)*. Among younger obese adults, decreased life expectancy is increased *(3)*. Social and economic costs of obesity and obesity-related diseases are enormous, accounting for approx 9.4% of US health care expenditures *(4)*.

3.1.1. OBESITY

Obesity is defined as excessive body fat, and typically assessed by evaluating the weight for height relationship expressed as the body mass index (BMI; e.g., weight in kg/ height in m^2). National Heart, Lung and Blood Institute (NHLBI) guidelines diagnose obesity using the BMI of 25–29.9—overweight; 30–34.9—class I obesity; 35–39.9—class II obesity, and over 40—class III obesity *(5)*. Energy consumed in excess of requirements is converted to fat and stored in adipocytes or fat cells. Adipocyte capacity is limited; once full, preadipocytes differentiate, increasing adipocyte numbers. During weight loss, adipocytes may decrease in size, but do not go away, making weight loss difficult *(6)*. Obesity-related diseases are more closely associated with adipocyte size and location (e.g., central deposition) than with total body fat, thus reduction of adipocyte size is an appropriate weight-loss goal *(7)*.

Weight loss is achieved when energy expenditure exceeds energy intake. Achievement and maintenance of ideal body weight (i.e., a return to both normal number and size of adipocytes) is virtually impossible and not an appropriate goal for most obese individuals. Contemporary research suggests that a 10% weight loss is sufficient to decrease risk of obesity-related diseases, and is reasonable to achieve and maintain *(8)*. Because loss of all excess body fat is not realistic, prevention of obesity through the establishment of appropriate dietary and activity patterns early in life is important. Food characteristics (e.g., energy-dense, processed), eating behaviors (e.g., binging, compulsive overeating), and environmental factors (e.g., marketing, portion sizes, accessibility) contribute to increased energy intake, whereas sedentary leisure activities (e.g., television, video games), safety issues (e.g., latch-key kids, absence of sidewalks or parks), and technological advances (e.g., automobiles, labor-saving devices) are thought to be responsible for lower energy requirements. A diet based on low-fat, minimally processed foods consistent with the US Department of Agriculture (USDA) Food Guide Pyramid *(9)* described in Table 1, and regular physical activity are recommended for prevention and treatment of obesity.

3.1.2. INSULIN RESISTANCE

Insulin resistance is characterized by impaired insulin function. Removal of glucose and free fatty acids from serum is reduced with insulin resistance; excess insulin is secreted to compensate and maintain normal serum glucose and free fatty acid concentrations. If resistance reaches the threshold where compensation is lost, serum glucose levels increase and the individual meets criteria for type 2 diabetes *(10)*. Insulin resistance without elevated glucose is not benign; resulting hypertension and dyslipidemia (e.g., small, dense low-density lipoprotein [LDL], hypertriglyceridemia and decreased high-density lipoprotein [HDL]) increase risk of cardiovascular disease (CVD). Individuals with central adiposity are at increased risk for insulin resistance and type 2 diabetes; reduction of adipocyte size has been shown to improve insulin response.

Insulin resistance is improved by weight loss and physical activity *(11)*. High carbohydrate diets, particularly those high in simple sugars, appear to aggravate insulin resistance. Therefore, diets moderate in both carbohydrate and fat, with emphasis on complex carbohydrate and unsaturated fats are recommended *(12,13)*.

3.1.3. HYPERLIPIDEMIA

Hyperlipidemias include a spectrum of disorders in which serum lipid levels are abnormal. Serum lipid levels are subject to genetic and environmental influences; both diet and physical activity can modify serum lipid levels. Hypercholesterolemia, particularly elevated LDL cholesterol and low HDL cholesterol, are associated with an increased risk of CVD *(14)*. Hypertriglyceridemia, which often presents with insulin resistance, is also associated with increased risk of CVD.

Weight loss and physical activity improve serum lipid levels. Additionally, a decrease in dietary total fat, saturated fat, and cholesterol will decrease serum cholesterol levels. Hypertriglyceridemia is improved by a diet containing moderate complex carbohydrates, low simple sugars, moderate fat, and limited alcohol *(14)*.

3.1.4. HYPERTENSION

High blood pressure is defined by the NHLBI as a systolic pressure of 140 mmHg or greater, diastolic pressure of 90 mmHg or greater, or use of antihypertensive medication *(6)*. As the BMI of individuals has risen in the United States, so has the prevalence of hypertension associated with insulin resistance and risk for CVD and stroke *(14)*.

Table 1
Daily Food Pattern Guides

Food Guide Pyramid for Americans[a]			DASH Food Guide[b]		
Food group	Serving size	No. of servings	Food group	Serving size	No. of servings
Fats, oils, and sweets	None specified	Use sparingly	Fats and oils	1 teaspoon soft margarine, 1 tablespoon low-fat mayonnaise, 2 tablespoons light salad dressing, 1 teaspoon vegetable oil	2–3
			Sweets	1 tablespoon sugar, jelly, or jam, 1/2 ounce jelly beans, 8 ounces lemonade	5 per week
Milk, yogurt, and cheese	1 cup milk or yogurt, 1 1/2 ounces natural cheese, 2 ounces process cheese,	2–3	Low-fat or fat-free dairy foods	8 ounces milk, 1 cup yogurt, 1 1/2 ounce cheese	3
Meat, poultry, fish, dry beans, eggs, and nuts	2 1/2–3 ounces cooked lean beef, pork, lamb, veal, poultry or fish. 1/2 cup cooked beans or egg or 2 tablespoons peanut butter or 1/3 cup nuts count as 1 ounce meat	2–3	Meat, poultry and fish	3 ounces cooked meats, poultry or fish	2
Fruit	1 piece fruit, 1/2 cup chopped, cooked or canned fruit, 3/4 cup fruit juice	2–4	Fruits	6 ounces fruit juice, 1 medium fruit, 1/4 cup dried fruit, 1/2 cup fresh, frozen, or canned fruit	5
Vegetable	1/2 cup raw leafy vegetables, 1/2 cup other vegetables, cooked or chopped raw, 3/4 cup vegetable juice	2–4	Vegetables	1 cup raw leafy vegetables, 1/2 cup cooked vegetables, 6 ounces vegetable juice	4–5
Bread, cereal, rice, and pasta	1 slice bread, 1 ounce ready-to-eat cereal, 1/2 cup cooked rice, pasta, or cereal	6–11	Grains and grain products	1 slice bread, 1 ounce dry cereal, 1/2 cup cooked rice, pasta, or cereal	8

[a] Source: From ref. 43, recommended values based on 1600–2800 calories per day.
[b] Source: From ref. 37, recommended values based on 2000 calories per day.
DASH, Dietary Approaches to Stop Hypertension Trial.

Lifestyle changes, including weight management, diet modification, and physical activity are recommended for management of hypertension *(1,15)*. Diets limited in sodium from processed foods, reduced in calories and saturated fat, but adequate in calcium, magnesium, and phosphorous may lower blood pressure *(16,17)*.

3.1.5. CARDIOVASCULAR DISEASE

CVD, the primary cause of mortality in the United States, has been the focus of nutrition and physical activity intervention trials since the 1940s. Beginning with the Framingham studies in 1967, physical activity was found to reduce the risk of heart disease, whereas obesity was found to increase the risk *(18)*.

CVD is characterized by atherosclerotic disease in the vessels supporting the heart. Associated risk factors include obesity, insulin resistance, hypertension, and dyslipidemia. Prevention and management of CVD targets risk factors and includes reduction of energy intake and increased physical activity *(19,20)*.

3.1.6. CANCER

Cancer, defined as a disease of deoxyribonucleic acid (DNA), is characterized by uncontrolled growth of cells secondary to initiating and promoting factors and failure of the body to inhibit the uncontrolled growth. Dietary factors have been associated with initiation (e.g., aflatoxin, nitrosamines) and promotion (e.g., salt, fat) *(1)*. Obesity and excessive alcohol intake increase risk of certain cancers. Antioxidants (e.g., vitamins A, C, and E) and folic acid found in fruits and vegetables and vitamin B_{12} found in animal products are thought to decrease risk of cancer. Dietary recommendations to prevent cancer include weight management, moderate energy and fat intakes, and a diet rich in fruits and vegetables *(21)*.

3.2. Dietary Deficiency and Diseases

Dietary deficiencies occur less frequently than dietary excesses in the United States, yet remain a significant public health burden, particularly for vulnerable populations. Poverty and environmental barriers are associated with insufficient food intake, reliance on highly processed foods, narrow food choices, and limited nutrient intakes. Young children and the elderly are particularly vulnerable *(22)*.

3.2.1. PROTEIN ENERGY MALNUTRITION

Protein energy malnutrition (PEM) is characterized by weight, stature, or weight for stature indices below the fifth percentile for age. PEM is the result of inadequate energy or protein to maintain weight and support growth. Diets characterized by insufficient energy and protein are typically deficient in multiple nutrients. The etiology of growth failure may be multifactorial. In addition to physical signs, individuals with PEM may exhibit cognitive delays, behavioral problems, and emotional problems secondary to PEM *(23,24)*.

Management of PEM includes identification and resolution of the underlying problem (e.g., access to food, dysphagia, food preparation barriers). Provision of appropriate and adequate foodstuff, including a variety of foods from all food groups, vitamin and mineral supplementation when food acceptance is severely limited, and limitation of energy-dense beverages with structured meals and snacks are recommended *(22)*.

Table 2
Dietary Sources of Iron, Folic Acid, and Vitamin B_{12}

Iron	Folic acid	Vitamin B_{12}
Meat	Green leafy vegetables	Meat
Egg yolk	Lean beef	Milk and dairy foods
Legumes	Wheat	Eggs
Whole or enriched grains	Eggs	
Dark green vegetables	Fish	
Dark molasses	Dry beans	
Shrimp	Asparagus	
	Broccoli	

3.2.2. ANEMIAS

Anemia is characterized by reduced red blood cell volume, insufficient hemoglobin, and reduced oxygenation of body tissues. Nutritional anemias are caused by inadequate iron, folic acid, or vitamin B_{12} intakes. Iron-deficiency anemia is a public health burden of infants, young children, and pregnant women, particularly those living in poverty. In addition to anemia, iron deficiency is associated with growth failure, impaired immune function, learning difficulties, and behavioral problems *(25)*. Folic acid deficiencies have been identified as a risk for neural tube defects and, through associations with elevated homocysteine levels, CVD *(26)*. Vitamin B_{12} deficiencies are associated with cognitive declines in the elderly and elevated homocysteine levels with increased risk of CVD *(27)*.

Management of nutritional anemias requires careful identification of the deficient nutrient; folic acid supplementation will correct a vitamin B_{12} deficiency anemia, but not concurrent neurological damage associated with the vitamin B_{12} deficiency. Iron-deficient anemia may be treated with supplemental iron and iron-containing foods *(28)*. Folic acid-deficient anemia is treated with supplemental folic acid and folic acid-containing foods. Supplemental folic acid is recommended for women at risk for pregnancy *(29)*. Vitamin B_{12} deficiency is treated with supplemental vitamin B_{12} and vitamin B_{12}-containing foods (e.g., animal products) if the diet is inadequate; supplemental vitamin B_{12} if gastric hydrochloric acid production is reduced; and by injection of vitamin B_{12} if intrinsic factor, which is required for absorption, is limited *(30)*. Table 2 lists dietary sources of iron, folic acid, and vitamin B_{12}.

3.2.3. OSTEOPOROSIS

Osteoporosis is characterized by decreased bone density and quality and is associated with an increased risk of fracture *(31)*. Although fractures do not typically occur until older ages, osteoporosis may be considered a pediatric disease because most bone accrual occurs during this life stage. Bone accrual is influenced by genetic and environmental factors, including diet, physical activity, and body size. Inadequate dietary calcium and insufficient vitamin D (either dietary or sunlight exposure) are associated with reduced bone density.

Maximization of bone density is a primary strategy for prevention of osteoporosis. Diets high in calcium and vitamin D (e.g., dairy products) and limited in low nutrient beverages (e.g., soft drinks) are recommended *(1)*.

3.2.4. IMMUNOCOMPROMISED

Nutrition and the immune system are intertwined; malnutrition increases the risk of infection and infection depletes nutrient reserves. During severe infection, both increased energy and protein requirements and decreased intakes contribute to PEM. Effects of micronutrient deficiencies are less obvious, but they also affect the function of the immune system. Specifically, deficiencies of iron, zinc, and vitamin A have been associated with altered immune functions *(23)*.

Diets providing adequate vitamins and minerals as well as sufficient protein and energy are necessary to support a functional immune system. During infection, nutrient requirements increase, and supplemental therapy may be required. Anorexia, secondary to the infection, may further compromise energy and nutrient intakes and nutritional status.

4. DIETARY GUIDELINES FOR OPTIMUM HEALTH

One of the greatest challenges in contemporary United States health care is the shift from the management of acute episodes of illness toward the management of chronic conditions. Although the health care provider manages acute episodes, effectiveness of chronic disease management ultimately depends on the patient's lifelong adherence to drug, diet, and exercise regimens and response to symptoms *(32)*. Five chronic diseases—heart disease, cancers, stroke, chronic obstructive pulmonary diseases, and diabetes—account for more than 66% of all deaths in the United States. Approximately 75% of health care costs each year are attributed to treatment of chronic diseases. In 2000, more than $76 billion in health care costs was associated with physical inactivity. More than $33 billion in medical costs and $9 billion in lost productivity have been attributed to poor nutrition and incidence of heart disease, cancer, stroke, and diabetes *(33)*.

Scientific evidence indicates that when clear and compelling health information is conveyed, the public is engaged. Communication strategies to inform and influence individual and community decisions on health promotion and disease prevention depend on documented evidence-based physical activity and dietary guidelines *(33)*. Longitudinal multicenter clinical trails, epidemiological evidence, and the expert opinion of government agencies, researchers, and academicians have lead to a better understanding of the role of dietary and physical activity in health promotion. Evolving guidelines serve as a framework and set policy for the interpretation and implementation of healthy choices.

4.1. Comparative Overview

Benchmarks used to determine the direction and framework for establishing dietary practices appropriate for decreasing risk for disease and health promotion have been expressed in a variety of formats. General guidelines or messages for making dietary choices are generally nonspecific but designed to increase awareness and establish guiding principles. Other guidelines are more targeted and prescriptive in nature. These fall into two categories: food pattern guides and targeted recommendations for specific nutrients that are associated with evidence from observational studies.

4.1.1. GENERAL GUIDELINES

Broad dietary and physical activity concepts based on significant population-based research have been published by a variety of government agencies and health-based organizations. Dietary Guidelines for Americans, the cornerstone for diet and nutrition

Table 3
Agency and Health-Based Organization Dietary Guidelines

Dietary Guidelines for Americans [a]	American Cancer Society [b]	National Cancer Institute [c]	American Heart Association [d]
Aim for Fitness by aiming for a healthy weight and being physically active each day.	Adopt a physically active life. Maintain a healthy weight throughout life.	Avoid obesity.	*A Healthy Body Weight* Match energy intake to energy needs, with appropriate changes to achieve weight loss when indicated.
Build a healthy base by using the Food Guide Pyramid to guide your food choices, choosing a variety of grain (especially whole grains), fruits, and vegetables daily and keeping food safe to eat.	Eat a variety of healthy foods, with an emphasis on plant sources.	Include a variety of fruits and vegetables in the daily diet.	*A Healthy Eating Pattern* Include a variety of fruits, vegetables, grains, low-fat to nonfat dairy products, fish, legumes, poultry, lean meats.
Choose sensibly by choosing a diet that is low in saturated fat, cholesterol, and sodium and moderate in total fat, as well as sugar from beverages and foods.		Minimize consumption of salt-cured, salt-pickled, and smoked foods.	*A Desirable Blood Cholesterol and Lipoprotein Profile* Limit foods high in saturated fat and cholesterol; and substitute unsaturated fat from vegetables, fish, legumes, nuts.
If you drink alcoholic beverages, do so in moderation.	If you drink alcoholic beverages, limit consumption.	Consume alcoholic beverages in moderation, if at all.	*A Desirable Blood Pressure* Limit salt and alcohol; maintain a healthy body weight and a diet with emphasis on vegetables, fruits, and low-fat/nonfat dairy products.

[a] Source: From ref. 43
[b] Source: From ref. 21
[c] Source: From ref. 44
[d] Source: From ref. 45

messages, was first published in 1980, followed by four intermittent revisions *(34)*. The most recent version, published in 2000, reflected recommendations based on current scientific knowledge from the Departments of Health and Human Services (HHS) and Agriculture (USDA) on how dietary intake may reduce risk for major chronic diseases and how a healthy diet may improve nutrition *(34)*. Table 3 represents the recent versions of the evolution of guidelines. Organizations focused on decreasing cancer or heart disease risk have chosen to express guidelines in a comparable format. These conceptual statements are designed to increase awareness and promote action related to associations between lifestyle behaviors and chronic disease risk. In some instances, they may represent suggested choices that are not yet fully substantiated by significant causal data.

4.1.2. FOOD PATTERN GUIDELINES

The clinician is encouraged to translate general guidelines to meet the needs of individuals. The Food Guide Pyramid for Americans *(9)* represents recommendations for selecting a variety of foods in amounts leading to successful implementation of the dietary guidelines. It is primarily a nutrition education tool and food guidance system used to illustrate balance and variety within the realm of scientific nutrition evidence. Over time, it has been modified and adapted for special groups, like children and the elderly, based on new knowledge and needs and will likely continue to change as new findings identify the role of foods in health promotion *(35)*. When similar pictorial representations of various international dietary guidelines were compared, it was concluded that recommendations for individuals to consume larger amounts of fruits, vegetables, and grains and moderate amounts of meats, milk, and dairy products were consistent. Major differences in suggested dietary patterns were attributed to cultural differences *(36)*. Table 1 describes the components of the Food Guide Pyramid for Americans *(9)*.

Attempts to further assist the public in interpreting dietary behaviors research efforts have focused on the role of daily dietary patterns. In Table 1, recommendations for managing hypertension were outlined according to findings from the Dietary Approaches to Stop Hypertension trial *(15)*. The trial was designed to test eating patterns rather than specific nutrient intake related to hypertension because so many nutrients play an interdependent role in maintenance of nutritional status *(37)*.

4.1.3. NUTRIENT INTAKE RECOMMENDATIONS

Dietary quality is further expressed in terms of nutrient composition. The evidence to support recommendations for both macronutrients and micronutrients represents a growing body of knowledge specifically targeting a variety of diseases.

The Institute of Medicine of the National Academy of Sciences *(38)* and the World Health Organization *(1)* have published extensive documents in support of dietary recommendations for health promotion. A summary of guidelines for caloric distribution from energy nutrients and additional nutrients of major concern are listed in Table 4 along with similar recommendations from other health-based agencies. Recommendations for protein, carbohydrate, and fat distribution in the daily diet are similar. Additionally, recommendations for specific nutrients like simple sugars and types of fat are not specified by all agencies. The unequivocal scientific evidence to clearly define what is optimum nutrition remains undefined. However, findings do support food guide recommendations broader in scope. Essentially, diets need to provide adequate protein

Table 4

Daily Recommendations for Major Nutrient Intakes by Percentage of Calories and for Dietary Cholesterol, Dietary Fiber, and Sodium Chloride

Nutrient	Institute of Medicine[a]	World Health Organization[b]	National Cholesterol Education Program[c]	American Heart Association[d]	American Diabetes Association[e]
			Percentage calories		
Protein	10–35	10–15	15	15	15–20
Carbohydrate	45–65	55–75	50–60	55 or <	60–70
Simple sugar	<25	<10			
Dietary fat	20–35	15–30	25–35	<30	
Monounsaturated			≤20	≤15	
Polyunsaturated		6–10	>10	<7	15–20
N-6 polyunsaturated	5–10	5–8			
N-3 polyunsaturated	6–1.2	1–2			
Saturated		<10	<7	<7	7–10
Trans-fatty acids		<1			
			Daily values		
Dietary Cholesterol		<300mg	<200 mg	<200 mg	200–300 mg
Dietary Fiber	25–38g		20–30 g		
Sodium Chloride		2–5g		<6 g	<6 g

[a] Source: From ref. 38
[b] Source: From ref. 1
[c] Source: From ref. 14
[d] Source: From ref. 45
[e] Source: From ref. 13

for tissue regeneration and maintenance plus a variety of carbohydrates to support cellular and systemic functions. Dietary fat intake determinations define the importance of the unsaturated fatty acids in health promotion.

The Dietary Reference Intakes offer standards for recommended amounts of specific elements, macronutrients, and vitamins to be included in a dietary pattern *(38–42)*. These multiple sets of values include (Estimated Average Requirements, Recommended Dietary Allowances, Adequate Intakes, and Tolerable Upper Intake Levels) for designated age groups, physiologic states, and sexes. Like the former Recommended Dietary Allowances these values replace, they are intended to meet the needs of healthy individuals over time. A detailed explanation of these values for individuals at different life stages is found in Appendix C.

5. SUMMARY

General health status can have an impact on dental diagnosis and treatment outcomes. Diet and nutrition are major indicators of status and can mediate the course of oral health outcomes. Likewise, oral health status has an impact on nutritional status. The synergy between oral health, general health, and nutrition is dynamic and should be viewed from a global perspective to provide clinical and community interventions targeted toward health promotion. The similarities among dietary guidelines and recommendations specific to the major chronic conditions and diseases help to create oral health and nutrition messages with multiple intents and outcomes.

Guidelines for Practice

	Oral Health Professional	*Nutrition Professional*
Prevention	• Assess dietary patterns and body mass index in identifying routine medical history for patients	• Include oral health screening in routine physical assessment
		• Provide messaging to patients about the synergy between general and oral health
Intervention	• Provide guidelines that promote oral health and support dietary changes necessary to decrease risk for chronic and disabling diseases	• Conduct dietary assessment and nutrition education with dental patients/clients
	• Develop a referral protocol to a nutrition professional for comprehensive dietary counseling and follow-up	• Tailor dietary counseling to include guidelines to promote optimum oral health and disease risk reduction
		• Develop a referral protocol to a dental professional for oral health maintenance

REFERENCES

1. World Health Organization. Diet, Nutrition, and the Prevention of Chronic Diseases. Report of a WHO/ FAO Consultation. Geneva:WHO Technical Report Series 916, 2002.
2. Task Force of the American Society for Clinical Nutrition. The evidence relating six dietary factors to the nation's health. Am J Clin Nutr 1979; 32(Suppl.):2621–2748.
3. Mokdad AH, Ford ES, Bowman, BA, et al. Prevalence of obesity, diabetes, and obesity-related health risk factors. JAMA 2003; 289(1):76–79.
4. Fontaine KR, Redden DT, Wang C, Westfall AO, Allison DB. Years of life lost due to obesity. JAMA 2003; 289(2):187–193.
5. Colditz GA. Economic costs of obesity and inactivity. Med Sci Sports Exerc 1999; 31(11S):S663–S667.
6. National Institutes of Health, National Heart, Lung and Blood Institute Obesity Education Initiative Expert Panel. Clinical Guidelines on the Identification, Evaluation, and Treatment of Overweight and Obesity in Adults: The Evidence Report. NIH Publication No. 98-4083, 1998.
7. Spiegelman BM, Flier JS. Adipogenesis and obesity: rounding out the big picture. Cell 1996; 87:377–389.
8. Yajnik CS. The lifecycle effects of nutrition and body size on adult adiposity, diabetes and cardiovascular disease. Obesity Reviews 2002; 3(3):217–224.
9. U.S. Department of Agriculture. Human Nutrition Information Service. The Food Guide Pyramid. 1992. Home and Garden Bull. No. 252, (updated 1996).
10. Oster G, Thompson D, Edelsberg J, Bird AP, Colditz GA. Lifetime health and economic benefits of weight loss among obese persons. Am J Public Health 1999; 89(10):1536–1542.
11. Expert Committee. Report of the Expert Committee on the Diagnosis and Classification of Diabetes Mellitus. Diabetes Care 2003; 26:S5–S20.
12. Diabetes Prevention Program Research Group. Reduction in the incidence of type 2 Diabetes with lifestyle intervention and metformin. N Engl J Med 2002; 346(6):393–403.
13. American Diabetes Association. Evidence-based nutrition principles and recommendations for the treatment and prevention of diabetes and related complications. Diabetes Care 2003; 26(Suppl. 1): S51–S52.
14. National Cholesterol Education Program (NCEP) Expert Panel. Third Report of the National Cholesterol Education Program (NCEP) Expert Panel on Detection, Evaluation, and Treatment of High Blood Cholesterol in Adults (Adult Treatment Panel III) final report. Circulation 2002; 106(25):3143–3421.
15. Lopes HF, Martin KL, Nashar K, Morrow JD, Goodfriend TL, Egan BM. DASH diet lowers blood pressure and lipid-induced oxidative stress in obesity. Hypertension 2003; 41(3):422–430.
16. Sacks FM, Katan M. Randomized clinical trials on the effects of dietary fat and carbohydrate on plasma lipoproteins and cardiovascular disease. Am J Med 2002; 113(Suppl. 9B):13S–24S.
17. The Trials of Hypertension Prevention Collaborative Research Group. Effects of weight loss and sodium reduction intervention on blood pressure and hypertension incidence in overweight people with high-normal blood pressure. The Trials of Hypertension Prevention, phase II. Arch Intern Med 1997; 157: 657–667.
18. Kannel WB. Habitual level of physical activity and risk of coronary heart disease: the Framingham study. Can Med Assoc J 1967 96(12):811–812.
19. Neuhouser ML, Miller DL, Kristal AR, Barnett MJ, Cheskin LJ. Diet and exercise habits of patients with diabetes, dyslipidemia, cardiovascular disease or hypertension. J Am College Nutr 2002; 21(5): 394–401.
20. Lalonde L, Gray-Donald K, Lowensteyn I, et al. The Canadian Collaborative Cardiac Assessment Group. Comparing the benefits of diet and exercise in the treatment of dyslipidemia. Preventive Medicine 2002; 35(1):16–24.
21. Byers T, Nestle M, McTiernan, A., et al. American Cancer Society 2001 Nutrition and Physical Activity Guidelines Advisory Committee. American Cancer Society guidelines on nutrition and physical activity for cancer prevention: Reducing the risk of cancer with healthy food choices and physical activity. Cancer J Clin 2002; 52(2):92–119.
22. Reilly JJ. Understanding chronic malnutrition in childhood and old age: role of energy balance research. Proc Nutr Soc 2002; 61(3):321–327.

23. Keusch GT. The history of nutrition: malnutrition, infection and immunity J Nutr 2003; 133(1): 336S–340S.
24. Caballero B. Global patterns of child health: the role of nutrition. Ann Nutr Metab 2002; 46(Suppl 1): 3–7.
25. Beard J. Iron deficiency alters brain development and functioning. J Nutr 2003; 133(5 Suppl. 1):1468S–14672S.
26. Remacha AF, Souto JC, Ramila E, Perea G, Sarda MP, Fontcuberta, J. Enhanced risk of thrombotic disease in patients with acquired vitamin B12 and/or folate deficiency: role of hyperhomocysteinemia. Ann Hematol 2002; 81(11):616–621.
27. Bender DA. Megaloblastic anaemia in vitamin B12 deficiency. Br J Nutr 2003; 89(4):439–441.
28. Viteri F. Iron supplementation for the control of iron deficiency anemia in populations at risk. Nutr Rev 1997; 55:189–203.
29. Honein MA, Paulozzi LJ, Mathews TJ, Erickson JD, Wong LC. Impact of folic acid fortification of the US food supple on the occurrence of neural tube defects. JAMA 2001; 285:2981–2986.
30. Elia M. Oral or parenteral therapy for B12 deficiency. Lancet 2003; 352(9142):1721–1722.
31. Harvey N, Cooper C. Determinants of fracture risk in osteoporosis. Current Rheumatology Reports 2003; 5(1):75–81.
32. DeBusk RF, West JA, Miller NH, Taylor CB. Chronic disease management: treating the patient with disease(s) vs treating disease(s) in the patient. Arch Int Med 1999; 159(22):2739–2742.
33. Centers for Disease Control and Prevention. The Promise of Prevention. Reducing the Health and Economic Burden of Chronic Disease. Atlanta, GA: Department of Health and Human Services, Centers for Disease Control and Prevention, 2003.
34. Keenan DP, Abusabha R. The fifth edition of the Dietary Guidelines for Americans: Lessons learned along the way. J Am Diet Assoc 2001; 101(6):631–634.
35. Davis CA, Britten P, Myers EF. Past, present, and future of the food Guide Pyramid. J Am Diet Assoc 2001; 101(8):881–885.
36. Painter J, Rah J, Lee Y. Comparison of International Food Guide pictorial representations. J Am Diet Assoc 2002; 102(4):483–489.
37. Vogt TM, Appel LJ, Obarzanek E, et al. Dietary Approaches to Stop Hypertension: rationale, design and methods. JADA 1999; 99(Suppl.):S12–S18.
38. Institute of Medicine. Dietary Reference Intakes for Energy, Carbohydrates, Fiber, Fatty Acids Cholesterol, Protein and Amino Acids. Washington DC: National Academy Press, 2002.
39. Institute of Medicine. Dietary Reference Intakes for Calcium, Phosphorus, Magnesium, Vitamin D, and Fluoride. Washington DC: National Academy Press, 1997.
40. Institute of Medicine. Dietary Reference Intakes for Thiamin, Riboflavin, Niacin, Vitamin B_6, Folate, Vitamin B_{12}, Pantothenic Acid, Biotin, and Choline. Washington DC: National Academy Press, 1998.
41. Institute of Medicine. Dietary Reference Intakes for Vitamin C, Vitamin E, Selenium, and Carotenoids. Washington DC: National Academy Press, 2000.
42. Institute of Medicine. Dietary Reference Intakes for Vitamin A, Vitamin K, Arsenic, Boron, Chromium, Copper, Iodine, Iron, Manganese, Molybdenum, Nickel, Silicon, Vanadium, and Zinc. Washington DC: National Academy Press, 2001.
43. Nutrition and Your Health: Dietary Guidelines for Americans, 5th Ed. Home and Garden Bulletin No. 232. Washington, DC: U.S. Department of Agriculture and U.S. Department of Health and Human Services, 2000.
44. National Cancer Institute. Action Guide For Healthy Eating. NIH Publication No. 96-3877, 1996.
45. Krauss RM, Eckel RH, Howard B, et al. AHA Dietary Guidelines: Revision 2000: A statement for healthcare professionals from the Nutrition Committee of the American Heart Association. Circulation 2000; 102(18): 2284–2299.

2 Pregnancy, Child Nutrition, and Oral Health

Connie C. Mobley and Elizabeth Reifsnider

1. INTRODUCTION

Growth and development begin with pregnancy and continue through adolescence and early adulthood. Growth is defined as increases in cell size caused by processes of cell multiplication involving hyperplasia, hypertrophy, and accretion. Development involves a progressive maturation, differentiation, or specialization that results in a final physical, emotional, psychological, and cognitive biological state. The effects of nutrition are manifested throughout this process and in all tissues and structures in the body *(1)*.

Both general nutrition and dietary intake of specific nutrients have been associated with oral growth and development. Dietary choices throughout life can have a primary effect on the tooth structure, whereas nutritional status exerts a systemic effect on the integrity and maintenance of other oral tissue *(2)*. However, research in this area has been limited to animal studies and a few preliminary human investigations. Lack of an extensive body of evidence to identify associations between specific nutrients and optimum oral growth and development has resulted in limited interpretations of the precise interactions.

The purpose of this chapter is to examine the synergy between oral health development and nutritional status from conception to adolescence and to review past, present, and future research in this area according to stages of development that include pregnancy, infancy, early childhood, and school-aged children. Finally, this chapter identifies issues in managing oral health and promoting nutrition for special-needs individuals during pregnancy and childhood.

2. PRENATAL AND PERINATAL NUTRITION AND TOOTH DEVELOPMENT

The nutritional intake of the pregnant woman has specific and global effects on the dentition of her child. The specific effects are related to the formation of the enamel and dentin of the primary and permanent teeth during fetal development. The global effects are related to the amount of weight she gains, her diet's overall nutritional quality, how much her infant weighs at birth, and the gestational age of her infant—that is, whether

From: *Nutrition and Oral Medicine*
Edited by: R. Touger-Decker, D. A. Sirois, and C. C. Mobley © Humana Press Inc., Totowa, NJ

the infant is delivered at term or preterm. Primary teeth begin to form at 6 wk of gestational age when cells in the fetal oral cavity begin to differentiate and form tooth buds. The dentin layer forms first and then the enamel layer is deposited *(3)*. Mineralization begins at 4 mo *in utero*, and central incisors (the teeth that erupt first) have 83% of their enamel formed by the time of birth *(3)*. Insults from teratogens or lack of crucial nutrients during pregnancy can have significant impact on the nearly developed primary teeth and the beginnings of the permanent teeth. Infants are born with all the primary teeth and many permanent unerupted teeth in varying stages of development *(4,5)*. A review of early childhood caries (ECC) and hypoplasia in infants and children in developing countries revealed that these conditions were most closely associated with a general underlying nutritional deficiency state (malnutrition or undernutrition) in the perinatal period *(6)*. A clear relationship has been found between specific dietary nutrients during critical periods of calcification and poorly calcified teeth, which reduces caries resistance *(7)*.

2.1. Maternal Protein Energy Malnutrition

Maternal malnutrition, specifically protein energy malnutrition (PEM), has global effects. A pregnant woman needs to gain enough weight to support the fetus, placenta, and associated gain in maternal tissues to support pregnancy and lactation. Generally, a weight gain of 27.5 lbs (12.5 kg) is considered adequate, but the recommended weight gain for a specific woman depends on her prepregnancy body mass index (BMI) *(8,9)*. The requirement for protein increases by 20%, to a total of approx 60 g per day *(10)* depending on body weight and age. A woman who enters pregnancy underweight with low protein stores and who does not gain sufficient weight during pregnancy to support the fetus and her increased metabolism is at risk of delivering a low birth weight (<2500 g) and/or preterm infant *(11)*.

Low birth weight and preterm delivery are associated with enamel hypoplasia of the primary and permanent teeth. Nutritional deficiencies during pregnancy can affect tooth size, timing of tooth eruption, defects in enamel mineralization, and salivary gland formation and can create increased susceptibility to caries *(12,13)*. Furthermore, developmental defects of enamel and enamel hypoplasia are seen as a result of malnutrition during pregnancy and early childhood *(14–16)*. When nutritional deficiencies or toxicities occur during "critical periods" of oral tissue development, consequences can be permanent and irreversible *(17)*. Turnover time for oral soft tissue is between 3 and 7 d. This is more rapid than in other tissue and may increase oral tissue needs for nutrients beyond those in tissue with longer turnover rates *(3)*. Female rats fed a low-protein diet gave birth to rats with smaller molars, impaired salivary gland function (which affects caries resistance), and delayed eruption of the first and second molars *(7)*. When female rats consumed protein- and calorie-deficient diets, the molars and incisors of the offspring weighed less than than those of the normally fed control group *(18)*. These defects can be permanent and irreversible because of the absence of enamel and dentin regenerations once tooth eruption occurs *(19,20)*. Eruption of primary teeth has been delayed in longitudinal studies of stunted infants compared to healthy infants and associated with a risk of caries later in life *(21)*.

2.2. Maternal Micronutrient Malnutrition

Deficiencies in micronutrients such as vitamins A, C, and D and minerals such as calcium, phosphorus, fluoride, iron, and iodine have an effect on developing dentition *(22)*.

Vitamin A deficiency is widespread and often accompanies protein–calorie malnutrition. It is especially prevalent when dairy product and fresh fruit and vegetable intakes are limited *(23)*. It can exert its effect on dentition through the global effect of malnutrition as well as from a specific deficiency. Vitamin A deficiency can increase the risk of maternal mortality and is associated with preterm birth, intrauterine growth retardation, and low birth weight *(24)*. A vitamin A deficiency that occurs during gestation results in decreased epithelial tissue development, tooth morphogenesis dysfunction, and decreased odontoblast differentiation in fetal development *(3)*. It is thought that a lack of vitamin A produces chemical changes in the dentin that reduce the extent of mineralization *(25)*. However, vitamin A can be teratogenic when ingested in the form of retinoic acid analogs, given to treat severe cases of acne vulgaris. The β-carotene form of vitamin A found in fruits and vegetables is not teratogenic *(26)*.

Vitamin C plays a role in the integrity of osteoblasts, fibroblasts, chondroblasts, and odontoblasts *(27–29)*. It is necessary for synthesis of collagen, which contributes to the organic matrix for the deposition of calcium phosphate crystals that occurs during bone mineralization *(27,30)*. In vitro odontogenesis is constrained by vitamin C deficiency caused by dedifferentiation of odontoblasts, which leads to a cessation of dentin production *(27,30)*. A positive correlation ($r = 0.245$, $p = 0.033$) was reported between higher intakes of vitamin C and changes in bone density in 76 subjects at 10–20 wk gestation *(31)*. Ogawara *(30)* studied vitamin C deficiency in rats and concluded that it causes a marked reduction in dentin formation. The recommended dietary intake (RDI) for vitamin C is increased by 67% during pregnancy and requires daily ingestion because it is a water-soluble vitamin. Many fresh fruits and vegetables provide excellent sources. A long-term deficiency of vitamin C leads to scurvy, which can cause swollen, bleeding gums and loss of teeth. Vitamin C also works in concert with vitamin A, as collagen and calbindin (a product of vitamin A), to promote mineralization and development of teeth *(27)*.

Vitamin D deficiency most often occurs when the dietary intake of vitamin D-fortified milk is deficient or when pregnant women choose clothing that inhibits exposure to sunlight *(32)*. Effects of vitamin D deficiency by itself are difficult to separate from the effects of calcium and phosphorus deficiency because vitamin D causes the effect of hypomineralization through lowering plasma calcium levels *(3,33)*. The effects of calcium, phosphorus, and vitamin D deficiency result in lowered levels of plasma calcium, hypoplastic effects/hypomineralization, compromised tooth integrity, and a delay in tooth eruption. Permanent as well as primary teeth are affected. Likewise, animal and human studies indicate that excess vitamin D can result in disturbances in tooth calcification and hypoplasia that are not reversible *(17)*.

The demands of calcification of the fetal skeleton and mineralization of the primary teeth result in an increased need for calcium during gestation. The permanent teeth begin mineralization just before fetal maturity is reached *(7)*. The RDI for calcium increases to 1000 mg per day for pregnant women *(33)*. Yet, many women do not ingest this amount, even though calcium is found in all dairy foods, many fruits and vegetables, and some dietary sources of protein *(34)*. Hypomineralization of primary teeth from deficiencies of vitamin D, calcium, and phosphorus can contribute to increased susceptibility to ECC *(35,36)*.

Fluoride increases the resistance of teeth to decay by increasing mineralization. Fluoride supplementation does not seem to benefit the developing fetus *(37)* even though it diffuses across the placental barrier and is incorporated into fetal bones and teeth. The uptake of fluoride into calcified teeth is most dramatic during infancy but decreases with age (3).

Iron and iodine are minerals closely associated with promoting oral health because of their effect on the development of fetal dentition (22,38). They are crucial for the health of the developing fetus. Iron-deficiency anemia is a serious condition for a pregnant woman (11). It can result in reduced oxygen-carrying capacity in the mother, leading to hypoxia for developing fetal tissues and reduced iron deposition in these tissues. Iodine is critical for the formation of thyroid hormones, and its deficiency can cause mental retardation in a fetus. Because it may be difficult for a pregnant woman to meet the dietary reference intake for iron exclusively from foods, iron supplementation of 30–60 mg is recommended (11). Iodine consumption can be easily accomplished through inclusion of iodized salt in the diet. However, for women on salt-restricted diets because of hypertension, elemental iodine is available in selected prenatal supplements.

Table 1 lists vitamin and mineral recommendations for promotion of fetal and infant health (39,40). Dietary sources are listed, and recommendations for supplementation are noted. A prenatal vitamin and mineral supplement has become part of routine prenatal care for women planning a pregnancy.

3. INFANT AND EARLY CHILDHOOD FEEDING PRACTICES AND ORAL HEALTH

Rate of growth during both fetal life and infancy has been associated with long-term consequences for bone health as well as cardiovascular risk and brain development in infants (41). Dietary and feeding practices have a primary influence on infant growth. The World Health Organization (WHO) recommended exclusive breastfeeding up to or beyond 2 yr of age (42). Recommendations were not given on introduction of solid foods for formula-fed infants even though there is evidence that introduction before 4 mo of age may be associated with increased body fat, higher BMI, increased incidence of respiratory illness in later childhood, and increased risk for ECC. A report including several cohorts of greater than 2000 infants born in the United Kingdom in the mid-1990s noted that weaning occurred on average 4 mo earlier than recommendations from the Department of Health and that this earlier weaning was associated with less positive health behaviors and significantly higher infant body weights at 6 mo of age (41). A significant relationship was identified between reported weaning practices and ECC in more than 1000 Hispanic children of women participating in the Women, Infants, and Children (WIC) Supplemental Feeding Program in south Texas, which suggests that feeding practices may modulate the incidence of ECC (43).

The fluoride content of breast milk is low (3,44). Fluoride inhibits demineralization, encourages remineralization, and increases the stability of the tooth enamel (3). Fluoride is most effective when ingested during infancy beginning at 6 mo of age through supplemented community water or through the use of infant formula constituted with fluoridated water that contains less than allowable optimal amounts of fluoride (0.3 ppm). Fluoride supplementation (in the form of drops) is not recommended during the first 6 mo of life (45). In the absence of access to fluoridated water, the infant's or child's physician may prescribe fluoride-containing vitamin supplements. Guidelines for fluoride supplementation have been established for children between 6 mo and 16 yr of age, based on the fluoride ion level in the drinking water and the use of other fluoride sources (46).

Table 1
Daily Vitamin and Mineral Recommendations During Pregnancy

Vitamin	Recommended intake [a]	Quantity in standard prenatal supplement	Some recommended food sources	Supplementation recommended?
A	770 RE		Fish oils, dark-green vegetables, and deeply colored fruits	No
B_1	1.4 mg		Green leafy vegetables, lean pork, soy milk, enriched whole grain breads and cereals	No
B_2	1.4 mg		Green vegetables, eggs, milk, meats	No
B_6	1.9 mg	2 mg	Wheat germ, pork, cereals, legumes	No
B_{12}	2.6 µg		Meats, poultry, fish, shellfish, milk, eggs, cheese	No
C	85 mg	50 mg	Dark-green vegetables, citrus fruits	No
D	5 µg	5 µg	Fortified milk, egg yolks, fatty fish	No
E	15 mg		Polyunsaturated plant oils, wheat germ, tofu, avocado, sweet potatoes	No
K	90 mg		Leafy green vegetables, cabbage, cheese	No
Folate	600 µg	400–600 µg	Dark-green leafy vegetables, beans, peas, lentils	Yes
Niacin	18 mg NE		Peanut butter, lean ground beef, chicken, tuna, shrimp	No
Mineral				
Iron	27 mg	30 mg	Spinach, broccoli, tofu, shrimp, iron-fortified cereals	Yes
Calcium	1000–1300 mg	250 mg	Dairy products including milk, yogurt and cheese; leafy green vegetables; almonds; calcium-fortified foods	No [b]
Phosphorus	700–1250 mg		All animal foods (meats, fish, poultry, eggs, milk)	No
Zinc	11–13 mg	15 mg	Lentils, shrimp, crab, turkey, pork, lean ground beef, eggs, tofu	No [c]

[a] Source: Institute of Medicine, refs. *33,40*.
[b] Supplementation is recommended if foods high in calcium are not consumed.
[c] Both iron and copper compete with zinc at absorption sites; therefore, zinc supplementation is recommended when elemental iron supplementation exceeds 60 mg/d.
RE, retinol equivalents; NE, niacin equivalents.

3.1. Health Consequences of Early Childhood Caries (ECC)

The simultaneous presence of cariogenic microorganisms, fermentable carbohydrate, and a susceptible tooth and host initiate the infectious and transmissible disease known as dental caries in adults and ECC in children. At a microscopic level, the biology of caries is the same for adults and children. However, in children this disease can have a negative impact on a child's diet, nutritional status, sleep patterns, psychological status, and, later on, school attendance. Children have been reported to experience pain with ECC that adults would not endure. ECC has been described as a virulent form of caries that starts soon after teeth erupt, and it proceeds rapidly to involve primary molars and canines *(6)*.

Children who develop ECC are more likely to experience delayed development. Several ECC interventions have been identified in the literature as important for the amelioration of a commonly coexisting condition of ECC and the condition of growth faltering *(45,47,48)*. Acs et al. *(49)* found that correcting ECC could lead to an accelerated velocity of weight gain, resulting in the improvement of the growth faltering. Long-term effects of reversed growth faltering on health status or, conversely, prevention of childhood obesity are unknown. Because ECC has been closely associated with underlying nutritional deficiencies in the perinatal period *(6)*, it is likely, as the disease progresses, that developmental eating behaviors and nutritional status are threatened.

3.2. Recommended Infant and Early Childhood Feeding Practices to Promote Oral Health

Nutrient- and energy-dense liquids are supplemented and partially replaced with solid foods in the infant's diet when developmental readiness occurs. Thus, introduction of pureed and solid foods is recommended to parallel physiological, emotional, and cognitive development. Guidelines to ensure maintenance of adequate nutrient intake to support growth, development, and oral health are in sync. Introduction of foods to the diet to diminish the transmission of oral bacteria from the caregiver to the child and to include a variety of textures and consistency may be important to craniofacial and occlusal development. Animal studies have shown that animals fed only soft diets had smaller maxillary and mandibular arch widths and lengths than those fed hard diets *(50)*. A variety of foods further supports nutrient needs and enhances mastication, which leads to salivary production beneficial in decreasing caries risk. Table 2 outlines recommendations for oral health promotion among infants and young children based on policy statements of the American Academy of Pediatric Dentists and the American Academy of Pediatrics *(51,52)*.

4. SCHOOL-AGE CHILDREN AND ORAL HEALTH

Approximately 50% of children have experienced dental decay or caries by the age of 8 despite the fact that oral health has improved in the past few decades. This diet-dependent infectious bacterial disease remains one of the most common diseases of childhood. According to the Surgeon General's Report on Oral Health in America, it is five times as common as asthma and seven times as common as hay fever. Some racial or ethnic minorities, homeless and migrant populations, children with disabilities, and those with human immunodeficiency virus (HIV) infection often present with the most advanced forms of caries. If those with dental caries remain untreated, serious general

Table 2
Recommended Dietary Guidelines and Practices
for Oral Health Promotion of Infants and Young Children

Birth to 6 mo	• Whether breast- or bottle-feeding is the method of choice, infant feeding schedules should encourage routine consumption of milk rather than on-demand feeding.
	• Discourage bedtime bottles and nocturnal feeding after eruption of first tooth.
	• Diminish transmission of bacteria from caregiver to infant by wiping the gums after feedings and implementing oral hygiene when the first tooth erupts.
	• Promote introduction of water in bottles as appropriate but not until routine feeding is well established.
	• Instruct mothers to avoid introduction of food until the infant doubles the birth weight or weighs at least 13 lbs or reaches 6 mo of age.
6–12 mo	• Promote weaning from the bottle in combination with the introduction of a cup and spoon.
	• Promote introduction of food to encourage self-feeding.
1–3 yr	• Stress the value of mealtime and snacks and the importance of variety and moderation. Offer no more that 1 cup/d of fruit juices and only at meals and avoid all carbonated beverages during the first 30 mo of life.

From refs. *51,52.*

health problems can result. It has been reported that among low-income children, almost 50% of caries remain untreated. Thus, these children may experience pain, inability to chew well and eat, failure to gain weight, and embarrassment because of discolored and damaged teeth. These circumstances can reduce a child's capacity to succeed in school and can alter self-esteem and health behavioral self-efficacy. Dental-related illness results in more than 51 million lost school hours each year. Likewise, head, neck, and mouth trauma resulting from violence, sports, falls, and motor vehicle crashes create additional oral health problems for children *(22)*.

4.1. Food Choices and Frequency of Dietary Intake

Caries risk throughout childhood remains dependent on the synergy existing among oral bacterial count, general health status, fluoride exposure, and dietary patterns. Diet is one of the significant factors in modulating the direction of the dynamic demineralization and remineralization process of the tooth enamel. Diet cannot alter the percentage of acidogenic bacteria in dental plaque, but the dietary composition and frequency of exposure can alter the pH of the environment adjacent to the tooth as well as promote saliva production *(53)*. Saliva buffers dental plaque pH and promotes tooth remineralization and oral clearance. When plaque pH is measured following the consumption of a fermentable food or beverage, it can drop from neutral (pH 7.0) to a critical level below 5.7 within a 5-min time frame. It takes approx 40–60 min and a maximum of 120 min to return to neutral, particularly if interventions such as oral hygiene or xylitol/sorbitol sugar-free gums are not introduced *(54)*. Thus, food choices and frequency of dietary intake are major determinants of caries risk.

4.2. Snacking and School Environments

The school environment provides a venue for a significant portion of a child's experiences with lifestyle behaviors that effect health. Using well-defined protocols to distinguish snack and meal consumption patterns, nationally representative data from three large surveys conducted between 1977 and 1996 described increased snacking prevalence in US children *(55)*. Groups of foods eaten within a 15-min time span were counted as one snack. Children between the ages of 2 and 5 yr and 6 and 11 yr reported significant increases in the number of snacks eaten daily as well as the kilocalories from those snacks. In 1996, 90% of children snacked, whereas only 80% did so in 1977. Total daily energy intake from snacks rose from about 18% to 25% during this time frame. Snack intake reflected an increased consumption of soft drinks, potato and corn chips, and other kinds of salty snacks and a simultaneous drop in fruit, vegetable, and milk consumption. Energy consumption from meals remained constant over time, and children between 6 and 11 yr decreased their intake of calcium and protein; however, there was no change in vitamin A and fiber intake from these foods. Although it was reported that the average size of snacks and the energy per snack remained relatively constant, the number of snacking occasions had increased significantly. These trends are related to both childhood obesity and dental health status *(55)*.

A smaller study conducted in Finland reported that children who had candy and juice more than once a week when they were 3 yr old generally consumed more sucrose 3 yr later and had more visible plaque, leading to a higher incidence of carious lesions by the age of 6 yr *(56)*. Those who had sweets once a week or less had less plaque and fewer lesions at 6 yr of age.

Snacking is essential to the dietary pattern of children for adequate nutritional support. Because both the food and beverage snack choices and the frequency of their consumption have implications for caries risk, guidelines for nutrition educators can augment and enhance their role in the promotion of children's overall health and well-being. Table 3 *(2,20,55–61)* suggests specific guidelines for children between the ages of 3 and 10 yr.

5. SPECIAL NEEDS CHILDREN, NUTRITION, AND ORAL HEALTH

5.1. Cleft Lip and Palate

Studies suggest that the development of cleft lip and palate are related to a gene–environment interaction *(62)*. Studies have shown that maternal multivitamin supplement use protects against cleft lip and palate *(63,64)*. In a Danish population, higher levels of vitamin A intake from multivitamins and liver sources also seemed to protect against cleft lip and palate *(65)*. Further studies have suggested that the protection was not entirely explained by multivitamin use, indicating that adequate levels of vitamin A may be required for normal development of the primary palate *(62)*. Other authors have identified other risk factors, including cigarette smoking and alcohol consumption, use of anticonvulsant drugs, and exposure to organic solvents. A protective effect has been shown for supplementation with folic acid *(66)*. Maternal diabetes has also been implicated as an etiologic agent in cleft lip and palate. Mothers with diabetes were found to be 1.352 times (95% confidence interval, 1.004–1.821; $p < 0.05$) more likely than nondiabetic mothers to have a newborn with cleft lip or palate *(67)*. Early glycemic control by expectant mothers may be an important factor in decreasing the incidence of this congenital anomaly.

Table 3

Oral Health Nutrition Messages for 3- to 10-Yr-Old Children and Their Caregivers

Message	Rationale	Reference
Starchy, sticky, or sugary foods should be eaten with nonsugary foods.	The pH will rise if a nonsugary item that stimulates saliva is eaten immediately before, during, or after a challenge.	55
Combine dairy products with a meal or snack.	Dairy products (nonfat milk, yogurt) enhance remineralization and contain calcium.	56
Combine chewy foods such as fresh fruits and vegetables with fermentable carbohydrates.	Chewy, fibrous foods induce saliva production and buffering capacity.	2
Space eating occasions at least 2 h apart and limit snack time to 15 min.	Fermentable carbohydrates eaten sequentially one after another promote demineralization.	20
Limit bedtime snacks	Saliva production declines during sleep.	57
Limit consumption of acidic foods such as sports drinks, juices, and sodas.	Acidic foods promote tooth erosion that increases risk for caries.	58
Combine proteins with carbohydrates in snacks. Examples: tuna and crackers, yogurt and berries, apples and cheese, cookies and milk.	Proteins act as buffers and are cariostatic.	2,60
Combine raw and cooked or processed foods in a snack.	Raw foods encourage mastication and saliva production, whereas cooked or processed foods may be more available for bacterial metabolism if eaten alone.	2,60
Encourage use of xylitol/sorbitol-based chewing gum and candies immediately following a meal or snack.[a]	5 min exposure is effective in increasing saliva production and dental plaque pH. Excessive use may cause gastrointestinal distress.	59,61
Sugar-free chewable vitamin–mineral supplements and syrup-based medication should be recommended.	Sugar-free varieties are available and should be suggested for high-caries risk groups.	
Encourage children with pediatric GERD to adhere to dietary guidelines.	GERD increases risk for dental erosion.	

[a] Not recommended for children under the age of 4 yr.
GERD, gastroesophageal reflux disease.

25

All of the above studies of possible etiology reveal that adequate preconceptual and prenatal nutrition has an important role in the primary prevention of cleft lip and palate.

Dietary recommendations for infants born with a cleft are no different from those for other infants. The delivery method of breast milk or formula can be altered to ensure adequate nutrient intake in preparation for successful future surgical outcomes *(69)*. Chappelle and Nunn *(68)* showed that only 34% of 12-yr-old children with cleft lip and palate were free of caries. All the 4-yr-olds examined in their investigation had evidence of erosion of enamel in the primary teeth (incisors and first molars) and 56% of the 12-yr-olds had erosion of permanent teeth (incisors and first permanent molars). Lin and Tsai *(70)* found that children with clefts who took a bottle to bed showed an increased risk of developing ECC. The parents or caretakers of bottle-fed children allowed use of the bottle beyond 1 yr of age and also showed a lack of motivation to perform regular preventive dental home care for their children. This suggests that oral health promotion programs should begin in infancy for children with clefts and their parents, teaching them to wean their children from a bottle by age 1 yr, avoid nocturnal nursing bottles, and practice good oral hygiene from infancy.

5.2. Neural Tube Defects

The etiology of neural tube defects (NTDs) is unknown, although it is thought to be the result of a genetic predisposition manifested by the environment. It results from the disruption of the orderly formation of the vertebral arches and spinal cord that occurs between the fourth and sixth week of embryogenesis. According to recent evidence, NTDs may be related to the interaction of a genetic propensity for the defect and a deficiency of folic acid or poor metabolism of folic acid. Multivitamins containing folic acid taken during the first 6 wk of pregnancy can prevent more than 50% of NTD occurrence *(71)*.

There are two common forms of NTDs: spina bifida occulta and myelomeningocele (meningomyelocele) *(72)*. The form of NTD expressed as myelomeningocele has many associated problems, such as hydrocephalus, paralysis, orthopedic deformities, and genitourinary abnormalities. Children with closed spina bifida present with skin covering the area. The defect occurs in the vertebral column with tissue protrusion through a bony cleft. It usually is observed as a tuft of hair, a dimple, or a pigmented area above a defect. Sometimes with growth, children with this condition may develop foot weakness or bowel and bladder sphincter disturbances *(73)*.

Children with NTDs often are on long-term liquid medications to manage these conditions. When these medications have high sucrose content, caries may result *(74)*. Children with spina bifida have associated circumstances that make them prime candidates for dental caries. Many of these children tend to be overweight, which can be attributed to frequent snacking and impaired mobility because of the nature of their disability *(73)*. Caloric intake for these children often exceeds energy expended and is coupled with a lack of stimulation from physical activities. Caregivers may use food as a demonstration of affection or as a reward. Without good oral hygiene, this creates a perfect environment for oral bacteria, making the teeth susceptible to decay. These children often are seen for extensive dental rehabilitation *(75)*.

Few reliable statistics on how many children with spina bifida experience dental caries can be found. These children, however, are at greater risk for periodontal disease than the general population because of their disabilities and potential defects in the developmental formation of their enamel *(76)*.

5.3. *Mentally and Physically Handicapped*

Children with mental retardation may be prone to childhood dental caries because their neurological impairment can make dental care difficult or impossible. Often, children with this disability need assistance with eating, clothing, and toileting from caregivers. Given all of these needs, diligent oral hygiene may be considered less important and thus may be neglected *(71)*. Dental health in children with special needs is as essential as immunizations, regular physical examinations, and attention to injury prevention. Children with mental retardation may acquire dental caries because of poor dental hygiene, poor nutritional intake, and long-term medication therapy *(77)*.

The dental status and treatment needs of Israeli children and adults with mental retardation were studied in a random sample of 387 subjects. Findings confirm high dental morbidity such as decayed and missing teeth and significant oral health differences by level of retardation, age, and dental clinic status. Specialized training designed to address treatment issues with handicapped populations is recommended for dental providers and the staffs of institutions to enhance oral health outcomes *(78)*.

Parents and caregivers of handicapped children should be educated to clean the gums and mouths of children who do not have teeth yet with moist gauze. Children with disabilities need an appropriately sized toothbrush and require assistance with brushing. The use of an electric toothbrush can be beneficial for children who have poor plaque removal technique because of their lack of manual dexterity *(79)*.

6. SUMMARY

Nutrition and diet are significant determinants of oral health status during pregnancy, infancy, and childhood. Adequate nutrition of the fetus during pregnancy that is extended into childhood increases the likelihood of establishing health behaviors that promote positive outcomes. Conversely, malnutrition can contribute to low birthweight, preterm delivery, failure to thrive, obesity, and altered growth patterns associated with increased risks for oral diseases. Dental professionals should address oral health issues specific to stages of growth and development and promote parenting behaviors in keeping with achieving good health.

Guidelines for Practice

	Oral Health Professional	*Nutrition Professional*
Prevention	• Educate women who are planning pregnancies, are pregnant, or are parenting about the role of nutrition in the oral health of infants and children	• Include oral health screening in routine prenatal, infant, and child dietary assessment activities • Provide messaging to parents about the synergy between nutrition and risk for oral disease
Intervention	• Provide guidelines that promote oral health and support dietary changes necessary to decrease risk for ECC • Develop a referral protocol to a nutrition professional for comprehensive dietary counseling and monitoring	• Conduct dietary assessment and nutrition education with dental patients/clients who are parenting • Tailor dietary counseling to include guidelines to promote optimum oral health and disease risk reduction • Develop a referral protocol to a dental professional for oral health maintenance

REFERENCES

1. Marshall TA. Diet and nutrition in pediatric dentistry. Dent Clin North Am 2003; 47:279–303.
2. Mobley CC. Nutrition and dental caries. Dent Clin North Am. 2003; 47:319–336.
3. DePaola DP, Faine M, Palmer C. Nutrition in relation to dental medicine. In Shils M, Olson J, Shike M, Ross AC, eds.. Modern Nutrition in Health and Disease, 9th Ed. Baltimore, MD: Williams and Wilkins, 1999:1099–1124.
4. Fitzsimons D, Dwyer JT, Palmer C, Boyd LD. Nutrition and oral health guidelines for pregnant women, infants and children. J Am Diet Assoc 1998; 98:182–186.
5. Jontell M, Linde A. Nutritional aspects of tooth formation. World Rev Nutr Diet 1986; 48:114–136.
6. Davis GN. Early childhood caries: a synopsis. Community Dent Oral Epidemiol 1988; 26:106–116.
7. DePaola DP, Kuftinec MM. Nutrition in growth and development of oral tissues. Dent Clin North Am 1976; 20:441–459.
8. Institute of Medicine. Nutrition During Pregnancy. Washington DC: National Academy Press, 1990.
9. Rossner S. Obesity and pregnancy. In Bray G, Bouchard C, James W., eds. Handbook of Obesity New York, NY: Marcel Dekker, 1998, 775–790.
10. Luke B, Johnson T, Petrie R. 1993 Clinical Maternal–Fetal Medicine. Boston: Little, Brown, 1993.
11. Reifsnider E. Gill SL. Nutrition for the childbearing years. J Obstet Gynecol Neonatal Nurs 2000; 29: 43–55.
12. Bailit HL. Dental variation among populations: an anthropologic view. Dent Clin North Am 1975; 19(1):125–139.
13. Dorsky R.Nutrition and oral health. Gen Dent 2001; 49(6):576–582.
14. Li Y, Navia JM, Bian J-Y. Prevalence and distribution of developmental enamel defects in primary dentition of Chinese children 3–5 years old. Community Dent Oral Epidemiol 1995; 23(2):72–79.
15. Rugg-Gunn AJ, Al-Mohammadi SM, Butler TJ. Effects of fluoride level in drinking water, nutritional status, and socio-economic status on the prevalence of developmental defects of dental enamel in permanent teeth in Saudi 14 year old boys. Caries Res. 1997; 31:259–267.
16. Seow WK. Enamel hypoplasia in the primary dentition: a review. J Dent Child 1991; 58:441–452.
17. Giunta J L. Dental changes in hypervitaminosis D. Oral Surg Oral Med Oral Pathol Oral Radiol Endod 1998; 4:410–413.
18. Nakamoto T, Mallak H M, Miller SA. The effect of protein-energy malnutrition on the growth of tooth germs in newborn rats. J Dent Res 1979; 58(3):1115–1122.
19. Dreizen S. The importance of nutrition in tooth development. J Sch Health 1973; 63(2):114–115.
20. Tinanoff N. Palmer CA. Dietary determinants of dental caries and dietary recommendations for preschool children. J Public Health Dent 2000; 60(3):197–209.
21. Ismail A I. The role of early dietary habits in dental caries development. Spec Care Dentist 1998; 18(1):40–45.
22. U.S. Department of Health and Human Services. Oral Health in America: A Report of the Surgeon General—Executive Summary. Rockville, MD: U.S. Department of Health and Human Services, National Institute of Dental and Craniofacial Research, National Institutes of Health, 2000.
23. Ladipo O.A. Nutrition in pregnancy: mineral and vitamin supplements. Am J Clin Nut 2000; 72: 280S–290S.
24. Ramakrishnan U, Manjrdkar R, Rivera J, Gonzalez-Cossio T, Martorell R. 1999 Micronutrients and pregnancy outcome: a review of the literature. Nutr Res 2000; 19:103–159.
25. Harris SS, Navia JM. In vivo and in vitro study of the effects of vitamin A deficiency on rat third molar development. J Dent Res 1986; 65(12):1445–1448.
26. Worthington-Roberts B. The role of maternal nutrition in the prevention of birth defects. Perinatal Nutr Rep 1996; 2(3):12.
27. Fontana M. Vitamin C (ascorbic acid): clinical implications for oral health—a literature review. Compend Contin Educ Dent 1994; 15(7):916–929.
28. Dixon SJ, Wilson JX. Adaptative regulation of ascorbate transport in osteoblastic cells. J Bone Miner Res 1992; 17(6):675–681.
29. Nizel AE, Papas AS. Nutrition in Clinical Dentistry, 3rd Ed. Philadelphia, PA: W.B. Saunders, 1989.
30. Ogawara M, Aoki K, Okiji T, Suda H. Effect of ascorbic acid deficiency on primary and reparative dentinogenesis in non-ascorbate-synthesizing ods rats. Arch Oral Biol 1997; 42(10):695–704.

31. Clark DE, Navia JM, Manson-Hing LR, Duncan HE. Evaluation of alveolar bone in relation to nutritional status during pregnancy. J Dent Res 1990; 69(3):890–895.
32. Bawden JW. Calcium transport during mineralization. Anat Rec 1989; 224(2):226–233.
33. Institute of Medicine. Dietary Reference Intakes for Calcium, Phosphorus, Magnesium, Vitamin D, and Fluoride. Washington DC: National Academy Press, 1997.
34. Giddens JB, Krug SK, Tsang RC, Guo S, Miodovnik M, Prada JA. Pregnant adolescent and adult women have similarly low intakes of selected nutrients. J Am Diet Assoc, 2000; 100(11):1334–1340.
35. Alvarez JO. Nutrition, tooth development, and dental caries. Am J Clin Nutr 1995; 61:410S–416S.
36. Jontell M, Linde A. Nutritional aspects of tooth formation. World Rev Nutr Diet 1986; 48:114–136.
37. Leverett DH, Adair SM, Vaughan BW, Proskin HM, Moss ME. Randomized clinical trial of the effect of prenatal fluoride supplements in preventing dental caries. Caries Res 1997; 31(3):174–179.
38. Dorsky R. Nutrition and oral health. Gen Dent 2001; 49(6):576–582.
39. National Research Council. Recommended Dietary Allowances. 10th Ed. Washington DC: National Academy Press, 1989.
40. Institute of Medicine. Dietary Reference Intakes: Thiamine, Riboflavin, Niacin, Vitamin B-6, Folate, Vitamin B-12, Pantothenic Acid, Biotin, and Choline. Washington DC: National Academy Press, 1998.
41. Fewtrell MS, Lucas A, Morgan JB. Factors associated with weaning in full term and preterm infants. Arch Dis Child Fetal Neonatal Ed 2003; 88(4):F296–301.
42. World Health Organization. Diet, Nutrition, and the Prevention of Chronic Diseases. Report of a WHO/ FAO Consultation. WHO Technical Report Series 916, 2002.
43. Garcia-Godoy F, Mobley CC, Jones DL. Caries and Feeding Patterns in South Texas Preschool Children. San Antonio, TX: University of Texas Health Science Center at San Antonio, 1995
44. van Palenstein Helderman WH, Mabelya L, Van't Hof MA, Konig KG. Two types of intraoral distribution of fluorotic enamel. Community Dent Oral Epidemiol 1997; 25(3):251–255.
45. Fitzsimons D, Dwyer JT, Palmer C, Boyd LD. Nutrition and oral health guidelines for pregnant women, infants and children. J Am Diet Assoc 1998; 98:182–186.
46. American Dietetic Association. The impact of fluoride on health. J Am Diet Assoc 2000; 100:1208–1213.
47. Acs G, Lodolini G, Shulman R, Chussid S. The effect of dental rehabilitation on the body weight of children with failure to thrive: case reports. Compend Contin Educ Dent 1998; 19(2):164–168, 170–171.
48. Elise CE, Fields HW. Failure to thrive: review of the literature, case reports, and implications for dental treatment. Pediatr Dent 1990; 12(3):185–189.
49. Acs G, Shulman R, Ng MW, Chussid S. The effect of dental rehabilitation on the body weight of children with early childhood caries. Pediatr Dent 1999; 21(2):109–113.
50. Beecher RM, Corruccini RS, Freeman M. Craniofacial correlates of dietary consistency in a nonhuman primate. J Craniofac Genet Dev Biol 1983; 3(2):193–202.
51. American Academy of Pediatrics. Policy statement: oral health risk assessment timing and establishment of the dental home. Pediatrics 2003; 111(5):1113–1116.
52. American Academy of Pediatric Dentistry. Journal of the American Academy of Pediatric Dentistry Reference Manual 1996–97. Pediatric Dentistry 1996; 18(6): 25–30.
53. Konig KG. Diet and oral health. Int Dent J 2000; 50:162–174.
54. Newbrun E. Cariology. Chicago: Quintessence, 1989
55. Jahns L, Siega-Riz MS, Popkin BM. The increasing prevalence of snacking among US children from 1977 to 1996. J Pediatr 2001; 138:493–498.
56. Karjalainen S, Soderling E, Sewon L, Lapinleimu H, Simell O. A prospective study on sucrose consumption, visible plaque and caries in children from 3 to 6 years of age. Community Dent Oral Epidemiol 2001; 29(2):136–142.
57. Geddes DAM. Diet patterns and caries. Adv Dent Res 1994; 8:221–224.
58. Dairy foods and oral health. In Miller GD, Jarvis JK, McBean LD. Handbook of Dairy Foods and Nutrition. 2nd Ed. Washington DC: CRC Press 2000: ,291–310.
59. Edgar WM, O'Mullane. Saliva and Oral Health. London, UK: British Dental Association, 1996.
60. Rugg-Gunn AJ. Nutrition and Dental Health. Oxford, UK: Oxford University Press, 1993.
61. Machiulskiene V, Nyvad B, Baelum V. Caries preventive effect of sugar-substituted chewing gum. Community Dent Oral Epidemiol 2001; 29:279–288.

62. Mitchell LE, Murray JC,, O'Brien S, Christensen K. Retinoic acid receptor alpha gene variants, multi-vitamin use, and liver intake as risk factors for oral clefts: a population-based case-control study in Denmark, 1991–1994. Am J Epidemiol 2003; 158(1):69–76.

63. Mastroiacovo P, Mazzone T, Addis A, et. al. High vitamin A intake in early pregnancy and major malformations: a multicenter prospective controlled study. Teratology 1999; 59:7–11.

64. Mills JL, Simpson JL, Cunningham GC, Conley MR, Rhoads GG. Vitamin A and birth defects. Am J Public Health 1997; 177:31–36.

65. Shaw D, Ray A, Marazita M, Field L. Further evidence of a relationship between the retinoic acid receptor alpha locus and nonsyndromic cleft lip with or without cleft palate (CL +/– P) Am J Hum Genet 1993; 53(5):1156–1157.

66. Leite IC, Paumgartten FJ, Koifman S. Chemical exposure during pregnancy and oral clefts in newborns. Cadernos de Saude Publica 2002; 18(1):17–31.

67. Spilson SV, Kim HJ, Chung KC. Association between maternal diabetes mellitus and newborn oral cleft. Ann Plast Surg 2001; 47(5):477–481.

68. Chapple J, Nunn J. Abstracts from other journals. Int J Paediatr Dent 2001; 11(6):457.

69. Redford-Badwal DA, Mabry K, Frassinelli JD. Impact of cleft lip and/or palate on nutritional health and oral–motor development. Dent Clin North Am 2003; 47:305–317.

70. Lin YT, Tsai CL. Caries prevalence and bottle-feeding practices in 2-year-old children with cleft lip, cleft palate, or both in Taiwan. Cleft Palate Craniofac J 1999; 36(6):522–526.

71. Milunsky A, Jick H, Jick SS, et. al. Multivitamin/folic acid supplementation in early pregnancy reduces the prevalence of neural tube defects. JAMA 1989; 262(20):2847–2852.

72. Hudson M. Dental surgery in pediatric patients with spina bifida and latex allergy. AORN J 2001; 74(1):56–57, 59–63, 65–66, 69–70, 72–78.

73. Farley J, Dunleavy MJ. Myelodysplasia. In Jackson P, Vessey J., eds. Primary Care of the Child with a Chronic Condition. 3rd Ed. St. Louis, MO: Mosby, 2000, 658–674.

74. Shaw L. The role of medications in dental caries formation: need for sugar-free medication for children. Pediatrician 1989; 16:153–155.

75. Haskins DR. Pediatric dental rehabilitation procedures in the OR. AORN J 1996; 64(4):573–579.

76. McDonald RE, Avery DR, Stookey GK. Dental caries in the child and adolescent. In McDonald RE, Avery DR, eds. Dentistry for the Child and Adolescent, 7th Ed. St. Louis, MO:Mosby, 2000, 221–222.

77. Helpin ML, Rosenberg HM. Beyond brushing and flossing. In Batshaw ML, ed. Children with Disabilities, 4th Ed. Baltimore, MD: Paul Brooks, 1977, 643–655.

78. Shapira J, Efrat J, Berkey D, Mann J. Dental health profile of a population with mental retardation in Israel. Spec Care Dent 1998; 18(4):149–155.

79. Dean JA, Hughes CV. Mechanical and chemotherapeutic home oral hygiene. In McDonald RE, Avery DR, eds. Dentistry for the Child and Adolescent, 7th Ed. St. Louis, MO: Mosby, 2000, 253.

3 Age-Related Changes in Oral Health Status

Effects on Diet and Nutrition

Carole A. Palmer

1. INTRODUCTION

The oral cavity is the vehicle through which the body receives and processes nourishment. Multiple oral tissues work together to support these vital functions. These oral tissues include muscles of mastication and deglutition (including the tongue), oral mucosa, teeth and periodontal tissues, salivary glands and their secretions, and taste and smell receptors. As a result, problems that occur in the oral cavity can affect the ability and desire to bite, chew, and swallow foods. For example, soft-tissue diseases and conditions can make it difficult and painful to masticate and swallow and, correspondingly, dental caries or missing teeth can make it difficult to bite and chew.

Compromised oral function has been linked to decreased self-esteem and a decline in the quality of life *(1)*. Adults with missing teeth or loose dentures may avoid certain social activities because they are embarrassed to speak, smile, or eat in front of others. Both systemic health and quality of life are compromised when oral conditions affect eating and food choices *(2)*. This chapter reviews how changes in oral soft and hard tissue effect diet and nutrition including life-cycle issues specific to aging.

2. DENTATE STATUS AFFECTS DIET AND NUTRITION

Of adults aged 25 and older, 11% have lost all of their natural teeth. This number increases to 30% for people over age 65 and is even higher for those living at the poverty level *(3)*. Despite this continued problem with tooth loss, most people are keeping an increasing number of their teeth into old age. Over the next three decades, the average number of teeth retained among the elderly is predicted to rise to 25.9 *(4)* from the current average of 20. Although the proportion of edentulous patients in the elderly population is declining, the total number of persons with no teeth in the United States is likely to remain constant at 9 million *(4)*.

Although more people are keeping their natural teeth longer in developed countries, a large number of people still depend on removable dentures. The third National Health and Nutrition Examination Survey (NHANES III), a US survey conducted between 1988 and 1994, reported that 44% of those aged 75 or older were missing all of their teeth *(5)*.

From: *Nutrition and Oral Medicine*
Edited by: R. Touger-Decker, D. A. Sirois, and C. C. Mobley © Humana Press Inc., Totowa, NJ

Half of all Americans aged 55 and older wore a partial or complete denture, whereas 60% of denture wearers reported one or more problems with their dentures (6).

2.1. Masticatory Ability

Research consistently has demonstrated that reduced chewing efficiency is associated with decreasing numbers of teeth, removable partial dentures as compared with a similar number of natural teeth, and complete dentures as compared with natural dentition (7). The position of natural teeth, the number of pairs of opposing tooth surfaces, and their function are thought to be more accurate indicators of masticatory ability than the total number of teeth in the mouth (8). Aging itself has little effect on chewing efficiency, but the reduced muscle mass associated with aging may cause reduced oral motor function (9,10).

2.1.1. NUMBER OF TEETH

Changes in dentition can have a profound impact on eating, although perceived chewing efficiency with dental prostheses may be a more likely determinant of food acceptance than measured function (11).

Compiled evidence from the 1950s to the 2000s indicated that tooth loss affects objective measures of masticatory performance. Early studies implied a significant decrease of masticatory efficiency in 75% of complete denture wearers compared to dentate subjects. Later research indicated that losses in masticatory efficiency because of tooth loss were closer to 30 to 40%. However, the data suffer from differences in research methods, test food choices, and test populations (12).

Masticatory ability is more a function of dentition status than of age (12). The Boston Veterans' Administration Dental Longitudinal Study showed that dentate status was the primary determinant of masticatory ability. The number of existing teeth affects masticatory performance and food selection (11,13–16). The presence of removable dentures and the possession of fewer than 20 teeth are both linked to reduced chewing ability. Chewing longer and swallowing larger food particles compensates for reduced chewing ability (17). As adults age, they tend to increase the number of chewing strokes and chew longer to prepare food for swallowing (15). Masticatory efficiency in wearers of a complete denture has been found to be approx 80% lower than in people with intact natural dentition (18).

The degree of dental impairment also determines chewing performance. When objective measures of chewing ability were assessed, individuals with intact dentitions chewed the best, followed in descending order by those with partially compromised dentitions (24–29 teeth) or compromised dentitions (20–26 teeth). People with one or two full dentures had the poorest chewing performance (18).

The Swallowing Threshold Test Index, an objective measure of chewing ability, assesses the number of chewing strokes required to reduce a hard food such as a raw carrot to a small enough particle size for swallowing and is used as a gold standard. When functional feeding skills were measured in 79 healthy adults aged 60–97 yr, these skills were not age dependent but were dependent on whether subjects wore full dentures (19).

2.1.2. FUNCTIONAL TOOTH UNITS

When Hatch et al. (20) tested a multivariate model of masticatory performance for dentate subjects, the number of functional tooth units and bite force were confirmed as

Table 1
Foods Difficult for Complete Denture Wearers to Chew

Foods with seeds and small particles	Hard foods	Sticky foods
Nuts	Meat (steak)	Chewing gum
Tomatoes	Apples (whole)	
Jam with seeds	Toast (crusts)	Soft bread
Pears	Raw fruit	Sticky candy
Figs	Salad (carrot, celery)	
Grapes	Corn on the cob	
Coconut		
Rice		
Seeds		
Crunchy peanut butter		

From ref. 7.

the key determinants of masticatory performance. Other investigators noted that older dentate adults reported difficulty chewing one or more of the following foods: steaks, chops, fibrous meats, raw carrots, celery, fresh apple, lettuce or spinach salad, and cooked vegetables (21).

Results from the British National Diet and Nutrition Survey (NDNS), conducted with 753 free-living British subjects aged 65 yr and older, found that 17% reported that their patterns of daily living, especially eating and speaking, on a regular basis were impacted by oral conditions. The impact levels were lowest in dentate subjects with the greater number of teeth. Among those whose dental status had an impact on eating, 25% said that the impact was severe and 42% said that they notice the impact on a daily basis. These perceptions were associated with inability to eat or difficulty in eating a range of 16 common foods (22). Approximately one in five dentate subjects said that they had difficulty eating or could not eat raw carrots, apples, well-done steak, or nuts. Perceived chewing ability increased with increasing numbers of natural teeth and pairs of opposing posterior teeth (23).

In summary, evidence to date has confirmed an association between food choices and masticatory efficiency by demonstrating that decreasing numbers of teeth leads to progressive alteration in food choices. The greatest effect is noted among those who are edentulous (7). Table 1 lists common foods that present difficulties among people with dentures. Table 2 provides guidelines for eating with dentures.

2.2. Diet Quality and Nutritional Status

Although oral conditions can exacerbate systemic conditions (e.g., diabetes), the extent to which tooth loss and dental disease alone can adversely affect nutritional health is not completely known (12). As the degree of dental impairment increases, the quality of the diet seems to decrease (24–26). This deterioration in diet quality is thought to increase risk for several systemic diseases (27). Among a sample of noninstitutionalized elders, those wearing one or two complete dentures had a 20% decline in the nutrient quality of their diets when compared to dentate peers (28). Indeed, the lifestyle factors linked most closely to inferior diets were low median family income, low educational

Table 2
Guidelines for Eating With Complete Dentures

Getting started

1. Begin with soft foods such well-cooked cereals, boiled eggs, and very tender or ground meats and gradually add firmer foods to the diet.
2. Chew small precut pieces of hard foods, such as apples, with the back teeth.
3. Divide food between both sides of the mouth and avoid chewing on only one side at a time.
4. Avoid holding liquids and beverages in the mouth before swallowing because this may loosen a lower denture.
5. Eat easy-to-bite foods, such as sandwiches, by applying pressure against the back of the front teeth as the mouth slowly closes.
6. Avoid sticky (peanut butter) or hard-to-chew (hard salami) sandwiches.

Food choices

1. Choose a variety of foods to provide an adequately balanced diet.
2. Carefully select leafy vegetables, such as lettuce, as they may adhere to the polished denture surface.
3. Replace fibrous or hard-to-chew meats with ground meats, poultry, fish, eggs, beans, or legumes.
4. Cream, stew, or roast tender cuts of meat.
5. Replace sticky foods with chewable high-fiber foods that will increase saliva and oral clearance.
6. Eat doughy foods, such as breads, with liquids to decrease their tendency to stick to dentures, or toast bread when possible.
7. Choose steamed or canned vegetables and chopped or shredded raw vegetables and fruit.

Adapted with permission from the University of Texas Health Science Center at San Antonio Dental School, Department of Community Dentistry

attainment, and wearing dentures. In the Nutrition and Oral Health Study (NOHS), 247 partially or fully dentate middle-aged and elderly subjects experienced declining intakes of vitamin A, fiber, and calcium with decreasing numbers of teeth *(29)*. This may be because dentate adults tend to eat more fruits and vegetables than full-denture wearers *(30,31)*.

Among 324 frail elders (mean age of 85) participating in a Swiss study, malnutrition as measured by serum albumin (<33g/L) and body mass index (BMI = < 21 kg/m^2) was most associated with either wearing dentures with defective bases or not wearing dentures at all. In the dentate subjects in this sample, corresponding identifiers were the number of occluding pairs of teeth (five or fewer, natural or prosthetic), the number of retained roots, and the presence of mobile teeth. In both groups, those with compromised oral functional status had a significantly lower BMI and serum albumin concentration than those with intact dentition *(32)*. Papas *(29)* and Lamy *(33)* both reported similar findings.

In 110 frail adults with an average age of 77 yr who were admitted to a rehabilitation unit, the number of oral problems, including limited chewing ability, was the most important predictor of weight loss *(34)*. Older adults with poor-fitting dentures may experience weight loss because of a low calorie intake or limited variety of foods *(35)*.

The US Department of Agriculture's Nutritional Status Study of 691 independent-living elders aged 60–98 yr found that poor diet quality was associated with self-report of partial or full dentures. In a random subsample of 181 subjects, significant correlations were found between quality of nutrient intake reported in 3-d food records and degree of tooth loss. Analysis of 53 nutrients showed that the dentate subjects had diets of signifi-

Table 3
Nutrition-Related Implications for Denture Wearers

- Diet quality decreases as the number of missing teeth increases.
- Dentures do not necessarily improve diet quality.
- Denture wearers present with higher serum cholesterol, higher body mass index, higher prevalence of type 2 diabetes, and higher sugar and carbohydrate intakes vs dentate people.
- Upper dentures can impair taste and swallowing function.
- Denture wearers experience accelerated alveolar bone resorption coupled with lower dietary calcium intake.

cantly higher nutritional quality than did those who were partially or totally edentulous (25). The denture wearers consumed more refined carbohydrates and sucrose than dentate adults (29). As the number of teeth declined, vitamin A, crude fiber, and calcium intakes declined, whereas dietary cholesterol intakes increased (29).

Subjects in the NDNS study who were edentate had intakes of most nutrients that were lower than in dentate subjects. Intakes of nonstarch polysaccharides, protein, calcium, nonheme iron, niacin, and vitamin C were significantly lower in edentate subjects. Individuals with 21 or more teeth consumed a greater amount of most nutrients (36).

Edentulous subjects in Connecticut and 10 European countries, without prosthetic replacements, had significantly reduced intakes of carbohydrate and vitamin B_6 when compared to dentate subjects (37). Intakes of vitamins B_1 and C, dietary fiber, calcium, and iron were also lower in the edentulous group.

Changes in food habits associated with denture wearing may ultimately affect general health. The Health Professionals Study reported that the diets of edentulous subjects contained fewer vegetables, less carotene and dietary fiber, and more dietary cholesterol, saturated fat, and total calories than diets of persons who had 25 or more teeth (38). Edentulous, middle-aged Swedish men and women were heavier and had lower levels of high-density lipoprotein (HDL) cholesterol than dentate adults, and edentulous women had significantly higher plasma total cholesterol and triglycerides than dentate women (39). Table 3 summarizes the implications of dentures on nutrition.

Nutritional deficiencies are not inevitable, however. Masticatory variables are not necessarily related to diet quality. Dietary quality indices defined by the Healthy Eating Index (40) were examined in a community-based sample of 731 subjects, aged 37–81 yr. Masticatory variables were not found to be related to differences in the indices, suggesting that chewing-related factors are not necessarily predictors of overall diet quality (41). Using analyses based on the same index, NHANES data from 5958 participants ages 50 yr and over showed that dental health is closely associated with nutritional status. Impaired dentition in this population was defined by number of posterior occluding pairs of teeth. Those wearing dentures and having fewer than five pairs of posterior teeth reported diets of poorer quality than those with increasing numbers of pairs of teeth. This was associated with lower fruit intake, higher fat intake, lower dietary fiber intake, and higher BMIs (42).

Some individuals compensate for decline in masticatory ability by choosing processed or cooked foods rather than fresh and by chewing longer before swallowing. Others, however, may eliminate entire food groups from their diet (11,15). Nutrient intakes of individuals with impaired dentition can fall below minimum recommendations, especially if the eating pattern is already marginal in quality and the patient is subjected to sudden insults such as illness, loss of taste, inability to chew, or changes in economic status and living situation *(12,38,43)*. In addition, a high number of smokers and former smokers is found among the edentulous, and adults who smoke generally have poorer diets *(38)*.

2.3. Sensory Perception

Taste buds on the tongue and oropharynx are responsible for the sensations of bitter, sweet, salty, and sour. Tactile and temperature sensations in the tongue help discern flavor. Depressed senses of taste and smell have been attributed to the aging process, disease, medications, smoking, lack of tongue cleaning, and other dental problems. Indeed, many oral conditions can directly or indirectly affect smell and taste. These include oral infections, oral lesions, salivary gland dysfunction, poorly fitting dentures, and systemic diseases *(44)*.

Diminished salivary secretions have an adverse effect on many oral functions such as chewing, tasting, swallowing, speaking, and wearing dentures successfully. There may also be burning or soreness of oral mucosa, increased susceptibility to oral candidiasis, and an increase in the incidence of severe caries *(45,46)*. Salivary gland dysfunction and/ or inadequate saliva contribute to the inability to obtain proper nutrition via difficulties in lubricating, masticating, tolerating, tasting, and swallowing food *(47)*. Elders with xerostomia experienced a reduction in taste and food perception, and these subjects also experienced significant ($p < 0.001$) deficiencies of dietary fiber, potassium, vitamin B_6, iron, calcium, and zinc as compared to the 1989 recommended dietary allowances *(47)*. Compared to people with normal salivary flow, those with xerostomia have been shown to have significantly lower caloric intake and inadequate intakes of fiber, potassium, vitamin B_6, iron, calcium, and zinc, despite the cause of the xerostomia *(47)*. Craniofacial and oral surgery, chemotherapy, and radiotherapy to head and neck regions can also cause temporary or permanent changes in taste and smell *(12)*.

A full upper denture can impede optimal taste and swallowing ability and may contribute to choking. Taste sensitivity can be reduced when an upper denture covers the hard palate (which contains taste buds). When the upper palate is covered, it is also difficult for a person to determine the location of food in the mouth, thus making swallowing less well coordinated *(48,49)*. Dentures are considered to be a major contributing factor to deaths from choking for this reason *(50)*.

Considerable differences exist between older and younger people regarding sensory perception and pleasantness of foods *(51)*. Several studies have also shown that people with poor odor perception have lower nutrient intakes than those with good odor perception. Dental status may be a contributing factor to odor perception in those who have other health conditions as well *(53)*. Tongue brushing can help increase taste sensation for older patients *(52)*.

2.4. Digestion and Gastrointestinal Function

The chewing of foods is important for the initiation of food digestion. Tosello showed that subjects with "a natural set of teeth" had significantly less gastrointestinal pathology than did partially edentulous subjects *(54)*. More specifically, poor oral function may lead to a semisolid or soft consistency of the alimentary bolus. This bolus, resulting from a low-fiber diet, may be the origin of gastric disorders (43). In support of this hypothesis, the use of gastrointestinal (GI) drugs appears to be higher in adult edentulous subjects with poor masticatory ability (55). Correcting the composition of the alimentary bolus may help avoid these GI pathologies (43).

In young and middle-aged adults, dental erosion and alterations in taste are associated with chronic vomiting, duodenal ulcer, and gastroesophageal reflux disease (GERD). Heartburn, chronic cough, hoarseness, asthma, and idiopathic pulmonary fibrosis have all been associated with GERD (56). Demineralization of the hard dental tissues, particularly at restoration margins, increases risk for dental caries and possibly tooth loss. Elevating the head of the bed, abstinence from alcohol and tobacco, avoidance of fatty and spicy foods, avoidance of foods and liquids 2–3 h before bedtime, and use of liquid antacids are generally recommended to control adverse effects.

3. ORAL HEALTH CARE INTERVENTION AND DIET AND NUTRITION

In 2000, the Surgeon General's Report on Oral Health in America stated (57): "Oral diseases are progressive and cumulative and become more complex over time. They can affect our ability to eat, the foods we choose, how we look, and the way we communicate. These diseases can affect economic productivity and compromise our ability to work at home, at school, or on the job. Health disparities exist across population groups at all ages." Oral health care includes interventions targeted to prolonging a positive oral health status and quality of life. However, these interventions can alter dietary intake and possibly nutritional status.

3.1. Oral Surgery and Maxillomandibular Fixation

Oral surgery and maxillomandibular fixation temporarily alter food intake and may contribute to weight loss. Nutritional requirements are increasing as a result of surgical stress simultaneous to the time when eating well becomes most difficult. After tooth extractions or gingival surgery, some patients will avoid eating because of local pain or fear that eating will cause pain. Oral surgical procedures may pose nutritional risks if patients are severely underweight; have had a recent loss of 10% of body weight or more; abuse alcohol or other substances; or take steroids, immunosuppressants, or antitumor agents that have catabolic properties (58). Reported weight loss may be an indicator of inadequate caloric intake. Fatigue, a common patient complaint following surgery, may also lead to skipping meals and reduced desire to eat.

Proactive diet suggestions may help prevent potential negative nutritional consequences of extensive oral surgery. For the first day or two after extensive oral surgery, a high-calorie liquid diet, including cool or cold foods (ice cream, milk shakes, eggnog, and chilled puddings) will help keep the local area comfortable. Adding snacks of fruit-juice popsicles, milk shakes, or liquid supplements provides additional calories The patient should consume eight or more glasses of fluids, water, fruit juices, or milk every 24 h. By the second or third day after surgery, the patient should be able to consume a soft diet. The typical oral surgery patient should be able to return to a normal diet within a week, but people with multiple extractions throughout the mouth may need to maintain a soft diet for a longer time. Table 4 includes suggestions that may be helpful to these patients.

Table 4
Dietary Guidelines for Biting or Chewing Difficulties Associated With Dental Procedures

Eating fruits and vegetables

- Turn fruits and vegetables into chopped salads.
    Fruit salad in bite-size pieces made from fresh cut-up fruit.
    Chopped greens, tomatoes, cucumbers.
    Corn salsa (take fresh corn off the cob and mix with salsa).
- Choose either very soft breads and crackers or very crisp ones (limit those that are "chewy" such as bagels, soft rolls, bread crusts).
- If raw vegetables are tough to chew even chopped, steam or stir fry for 5 min and then chop and chill for a salad.
- Pasta salads (pasta mixed with chopped vegetables or beans and chilled).

Snacks foods that are easy to eat

- Bite-size tortilla chips broken in half.
- Bite-size rice cakes.
- Fruit smoothies: frozen fresh fruit and yogurt or milk in the blender (high in calcium also).
- Frozen berries or grapes (great to suck on).
- Flour tortilla pizza strips (flour tortillas with a layer of salsa and cheese, microwave for 1 min, then cut in strips.

Drinking liquids

- Drink at least 8 cups of liquid (= amount of water) daily.

Adequate fiber

- Dietary fiber intake may decrease; using these tips for eating chopped and cut food will help maintain fiber intake.
- If needed or desired, try 1/2 to 1 cup of bran cereal daily and include high-fiber foods such as corn, blueberries, cooked dried beans.

Adapted with permission from University of Medicine and Dentistry of New Jersey.

Intermaxillary fixation (wiring the maxilla and mandible together) may be necessary after major reconstructive jaw surgery or to immobilize a fractured jaw and may last several weeks. During this period, patients may be at increased nutritional risk because of impaired eating ability. If the jaw wiring is prolonged, food intake may decrease dramatically. Weight loss is common after jaw fixation owing to the limited volume of food eaten. If patients have suffered injury, they will often be in negative nitrogen balance as well, indicating breakdown of body protein and increased risk for malnutrition.

A liquid or blenderized diet is generally indicated during jaw immobilization *(59)*, and six to eight small meals a day may be required to obtain adequate calories and protein. Blenderized liquid foods that can pass through a straw are generally well tolerated *(60)*. Liquid supplements given to healthy orthognathic surgery patients for 6 wk after surgery aided patients in maintaining nitrogen balance, body weight, and balanced nutrient intake *(61)*.

3.2. Tooth Replacement

The overall risk for caries in individuals aged 45 and older has not decreased appreciably. The increase in restorative care needed between 1990 and 2030 will be highest in adults over the age of 44 yr *(62)*. The prevalence of root caries and the number of restored teeth will be greatest in the elderly population, requiring caries risk management that includes dietary modification.

The effect of dentures on nutritional status is highly variable among individuals, and tooth replacement with complete upper and lower dentures does not completely restore masticatory function and sensory ability *(26,63,64)*. Replacing poorly fitting dentures with new ones does result in better retention, better stability, and improved occlusion. Replacing posterior teeth by fixed or removable prostheses increases masticatory muscle activity and reduces chewing time and the number of chewing strokes until swallowing. However, as previously discussed in this chapter, tooth replacement alone has not shown to markedly improve dietary intakes *(7,19,24,65,66)*.

Implant-supported mandibular dentures also improve masticatory function, particularly biting force. However, no significant improvement in food selection or nutrient intake has been noted in patients exchanging optimal complete dentures for implant-supported dentures *(62,67,68)*.

3.3. Temporomandibular Disorders

Dysfunction of the temporomandibular region, where the mandible joins the temporal bone, can result in pain, discomfort, and the inability to open the mouth widely. These impediments can limit biting and chewing ability *(69)* and may alter food choices. Although the exact causes of temporomandibular disorders (TMD) are not well understood, the most commonly documented causes include injury to the joints or muscles of the jaw, occlusal problems such as poor bite or misaligned jaw, and habits such as clenching, bruxing, or excessive gum chewing. TMD is more common among postmenopausal women receiving hormone replacement therapy and young women using oral contraceptives *(70)*.

3.4. Dysphagia

Dysphagia (difficulty in swallowing) is most commonly associated with stroke, but poor dentition (natural or artificial), head and neck radiation or other anticancer therapy, surgery involving oral structures, esophagitis, or severe trauma to the oral facial areas may also cause dysphagia *(15,71)*. Dysphagia, in turn, can result in reduced caloric intake and a decrease in important food components such as fiber. Chapter 5 discusses dysphagia in greater detail.

3.5. Special Populations

Throughout the life cycle, oral health status, promotion, and care are defined by special needs and concerns. Chapter 2 describes in detail considerations specific to the oral health and nutritional well-being of infants and children.

4. SUMMARY

Oral health status can affect food choices and ultimately impact dietary adequacy, nutritional status, and general health. Lack of teeth can affect chewing ability and food choices. However, research to date has not unequivocally shown an effect on nutritional status *(72)*. One major implication of dentures seems to be the life-threatening risk of choking *(50)*.

Inadequate methods for obtaining accurate diet data, including failure to control for confounding variables, have made research in the area of oral status and nutrition difficult to interpret. However, it is clear that oral status can affect food choices and quality of life.

Dental professionals should assess the dietary patterns of patients as a measure of successful oral health care. Changes in oral health status as a result of changes in general health or alteration in dentition necessitate the implementation of nutrition education to accommodate temporary or prolonged changes in mastication, salivation, and oral soft tissue health. These initiatives should include referral to a dietetic professional if merited and resources for dental patients that include nutrition education materials.

Allied health professionals in healthcare facilities and public health arenas should be assessing the adequacy of mastication, the presence of pain, and physical changes in oral tissue to initiate referral to a dental professional and nutrition education appropriate to facilitate optimum oral health and oral health care.

Guidelines for Practice

	Oral Health Professional	Nutrition Professional
Prevention	• Include routine dietary screening for patients who report difficulty chewing or swallowing or oral pain • Integrate nutrition education into oral health promotion messaging	• Include oral health screening in routine physical assessment • Provide messaging to patients about the interaction between nutrition and maintenance of oral health
Intervention	• Provide guidelines to support dietary changes necessary to accommodate dentition • Develop a referral protocol to a nutrition professional for comprehensive dietary counseling and follow-up	• Conduct dietary assessment and nutrition education with edentulous patients/clients • Tailor dietary counseling to include guidelines to promote optimum masticatory function for patients with compromised dentition or those recovering from dental treatment

REFERENCES

1. Gift HC, Redford M. Oral health and quality of life. Clin Geriatr Med 1992; 8(3):673–683.
2. Hollister MC, Weintraub JA. The association of oral status with systemic health, quality of life, and economic productivity. J Dent Educ 1993; 57(12):901–912.
3. U.S. Department of Health and Human Services. Oral Health in America: A Report of the Surgeon General. Rockville, MD: U.S. Department of Health and Human Services, National Institute of Dental and Craniofacial Research, National Institutes of Health, 2000.
4. Ettinger R. Changing dietary patterns with changing dentitions: how do people cope? Spec Care Dentist 1998; 18:33–39.
5. Marcus S, Drury TF, Brown LJ, Zion GR. Tooth retention and tooth loss in the permanent dentition of adults: United States, 1988–1991. J Dent Res 1996 ; 75(special issue):684–695.
6. Redford M, Drury TF, Kingman A, Brown LJ. Denture use and the technical quality of dental prostheses among persons 18–74 years of age: United States, 1988–1991. J Dent Res 1996; 75(special issue): 714–725.
7. Walls AW, Steelem JG, Sheiham A, Marcenes W, Moynihan PJ. Oral health and nutrition in older people. J Public Health Dent 2000; 60(4):304–307.
8. Hildebrandt GH, Dominguez BL, Schork MA, Loesche WJ. Functional units, chewing, swallowing, and food avoidance among the elderly. J Prosthet Dent 1997; 77:588–595.

9. Baum B, Bodner L. Aging and oral motor function: evidence for altered performance among older persons. J Dent Res 1983; 62:2–6.

10. Newton J, Yemm R, Abel RW, Menhinick S. Changes in human jaw muscles with age and dental state. Gerodontology 1993; 10:16–22.

11. Wayler A, Muench ME, Kapur K, Chauncy HH. Masticatory performance and food acceptability in persons with removable partial dentures, full dentures, and intact natural dentition. J Gerontol 1984; 39:284–289.

12. Ship JA, Duffy V, Jones JA, Langmore S. Geriatric oral health and its impact on eating. J Am Geriatr Soc 1996; 44(4):456–464.

13. Feldman R, Kapur KK, Alman JM, Muench MR, Chauncey HH. Aging and mastication: changes in performance and in the swallowing threshold with natural dentition. J Am Geriatr Soc 1980; 28:97–103.

14. Wayler A, Kapur KK, Feldman RS, Chauncey HH. Effects of age and dentition status on measures of food acceptability. J Gerontol 1982; 37:294–299.

15. Wayler A, Chauncey HH. Impact of complete dentures and impaired natural dentition on masticatory performance and food choice in healthy aging men. J Prosthet Dent 1983; 49:427–433.

16. Feldman R, Alman J, Muench MR, Chauncey HH. Longitudinal stability and masticatory function of human dentition. Gerodontol 1984; 3:107–113.

17. Budtz-Jorgensen E, Chung JP, Mojon P. Successful aging: the case for prosthetic therapy. J Public Health Dent 2000; 60(4):308–312.

18. Kapur K, Soman SD. Masticatory performance and efficiency in denture wearers. J Prosthet Dent 1964; 14:687–694.

19. Fucile S, Wright PM, Chan I, Yee S, Langlais ME, Gisel EG. Functional oral-motor skills: do they change with age? Dysphagia 1998; 13(4):195–201.

20. Hatch JP, Shinkai RS, Sakai S, Rugh JD, Paunovich ED. Determinants of masticatory performance in dentate adults. Arch Oral Biol 2001; 46(7):641–648.

19. Hatch JP. Oral function and diet quality in a community-based sample. J Dent Res 2001; 80(7):1625–1630.

21. Foerster U, Gilbert GH, Duncan P. Oral functional limitation among dentate adults. J Public Health Dent 1998; 58:202–209.

22. Sheiham A, Steele JG, Marcenes W, Tsakos G, Finch S, Walls AW. Prevalence of impacts of dental and oral disorders and their effects on eating among older people: a national survey in Great Britain. Community Dent Oral Epidemiol 2001; 29(3):195–203.

23. Sheiham A, Steele JG, Marcenes W, Finch S, Walls AW. The impact of oral health on stated ability to eat certain foods: findings from the National Diet and Nutrition Survey of Older People in Great Britain. Gerodontol 1999; 16(1):11–20.

24. Gunne H. The effect of removable partial dentures on mastication and dietary intake. Acta Odontol Scand 1985; 42:269–278.

25. Papas AS, Palmer CA, Rounds MC, Russell RM. The effects of denture status on nutrition. Spec Care Dent 1998; 18(1):17–25.

26. Krall E, Hayes C, Garcia R. How dentition status and masticatory function affect nutrient intake. J Am Dental Assoc 1998; 129:1261–1269.

27. Ritchie CS, Joshipura K, Hung H, Douglass CW. Nutrition as a mediator in the relation between oral and systemic disease: associations between specific measures of adult oral health and nutrition outcomes. Crit Rev Oral Biol Med 2002; 13(3):291–300.

28. Papas AS, Palmer CA, Rounds MC, et al. Longitudinal relationships between nutrition and oral health. Ann NY Acad Sci 1989; 561:124–142.

29. Papas AS, Joshi A, Giunta JL, Palmer CA. Relationships among education, dentate status, and diet in adults. Spec Care Dent 1998; 18(1):26–32.

30. Greska L, Parraga IM, Clark CA. The dietary adequacy of edentulous older adults. J Prosthet Dent 1995; 73:142–145.

31. Ranta K, Tuominen R, Paunio I, Seppanen R. Dental status and intake of food items among an adult Finnish population. Gerodontics 1988; 4:32–35.

32. Mojon P, Budtz-Jorgensen E, Rapin CH. Relationship between oral health and nutrition in very old people. Age and Aging 1999; 28(5);463–468.

33. Lamy M, Mojon PH, Kalykakis G, Legrand R, Butz-Jorgensen E. Oral status and nutrition in the institutionalized elderly. J Dent 1999; 27(6):443–448.
34. Sullivan DH, Martin W, Flaxman N, Hagen JE. Oral health problems and involuntary weight loss in a population of frail elderly. J Am Geriatr Soc 1993; 41(7):725–731.
35. Knapp A. Nutrition and oral health in the elderly. Dent Clin North Am 1989; 33:109–125.
36. Sheiham A, Steele JG, Marcenes W, et al. The relationship among dental status, nutrient intake, and nutritional status in older people. J Dent Res 2001; 80(2):408–413.
37. Fontijn-Tekamp FA, van 't Hof MA, Slagter AP, van Waas MA. The state of dentition in relation to nutrition in elderly Europeans in the SENECA Study of 1993. Eur J Clin Nutr 1993; 50:S117–122.
38. Joshipura K, Willett WC, Douglass CW. The impact of edentulousness on food and nutrient intake. J Am Diet Assoc 1996; 127:459–467.
39. Johansson I, Tidehag P, Lundberg V, Hallmans G. Dental status, diet, and cardiovascular risk factors in middle-aged people in northern Sweden. Community Dent Oral Epidemiol 1994; 22(6):431–436.
40. Bowman SA, Lino M, Gerrior SA, Basiotis PP. The Healthy Eating Index: 1994–96. CNPP-5. Washington, DC: USDA, Center for Nutrition Policy and Promotion, 1998.
41. Shinkai RS, Hatch JP, Sakai S, Mobley CC, Saunders MJ, Rugh JD. Oral function and diet quality in a community-based sample. J Dent Res 2001; 80(7):1625–1630.
42. Sahyoun NR, Lin CL, Krall E. Nutritional status of the older adult is associated with dentition status. J Am Diet Assoc 2003; 103:61–66.
43. Brodeur J, Laurin D, Vallee R, Lachapelle D. Nutrient intake and gastro-intestinal disorders related to masticatory performance in the edentulous elderly. J Prosthet Dent 1993; 70:468.
44. Ship J. Gustatory and olfactory considerations: examination and treatment in general practice. J Am Dent Assoc 1993; 124:55–62.
45. Rieke JW, Hafermann MD, Johnson JT, et al. Oral pilocarpine for radiation-induced xerostomia: integrated efficacy and safety results from two prospective randomized clinical trials. Int J Radiat Oncol Biol Phys 1995; 31(3):661–669.
46. Atkinson J, Fox PC. Salivary gland dysfunction. Clin Geriatr Med 1992; 8:499–511.
47. Rhodus NL, Brown J. The association of xerostomia and inadequate intake in older adults. J Am Diet Assoc 1990; 90(12):1688–1692.
48. Manley R, Pfaffman C, Lathrop DD, Keyser J. Oral sensory thresholds of persons with natural and artificial dentitions. J Dent Res 1952; 31:305–312.
49. Henkin R, Christianson RL. Taste thresholds in patients with dentures. J Am Dent Assoc 1967; 75: 118–120.
50. Anderson D. Death from improper mastication. Int Dent J 1977; 27:349–354.
51. Schiffman S. Perceptions of taste and smell in elderly persons. Crit Rev Food Sci Nutr 1993; 33: 17–26.
52. Winkler S, Garg AK, Mekayarajjananonth T, Bakseen LG, Khan E. Depressed taste and smell in geriatric patients. J Am Dent Assoc 1999; 130(12):1759–65.
53. Griep MI, Verleye G, Franck AH, Collys K, Mets TF, Massart DL. Variation in nutrient intake with dental status, age and odour perception. Eur J Clin Nutr 1996; 50(12):816–825.
54. Tosello A, Foti B, Sedarat C, et al. Oral functional characteristics and gastrointestinal pathology: an epidemiological approach. J Oral Rehabil 2001; 28:668–672.
55. Laurin D, Brodeur JM, Bourdages J, Vallee R, Lachapelle D. Fibre intake in elderly individuals with poor masticatory performance. J Can Dent Assoc 1994; 60:443–449.
56. Barron RP, Carmichael RP, Marcon MA, Sandor GKB. Dental erosion in gastroesophageal reflux disease. J Can Dent Assoc 2003; 69(2):84–89.
57. U.S. Department of Health and Human Services. Oral Health in America: A Report of the Surgeon General—Executive Summary. Rockville, MD: U.S. Department of Health and Human Services, National Institute of Dental and Craniofacial Research, National Institutes of Health, 2000.
58. Patten J. Nutrition and Wound Healing. Compend 1995; 16:200–212.
59. Nelson J, Moxness KE, Jensen MD, Gastineau CF. Mayo Clinic Diet Manual: Handbook of Nutrition Practices. Vol. 7th Ed. St. Louis, MO: Mosby, 1994.
60. Soliah L. Clinical effects of jaw surgery and wiring on body composition: a case study. Dietetic Currents 1987; 14:13–16.

61. Olejko R, Fonseca RJ. Preoperative nutritional supplementation for the orthognathic surgery patient. J Oral Maxillofac Surg 1984; 42:573–578.
62. Anusavice KJ. Dental caries: risk assessment and treatment solutions for an elderly population. Compend Cont Ed Dent 2002; 23:12–20.
63. Sandstrom B, Lindquist LW. The effect of different prosthetic restorations on the dietary selection in edentulous patients: a longitudinal study of patients initially treated with optimal complete dentures and finally with tissue-integrated prostheses. Acta Odontol Scand 1987; 45(6);423–428.
64. Norlen P, Steen B, Birkhed D, Bjorn A-L. On the relations between dietary habits, nutrients, and oral health in women at the age of retirement. Acta Odontol Scand 1993; 51:277–284.
65. Garrett N, Perez P, Elbert C, Kapur KK. Effects of improvements of poorly fitting dentures and new dentures on masticatory performance. J Prosthet Dent 1996; 75:269–275.
66. Gunne H, Wall AK. The effect of new complete dentures on mastication and dietary intake. Acta Odontol Scand 1985; 43:257–268.
67. Geertman ME, Boerrigter EM, Van't Hof MA, et al. Two-center trial of implant-retained mandibular overdentures: chewing ability. Community Dent Oral Epidemiol 1996; 24:79–84.
68. Sebring N, Guckes AD, Li S-H, McCarthy GR. Nutritional adequacy of reported intake of edentulous subjects treated with conventional or implant suppported mandibular dentures. J Prosthet Dent 1995; 74:358–363.
69. Stegenga B, de Bont LG, de Leeuw R, Boering G. Assessment of mandibular function impairment associated with temporomandibular joint osteoarthrosis and internal derangement. Orofacial Pain 1993; 7(2):183–195.
70. LeResche L, Saunders K, Von Korff MR, Barlow W, Dworkin SF. Use of exogenous hormones and risk of temporomandibular pain. Pain 1997; 69:153–160.
71. Galvan TJ. Dysphagia: going down and staying down. Am J Nurs 2001; 101(1):37–43.
72. Rugg-Gunn AJ. The value of teeth in nutrition. In Rugg-Gunn AJ, ed. Nutrition and Dental Health. New York, NY: Oxford University Press 1993, 322–337.

4 Impact of Environment, Ethnicity, and Culture on Nutrition and Health

Joanne Kouba

1. INTRODUCTION

The physiological response to hunger and taste preferences are powerful stimuli influencing food choices, but the environment combined with the individual's personal history likely has an equal influence *(1)*. In a contemporary society representing many cultures and differing demographics, it is important to understand how each of these variables interacts. Health professionals can best address the dietary and nutritional needs of the population when the mediating forces can be identified and accommodated in attempts to promote healthful food choices. This chapter considers the external influences of dietary patterns, nutrition, and health on dietary needs on the basis of cultural experiences associated with environments and ethnicity.

2. FOOD AND CULTURE

One set of characteristics that contributes to humanity is how food is managed, whether one considers large aggregates of a nation or a small grouping of a nuclear family. Distinct patterns of behavior related to eating have developed among population groups. Through the ages, people have managed to move from a pattern of locating food for one meal to cultivating plants and raising livestock to last through several seasons. Currently, sophisticated manufacturing systems that can produce and store food for years in many countries have expanded the food supply. Besides food production, social norms are cultural phenomena worthy of consideration within the health care context.

Maslow's hierarchy of needs theory provides a framework for understanding the external influences on nutritional status *(2)*. For example, physiological need for food for survival is at the bottom of the hierarchy. The next level addresses food security. Meeting needs for belonging to a group is at the subsequent level. Food not only fulfills physical needs but also may provide a sense of emotional or social nourishment. The complex rules of etiquette are used to demonstrate refinements in social norms related to food. Food habits are often used to illustrate social status within political or environmental situations. Self-realization or actualization is achieved when movement has occurred through all levels, at which point personal preference governs food choices.

From: *Nutrition and Oral Medicine*
Edited by: R. Touger-Decker, D. A. Sirois, and C. C. Mobley © Humana Press Inc., Totowa, NJ

Culture refers to beliefs, attitudes, values, customs, and habits accepted by a community. Commonly, cultural practices are outward expressions of daily life. Cultural influences also effect internal decision making and behaviors related to values, family roles, status, and nonverbal communication. Ethnicity defines cultural membership that is based on more than nation of origin or race *(2)*. Successive generations have changed traditional dietary patterns. This "acculturation" is often a result of food availability and change in work and school routines in a new country where societal influences change *(2)*. This frequently results in various ethnic groups adopting foods typifying choices in a new environment. Assimilation refers to the loss of cultural identify by immigrants or descendants with adoption of the majority culture *(2)*. Other factors that effect food habits are income, occupation, geographic area, religious considerations, education, food production and distribution systems, and access to food assistance programs.

3. INFLUENCE OF RELIGIOUS PRACTICES ON DIETARY PATTERNS

Spirituality, faith, and religion influence many people's lives. Food is an important part of religion whether during formal services or as part of one's daily habits. Judaism, Christianity, Islam, Hinduism, and Buddhism are religions with explicit dietary laws and practices. Because of the range of ethnic mixes within various religions, data have not been documented relating health status to religion. Understanding religious dietary practices is more useful in facilitating dietary practices to promote health within the religious dietary laws.

3.1. Judaism

Judaism is practiced by millions of individuals in the world. Most of the 6 million Jews living in the United States are Ashkenazi, with ancestors who came from Germany, eastern Europe, or France *(2)*. There are also Sephardim, whose ancestors migrated from the Middle East, Spain, or southern Europe. There are five sects including hasidism, orthodoxy, conservative, reformed, and reconstructionist. *Kosher* is the term that is used to refer to the Jewish dietary laws. The term literally means "fit."

Kosher dietary laws allow for including mammals that have cloven feet and chew their cud, along with the milk of that animal *(3)*. Dietary pattern laws include prohibiting combined meat (including poultry) and dairy product consumption *(4)*, as well as shell-fish or other fish without fins or scales. If dairy foods have been consumed, then at least 1 h must pass before meat can be eaten

In addition to the daily kosher dietary laws, there are special feast and fast days. The Sabbath is observed from sundown on Friday until sundown on Saturday *(5)*. *Challah*, a braided soft bread, is a part of the Sabbath meal. Apples dipped in honey or honey cakes are commonly served to symbolize wishes for a sweet year at the Jewish New Year celebration, Rosh Hashanah. Yom Kippur is a day of fasting and penitence 10 d after Rosh Hashanah. During the 8 days of Passover, no leavened bread or any other food that may rise is eaten. Matzoh, the unleavened bread, is consumed during this week and replaces flour *(3–5)*. There are other feast and fast days for those who strictly observe kosher dietary laws.

3.2. Christianity

There are three primary branches of the Christian religion: Roman Catholicism, Eastern Orthodox Christianity, and Protestant Christianity. The latter encompasses, among others, the Presbyterian, Methodist, Anglican, Episcopalian, and Lutheran denominations. Roman Catholicism incorporates guidelines for days of fast and abstinence. Most commonly, Catholics fast on Ash Wednesday (the first day of Lent), every Friday in Lent, and Good Friday before Easter Sunday. Fasting in the Catholic religion allows one full meal per day and additional small snacks. Abstinence prohibits consumption of meat or poultry, but fish, seafood, eggs, and dairy are allowed. Some Catholics may still observe the practice of abstinence every Friday, but this dietary law was eliminated in the United States in 1966 *(2)*.

The Eastern Orthodox religion proscribes many days for fasting when meat, fish, animal products, dairy, or eggs may not be eaten. Older or more devout members of the Eastern Orthodox religion sometimes eliminate olive oil on fast days as well. These include every Wednesday and Friday (except the week after Christmas, Easter, and Trinity Sunday) during the entire Advent and Lent seasons and several other holy periods.

Most Protestant denominations do not have specific dietary laws or fast days. Mormons, or members of the Church of Jesus Christ of the Latter Day Saints, prohibit the use of tobacco, alcoholic beverages, tea, and coffee and fast one day monthly. Seventh Day Adventists (SDAs) also observe the Sabbath, from sundown on Friday to sundown on Saturday, as a day of prayer and rest and follow an ovolacto vegetarian diet with nuts and beans. They avoid alcohol, tobacco, coffee, tea, and spicy seasonings such as pepper. Although not all SDAs are vegetarian, pork and shellfish are avoided by most.

3.3. Islamism

Members of the Islamic faith are called Muslims. It is estimated that 2 million Muslims live in the United States *(6)* and many more live throughout the world. As in other faiths, Muslims may be of African, Middle Eastern, Asian Indian, or any other ethnic descent. Comparable to that of other faiths, there is a range of how one practices the Islamic faith from very traditional to more liberal lifestyle patterns, including dietary laws. Food is considered important for good health and survival, whereas overeating, wasting food, and not sharing are considered improper. Haram are foods that are not permitted. This includes pork, shellfish, birds and animals of prey, improperly slaughtered animals, and alcoholic beverages *(2,7)*. Similar to the kosher labeling symbols, the Islamic Food and Nutrition Council of America labels foods with a symbol to indicate compliance with dietary laws. Fasting involves adults avoiding food, beverages, alcohol, smoking, and sexual intercourse from dawn to sunset. During the month of Ramadan, Muslim adults are required to fast during the day only. Fasting rules do not apply to those who are ill, traveling, pregnant or lactating women, the elderly, and those involved in strenuous labor.

3.4. Hinduism and Buddhism

Eastern religions include Hinduism and Buddhism. Many Hindu are vegetarian because, although the religion does not specifically prohibit consumption of meat, it is suggested that those who avoid it will be rewarded. The cow is considered sacred and taboo for human consumption. Pork and certain fish are generally avoided. Fasting is practiced monthly and on holy days. However, the extent and types of food avoided vary among individuals according to family and local customs. Many Buddhists follow an ovolacto vegetarian diet.

4. ETHNIC AND REGIONAL INFLUENCES ON DIETARY PATTERNS AND HEALTH

Ethnicity refers to aspects of relationships between groups who consider themselves, and are regarded by others, as being culturally distinctive. It is different from race based on genetics. The difficulty arises in trying to define race, given that worldwide interracial mingling blurs distinctions *(8)*. Yet, dietary patterns continue to be identified with ethnic groups who have maintained practices by virtue of their cultural origin or environmental influences. Likewise, persons throughout society have adopted ethnic cuisines based on taste and desirability. How these have specifically influenced health is still a question to be answered, but there appear to be significant associations between ethnic food ways and possible risk for chronic disease. Table 1 lists examples of specific popular foods associated with select ethnic groups.

4.1. European and Scandinavian Influences

With the considerable length of time in the United States and also intermarriage between various European and non-European ethnicities, there is widespread dispersion and intermingling of Americans from European ancestry throughout urban, suburban, and rural America. Some of the largest ethnic groups originated in Europe, influencing the majority culture in this country. What we may think of as "typical American" food habits actually originated in Europe. As Europeans moved to the Americas, the original cuisine was blended with native ingredients and other regional influences to an adopted fare.

About 45 million Americans claim northern European heritage, so it is not surprising that food ways of the British Isles and France have left a mark on meal patterns *(9)*. In addition, the popular Cajun and Creole American regional cuisines developed from French, Spanish, African, and Native American cooking in Louisiana *(10)*. In general, meal patterns included a breakfast of cereal, toast, breads, eggs, bacon, and sausages. The contemporary adaptation has resulted in lighter breakfasts during the week and larger breakfasts on weekends and light items for lunch. A template of meat, starch, vegetables, bread, and dessert for dinner still prevails in today's society.

Most immigration from southern Europe was from Italy with lesser numbers from Portugal and Spain. Italian cuisine varies greatly by region and locally available food items *(11)*. Core foods in the dietary patterns of Russia and the central European countries including Germany, Austria, Hungary, Romania, the Czech Republic, and Poland listed in Table 1 are those grown in cold climates *(10,12,13)*. Many adaptations of this cuisine are regular items in "American" foods exemplified in the popularity of pretzels, sticky buns, pickles, and hot dogs (wienerwurst).

The Scandinavian countries include Sweden, Norway, Denmark, and Iceland. Scandinavian food habits illustrate simple and hearty dishes. Pickling, curing, smoking, and salting were commonly used to preserve foods and these foods are still popular today.

4.1.1. RELATED NUTRITION AND HEALTH ISSUES

Information on the influences of dietary patterns of northern, southern, or central Europeans on food choices is minimal. The significant extent of assimilation into mainstream culture and intermarriage within successive generations and lower migration in recent decades than other minority groups make it difficult to sift through the limited

Table 1
Examples of Common Food Selections and Habits Associated With Dietary Practices of Selected Ethnic Groups

Ethnic group	Animal foods	Starches/vegetables	Unique foods	Related habits/practices
European and Scandinavian influences				
British Isles	Roast beef, ham, leg of mutton, sausage, bacon, eggs, cheese	Potatoes, white, leavened bread		
France			Sauces, imported cheese, quiche	Cajun/Creole cuisine noted for use of onions, tomatoes, peppers, celery, garlic, and spices in gumbos and jambalayas
Italy	Italian cheeses and sauce	Filled or unfilled pastas in various shapes, pizza, polenta	Olive oil, basil, garlic, and anchovy hot oil dip	
Central European[b,c,d,e] countries and Russia (Germany, Austria, Hungary, Romania, the Czech Republic, and Poland)	Eggs, dairy products, pork, beef, chicken, sausages (*kielbasa* and *wursts*), pickled and smoked fish	Potatoes, cabbage, rye, wheat, and barley grains Stuffed dumplings (*piergo* and *Pelmeni*), noodles	Foods flavored with paprika, poppy seeds, caraway, dill, garlic, horseradish, mace, marjoram, mustard, almonds, chestnuts, pecans, and walnuts	*Sauerbraten* is a classic, marinated beef roast
Scandinavian (Sweden, Norway, Denmark and Iceland)	Beef, pork, fish	Rye and buckwheat breads, oats, pancakes, pastries, noodles, barley, potatoes, cabbage, legumes, apples, berries	Flavoring with caraway, dill, fennel, garlic, horseradish, lemon, ginger, mustard, tarragon, allspice, cloves, vinegar, almonds, and other nuts	Pickled, cured, smoked, salted foods are commonly used; dairy is consumed daily
African influences[f]				
Angola, Nigeria, Senegal, Sierra Leone, and Liberia	Variety and smoked meats	Corn, millet, barley, wheat, rice, yams, legumes, okra	Allspice, cardamom, cayenne, cinnamon, cloves, cumin, ginger, nutmeg, nuts, and coconut	Diet is rich in fruit and vegetables; diet evolved into traditional southern American cuisine; pork fat and lard used for seasoning

Continued on next page

49

Table 1 (Continued)
Examples of Common Food Selections and Habits Associated With Dietary Practices of Selected Ethnic Groups

Ethnic group	Animal foods	Starches/vegetables	Unique foods	Related habits/practices
Mexican and Central American influences[g,h]				
Mexican	Beans, poultry, beef, goat, pork, seafood, cheese	Filled tortillas (enchiladas, tacos, quesadillas, burritos), cactus, chilies, jicama, yucca, squash, yeast, and sweet breads.	Dried chilies, cumin, cinnamon, cocoa, nuts, tropical fruits, and pumpkin seeds	Milk consumption is low; beans and rice are common staples; salsa is a popular condiment
Central American	Red and black beans, ground meat, sausage, cheese	Pickled vegetables, empanadas (fried, filled breads)	Coconut milk, sour orange juice mixed with peppers	
Asian influences[i]				
Chinese[j]	Legumes, poultry, fish, soy	Rice, egg rolls, spring rolls filled with vegetables, noodles	Soy sauce, spicy sauce, fiery chili pastes, nuts, seeds	Congee is a common breakfast gruel; dairy products are rare; vegetable oil use is common
Japanese	Fish, soybeans, tofu	Rice, noodles, seaweed, algae, mushrooms, gourds, bamboo shoots, radish	Wasabi (horseradish)	Pickling is popular; raw fish as sushi is popular; green tea is preferred
Korean	Fish, beef, poultry	Rice, noodles, seaweed, cabbage, eggplant, adzuki beans	Garlic, ginger, fish sauce	Kimchi is a pickle relish; dried fish is common
Asian Indians[k,l]	Legumes	Rice, flat bread, potatoes, mango	Curry, masalas, chutneys	Pureed lentils and curry side dishes are common; many are vegetarian; yogurt dishes are popular
Southeast Asia and Philippines	Fish, seafood, poultry, legumes, soy	Rice, noodles	Bamboo shoots, bean sprouts, cassava, heart of palm, water chestnut, fish pastes, soy sauce, lime, flavored chili, coconut milk	Fried rice and stir-fries are popular

[a] From ref. 2.
[b] From ref. 10.
[c] From ref. 11.
[d] From ref. 12.
[e] From ref. 13.
[f] From ref. 20.
[g] From ref. 33.
[h] From ref. 34.
[i] From ref. 67.
[j] From ref. 45.
[k] From ref. 79.
[l] From ref. 80.

50

data. It is assumed that diet, nutrition, and health concerns parallel those of the overall US population (2). The major adaptations that have occurred are a shift in the proportion of macronutrients in the diet to less complex carbohydrates from staple items such as bread, legumes, pasta, noodles, and vegetables to increased dietary sources of protein and fat from meat and cheeses. Information on the nutrition status of European and Scandinavian populations suggests inadequate dietary iron intakes associated with high phytate (fiber) and tea consumption and low intakes of vitamin C, which enhances iron uptake (14). Martinchik et al. reported low dietary intakes of riboflavin and calcium and major dental health problems in 10- to 15-yr-olds in Russia (15,16). Risk for cardiovascular disease (CVD) is a concern in middle-aged men in Russia because high fat and dietary cholesterol intakes are reported to be approx 500 mg/d on average (17,18).

4.2. African-American Influences

The majority of African Americans are descendants of West African countries including Angola, Nigeria, Senegal, Sierra Leone, and Liberia. Besides forced migration to the Americas, Africans were also transported to the Caribbean islands during the 17th and 18th centuries (19).

Core foods in the African diet include an array of complex carbohydrates with an abundance of vegetables and fruits (20). With the establishment of the African-American culture in the southern United States, the traditional African diet evolved to include corn product-based dishes (cornmeal grits, corn pone, spoon bread, hominy, hushpuppies, hoecake) as staple items, garden-grown vegetables, and variety of meat cuts such as feet, knuckles, chitterlings, and organs. Pork fat or lard replaced palm oil. Common dishes were hearty vegetable and bean stews, thickened with okra or sassafras and seasoned with small pieces of smoked meat. The dietary patterns of African Americans have been characterized as including a high intake of fried foods, cornbread, greens, sweet potatoes, and fruit drinks, with a lower intake of cereals and dairy products (2).

4.2.1. RELATED NUTRITION AND HEALTH ISSUES

Robinson and Hunter reported the nutrient intake of urban African Americans to include diets composed of 42.7% dietary fat from total calories, 14.6% saturated fat from calories (compared to the recommended maximum of 10%), a sodium intake that is 150% of recommendations, and a dietary fiber intake that is 30% of optimal (21). Significant heterogeneity exists in nutrient patterns among African Americans (22). Health concerns of the African-American population have changed as this population has moved from an agricultural-based lifestyle characterized by dietary patterns that were low in fat and high in fiber, fruits, and vegetables with frequent malnutrition to dietary patterns characterized by a high animal fat and refined food intake and overnutrition (19). Emerging problems include an increased prevalence of CVD, hypertension, kidney diseases, obesity, diabetes mellitus, and cancer (23). Infant mortality rate (IMR), based on the 1998 baseline data, is 13.8 per 1000 live births for the US African-American population compared to a rate of 7.2 for the overall US population (23).

Luke et al. identified the trend of body mass index (BMI) increasing in women living in West Africa, the Caribbean, and the United States from 22.6 to 23.5 to 30.8, respectively (19). Prevalence of obesity (defined as BMI ≥30) ranging from 5% in Nigerian men to 49% in US women is associated with increased risk of type 2 diabetes mellitus

(T2DM). Of the African-American adult population, 34% are at a healthy weight, compared to 42% of the overall US adult population *(23)*. Secondary complications of T2DM such as end-stage renal disease, retinopathy, and amputations in the African-American population are a major concern *(24–26)*.

Review of age-adjusted prevalence of hypertension for men from Nigeria, Jamaica, and the United States shows a pattern similar to that of obesity and T2DM *(27)*. Research has focused on the extent to which this is genetic compared to environmental, although nutritional factors are considered to account for a majority of these cases *(27–30)*. Although coronary heart disease (CHD) is the leading cause of death in the United States for both the African-American and white populations, the African-American population has experienced less of a decline in mortality associated with CHD. This differential may be caused by lifestyle factors related to lipid levels, hypertension, smoking, and physical activity.

4.3. Mexican and Central American Influences

It is projected that by 2050, the US Hispanic population will be 96.5 million, or 24% of the total US population, with Mexican Americans constituting about 64% of the US Hispanic population and the largest ethnic group in this country *(31)*. Similar to many other cultural and ethnic groups, there is a wide range of food habits in Hispanics related to the strength of cultural influences and degree of acculturation *(32)*.

Major contributions of this cuisine in terms of complex carbohydrate sources include the popular tortillas (flat bread made from a variety of corns or flour), a one-dish meal accompaniment *(33,34)*. Flour tortillas are more popular in the United States than the corn tortillas preferred in Mexico. Beans are a low-cost staple source of complex carbohydrate, fiber, water-soluble vitamins, and iron often combined with rice. The Mexican cuisine is rich in vegetables used as ingredients in many mixed dishes. Approximately 100 varieties of chilies are used as the basic flavoring in many dishes *(33,34)* and salsas made with fresh, raw chilies, tomatoes, tomatillos, onions, cilantro, citrus juice, or fruit accompany meals.

Mexican Americans are likely to adapt meal composition and cycle to the "typical" American pattern of a small breakfast and lunch with a large dinner compared to the traditional Mexican meal pattern of four to five meals daily, with the largest in the early afternoon.

Central America includes Belize, Guatemala, El Salvador, Honduras, Nicaragua, Costa Rica, and Panama. The cuisine includes many similarities with that of Mexico but there are specific regional differences in preferences for bean dishes.

4.3.1. RELATED NUTRITION AND HEALTH ISSUES

Nutritional concerns in the diets of Hispanic Americans have been reported to include higher intakes of fat, meat, cheese, sugar-sweetened beverages, butter, and dressings and lower intakes of protein, fruit, vegetables (including beans), compared to non-Hispanics *(2)*. Dixon et al. concluded that, in general, those born in Mexico consumed significantly less fat and more fiber; vitamins A, C, E, and B_6; folate; calcium; potassium; and magnesium than either group born in the United States *(35)*. Similarly, Polednak found that education and level of acculturation were not associated with fat intake in Hispanic adults in New York and Connecticut; although the male gender and younger individuals reported higher fat intakes from whole milk, red meat, and french fries *(36)*. Prevalence of iron-deficiency anemia, 6.2% compared to 2.3%, has been reported in Mexican American women compared to non-Hispanic whites despite comparable intakes in iron and vitamin C *(37)*.

Prevalence of obesity, overweight, and T2DM has been reported in Mexican Americans *(22)*. After adjustments for age and socioeconomic status, Winkleby noted that Mexican American women continued to exhibit significantly higher levels of BMI, blood pressure, T2DM, and physical inactivity than white women *(38)*. Higher levels of risk factors, not actual CVD morbidity and mortality, have been suggested among US Hispanics vs non-Hispanics *(39)*. Conversely, Pandey et al. and Goff et al. found higher levels of CVD mortality in Mexican Americans in Texas compared to the non-Hispanic white population *(40,41)*. After studying Hispanic Health and Nutrition Examination Survey (HHANES) data on hypertension in Mexican American, Cuban American, and Puerto Rican women, Goslar et al. found that age, BMI, and level of acculturation were significantly associated with hypertension in all three subgroups *(42)*.

Diabetes, particularly T2DM, was found to be 1.9 times more prevalent in the Mexican American population compared to non-Hispanic whites based on NHANES III data *(43)*. According to the Healthy People 2010 objectives, approx 30% of Mexican American adults are at a healthy weight compared to 42% for the overall population *(23)*.

Data are lacking for the total Hispanic population and other subgroups related to dental health. Based on Healthy People 2010 data, 57% of Mexican Americans aged 15 yr or more have experienced dental caries compared to 61% of the total US population. However, for younger ages, there are more dental caries among Mexican Americans than among all US children *(44)*.

4.4. Asian Influences

Asian cuisine encompasses the food of many nations including the People's Republic of China, Japan, the Republic of China (Taiwan), the Democratic People's Republic of Korea, the Republic of Korea, Thailand, Vietnam, India, and the Philippines *(8)*. There are commonalities in Asian dietary patterns.

Core foods in the Chinese diet vary by region but generally are carbohydrate-based and include rice and wheat. Rice is a symbol of prosperity, good fortune, health, and blessings of life *(45)* and is traditionally eaten from a small separate bowl, whereas fruits are not frequently eaten, but do provide an occasional snack or dessert. Soy is a significant source of protein and calcium in the Asian diet.

Japanese dietary patterns have parallels to Chinese patterns. Seaweed is used in sushi and soups and eaten as a dish by itself. Consumption of raw fish as sushi and sashimi is popular, whereas consumption of dairy has been typically low. One characteristic Japanese flavoring is wasabi, a green horseradish condiment that can be very hot and spicy.

The Korean diet includes kimchi, a pickled relish that is eaten along with rice and meats or mixed with soups. Garlic, ginger, peppers, toasted seeds and nuts, fish sauces, and spicy chilies are key flavorings in this cuisine *(2)*. The traditional Korean diet is low in fat, cholesterol, and calcium and high in carbohydrates and sodium.

There is a significant diversity within the Asian Indian population in terms of religions, languages, and dietary patterns. Many Asian Indian Americans observe vegetarian dietary practices that make intake of animal tissue, fish, and seafood taboo. Fermented dairy products, such as yogurt, are a common source of protein that is consumed almost daily in the traditional Indian diet.

The southeast Asian countries of Vietnam, Cambodia, the Philippines, and Laos have culinary influences of China and France, Spain, and other European countries (2). Flavorings and seasonings range from hot and spicy in the Thai diet, which uses a variety of chilies and curries, to relatively mild in the Cambodian diet. Dairy products are not consumed in high amounts in the traditional diets.

4.4.1. NUTRITION AND HEALTH ISSUES RELATED TO ASIAN INFLUENCES

Similar to other cultural groups, change in dietary patterns occurs in Chinese and Chinese Americans with increasing length of stay in the new country and with shifts to more "Americanized" diets (46). Wu et al. found tofu intake in Asian American women to be twice that of American women (62 times compared to 30 times per year) (47). Other shifts in eating patterns are noteworthy for increased intakes of soft drinks. Parallel to the changes in eating patterns, nutrient quality of the diet also changes. The traditional Chinese diet is low in fat and dairy, and high in complex carbohydrates and sodium. However, Chinese descendants report a shift to higher fat, protein, sugar, and cholesterol intakes with increasing length of time in the United States (48).

Other health concerns of Chinese Americans include lactose intolerance and increasing rates of colorectal and breast cancers compared to rates in China (48,49). Asian American women have been noted to have lower rates of breast cancer compared to those of the overall American population but higher than those of native Asian women (23,50). Obesity, CVD, infant mortality, and hypertension rates have been reported to be lower in populations of Chinese Americans. Baseline 1996 Healthy People 2010 objectives noted the IMR was lower for the Asian population than total IMR of 7.2 per 1000 live births (23).

The traditional Japanese diet is low in fat and cholesterol and higher in sodium and smoked or cured foods. When Kudo studied second- and third-generation Japanese American women, second-generation women reported consuming more total meats, fish, vegetables, and legumes than third-generation women, who reported consuming more American-type snack foods, sugar-sweetened soft drinks, and alcoholic beverages (51,52). Traditional Japanese have experienced higher rates of hypertension, cerebrovascular accidents (CVA), and stomach cancer, and lower IMR, colorectal and breast cancer, and CVD. Increased rates of certain cancers and T2DM have been associated with adoption of Western diets (53). Lauderdale et al. reported that Asian American women have lower bone density and more osteoporosis, although fewer hip fractures, than white women in the United States (54). Both colorectal and gastric cancer have increased dramatically in Japanese migrants to the United States (55), but rates have not been as high as the rates for those in Japan (56). The Japanese American population has a higher prevalence of T2DM than Japanese living in Japan (57–59).

Korean Americans experience a disproportionately higher incidence of stomach cancer compared to the total US population (60). Dietary etiological factors including frequent consumption of salted and fermented fish products, nitrates, sodium, and hot and spicy foods are thought to be related. Hypertension and hyperlipidemia have been found to be lower in Korean Americans (61).

On average, Asian Indians who have migrated to Western countries report diets with the macronutrient distribution for carbohydrate, protein, and fat to be approx 49%, 14%, and 36% of the total caloric intake, respectively *(62)*. This suggests higher fat intakes than is currently recommended and that is part of the traditional Indian diet *(62)*. CVD and T2DM occur at rates of one to four times that of the US population and higher than native Asian Indians in acculturated groups *(63)*.

Because of the frequent use of frying as a cooking method, the Filipino diet is traditionally higher in fat *(64)*. Hypertension and T2DM are prevalent in this group, although data are not available to support associations with dietary variables.

Vitamin and mineral deficiency states have been observed in recent immigrants from southeast Asia, including deficiencies of iron (particularly in children and refugees) and vitamins B_6, D, and E; folacin; calcium; phosphorus; potassium; and magnesium in pregnant women *(65,66)*. Nutritional problems are compounded by intestinal parasites, liver disease, tuberculosis, and dental problems *(66)*.

4.5. Other Cultural Influences

This discussion does not allow space for a detailed review of each specific cultural influence. With technology, the globalization of health has led to a better understanding of cultural practices related to health status.

4.5.1. Nutrition and Health Issues Related to Selected Cultural Influences

Health issues of interest among the Greeks include lower levels of CHD, which may be attributable to "Mediterranean" dietary patterns associated with high intakes of monounsaturated fatty acids (from olive oil), a generous antioxidant intake from a high fruit and vegetable intake, and fish, with lower intakes of red meat and saturated fat *(67)*.

Based on HHANES and Health and Nutrition Examination Survey II data for Cuban Americans and Puerto Ricans in New York City, lower rates of hypertension were noted compared to age-adjusted data for white and African-American populations *(68)*. However, Bauer et al. reported higher sodium, calcium, and potassium intakes in mainland Puerto Rican populations compared to African-American or EuroAmerican populations *(69)*. These conflicting results imply the need for additional studies designed to identify the profound effects of culture and ethnicity on dietary patterns and health outcomes.

5. SOCIETAL INFLUENCES ON DIETARY PATTERNS AND HEALTH

From an ethnographic perspective, cultural influences on diet and nutrition may not be as influential on dietary patterns and health as societal trends, mass media messages, and peer pressure. With advances in transportation systems including railroads, automobiles, and trucks, the variety and quantity of foods available to Americans have greatly increased and are not limited to seasonal availability from local farmers. Railroads, coupled with the invention of mobile refrigeration systems, allowed milk to be provided in abundance to children in New York City *(70)*. Citrus fruits became available to midwesterners in the winter. These advances improved diet quality. This increased mobility in the last century has led to the creation of "drive-in" and now "drive-through" restaurants. Additionally, the food manufacturing industry has created transportable foods made for busy lifestyles. Examples include prepackaged breakfast burritos, corn dogs on a stick, prepackaged bagel sandwiches, breakfast bars, and yogurt in a tube. It is easier than ever to eat a meal without sitting down at a table or using a dish or eating utensil.

5.1. Technological Influences on Dietary Patterns

The workplace influences our diets and nutritional health. During agrarian periods in history, the largest meal was eaten in the early afternoon after a morning of heavy labor. The second meal of the day was eaten in the late afternoon. With the industrial revolution, meal patterns shifted to a quick breakfast and lunch to accommodate the demands of the mechanized workplace. The last meal of the day was eaten in the home later in the day and became the larger meal. In the last several decades, more women have begun working outside of the home, which created a market for convenience foods for all family members. As a result, an abundance of innovative convenience food products from prepackaged lunches and stir-fry "kits" to french fries for the microwave have exploded for use in the home, in restaurants, and by personal chef services.

The food supply has expanded dramatically with the advent of the industrial revolution, technological improvements, and growth of nutritional science. Trends in food supply data in the United States indicated that overall energy, fat, fruit, vegetable, and soft drink (including vending machines) availability has increased in the last 25 yr (71). Added fat consumption doubled between 1908 and 1998 (71). American consumers frequented restaurants in increasing numbers (72). Brand-name identification (a regularly practiced concept in shopping), supermarkets, and advertisements have become big business and major industries. This has created new health promotion challenges. The practice of schools entering into contracts with food manufacturers to place soft drink or brand-name items into school cafeterias is an example of controversial practices with potential negative health consequences for America's youth (71,73).

A discussion of secular trends in diet cannot ignore the influential role of media, including radio, newspapers, magazines, signage, personal computers, and television. These modes of communication include featured articles or programs as well as advertisements. The phenomenon of television has sparked inventions such as the "TV dinner," created more reasons to snack, and may be changing the family dynamics of mealtimes in our society (70). Not only does television provide cues to eat, it is associated with limiting physical activity (71). In addition to persuasive messages from Madison Avenue, news segments of the media are vying for one's attention through reports of the latest cancer prevention nutrient, ways to reduce cholesterol, or a weight loss program. This has led to some degree of confusion and skepticism by the public about nutrition information (74–76). Of those surveyed in 1995, 78% responded that concepts of "healthy" foods were very likely to change completely within 5 yr (74). The need for health care practitioners, dietitians, and nutritional scientists to accurately convey diet and health messages will increase (74,77).

The internet has influenced dietary choices. Davison et al. examined dietary data available on the internet and determined that 45% of the dietary information was inconsistent with the principles of the Canadian Guidelines for Healthy Eating (78). Sources were largely private vendors or individual web pages. However, reliable health-promoting messages and campaigns also existed such as the "Five-A-Day for Better Health" initiative of the National Cancer Institute (71).

6. SUMMARY

Health care professionals recognize and work with the many influential facets that may determine dietary behaviors. These include individual factors such as taste preferences, religious practices, ethnicity, and societal factors such as those governed by work schedules, food industry practices, or mass media messages. Acknowledging the intricacies that determine the interaction among these influences will become increasingly important with the continued mobilization and globilization of societies and cultures.

REFERENCES

1. Glanz K, Basil M, Maibach E, Goldberg J, Snyder D. Why Americans eat what they do: taste, nutrition, cost, convenience, and weight control concerns as influences on food consumption. J Am Diet Assoc 1998; 98(10):1118–1126.
2. Kittler PG, Sucher KP. Food and Culture. Belmont, CA: Wadsworth, 2001, 199–225.
3. Greenberg B. How to run a traditional Jewish household. Northvale, NJ: Aronson, 1985.
4. Greenwald Z, Greenwald Z, Gonopolsky M. Vol. 3: The Kosher Kitchen. New York, NY: Philipp Feldheim 1997.
5. Hirsh A, Miksch A. Our Food: The Kosher Kitchen. New York, NY: Doubleday, 1993.
6. U.S. State Department. (Website: http://uninfo.state.gov/usa/islam/demograph.htm). Accessed 4/19/02.
7. McKennis, AT. Caring for the Islamic patient. AORN J 1999; 69(6):1185–1206.
8. Ericksen, TH. Ethnicity and Nationalism: Anthropoligical Perspectives. London, UK: Pluto Press, 2002.
9. U.S. Census Bureau.
10. Zibart E. Ethnic Food Lover's Companion. Birmingham, AL: Menasha Ridge Press, 2001.
11. Smith J. The Frugal Gourmet on Our Immigrant Ancestors. New York, NY: William Morrow 1990, 70–83, 100–152, 221–232, 484–492.
12. Brizova J. The Czechoslovak Cookbook. New York, NY: Crown , 1965, 1–59, 91–129.
13. Schargenberg H. The Cuisines of Germany. New York, NY: Poseidon Press, 1980, 280–321.
14. Kohlmeier L, Mendez M, Shalnova S, Martinchik A, Chakraborty H, Kohlmeier M. Deficient dietary iron intakes among women and children in Russia. Am J Public Health 1998; 88(4):576–580.
15. Martinchik AN, Baturin AK, Helsing E. Nutrition monitoring of Russian schoolchildren in a period of economic change: a World Health Organization multicenter survey, 1992–1995. Am J Clin Nutr 1997; 65(4): 1215S–1219S.
16. Turner C, Zagirova A, Frolova L, Courts FJ, Williams WN. Oral health status of Russian children with unilateral cleft lip and palate. Cleft Palate Craniofac J 1998; 35(6):489–494.
17. Cockerham WC. Health lifestyles in Russia. Soc Sci Med 2000; 51(9):313–324.
18. Charzewska J. Gaps in dietary survey methodology in Eastern Europe. Am J Clin Nutr 1994; 59(S):157S–160S.
19. Luke A, Cooper RS, Prewitt TE, Adeyemo AA, Forrester TE. Nutritional consequences of the African diaspora. Annu Rev Nutr 2001; 21:47–71.
20. Harris J. The African Cookbook: Tastes of a Continent. New York, NY: Simon and Schuster, 1998, 1–72.
21. Robinson ME, Hunter PH. Nutritional assessment of a predominantly African American inner city clinic population. Wis Med J 2001; 100(9):32–38.
22. Bronner YL, Harris E, Ebded TL, Hossain MB, Nowverl A. Historical assessment of nutrition studies using only African American study subjects: gender, socioeconomic status, and geographic location. Ethn Dis 2001; 11(1):134–143.
23. U.S. Department of Health and Human Services. Healthy People 2010. 2nd Ed. With understanding and improving health and objectives for improving health. 2 Vols. Washington, DC: U.S. Government Printing Office, November 2000.
24. Cowie CC, Port PK, Wolfe RA, Savage PJ, Moll PP, Hawthorne VM. Disparities in incidence of end-stage renal disease according to race and type of diabetes. N Eng J Med 1989; 321:1074–1079.

25. Harris EL, Feldman S, Robinson CR, Sherman S, Georgopoulos A. Racial differences in the relationship between blood pressure and risk of retinopathy among individuals with NIDDM. Diabetes Care 1993; 16:748–754.

26. Lavery LA, Ashry HR, vanHoutum W, Pugh JA, Harkless LB, Basu S. Variation in the incidence and proportion of diabetes-related amputations in minorities. Diabetes Care 1996; 19:48–52.

27. Cooper RS, Rotimi C, Ataman S, McGee D, Osotimehim B. The prevalence of hypertension in seven populations of West African origin. Am J Public Health 1997; 87:160–169.

28. Knuiman JT, West CE, Katan MB, Hautvast JGAJ. Total cholesterol and high density lipoprotein cholesterol levels in populations differing in fat and carbohydrate intake. Arteriosclerosis 1987; 7: 612–619.

29. Okosum IS, Forrester TE, Rotimi CN, Lsotimehim BO, Muna W, Cooper RS. Abdominal obesity in six populations of West African descent: prevalence and population attributable fraction of hypertension. Obesity Res 1999; 7:453–462.

30. Okosun IS, Cooper RS, Rotimi CN, Osotimehin B, Forrester T. Association of waist circumference with risk of hypertension and type 2 diabetes in Nigerians, Jamaicans, and African-Americans. Diabetes Care 1998; 21(11):1836–1842.

31. Day JC. Population projections of the United States by age, sex, race and Hispanic origin: 1995–2050. Washington, DC: U.S. Bureau of Census.

32. Wallendorf M, Reilly MD. Ethnic migration, assimilation, and consumption. J Con Res 1983; 10:292–302.

33. Kennedy D. The Cuisines of Mexico. New York, NY: Harper and Row, 1972, 3–49, 59–106, 278–295.

34. Bayless R. Mexico One Plate at a Time. New York, NY: Scribner, 2000, 139–293; 353–360.

35. Dixon LB, Sundquist J, Winkleby M. Differences in energy, nutrient, and food intakes in a U.S. sample of Mexican American women and men: findings from the Third National Health and Nutrition Examination Survey, 1998–1994. Am J Epidemiol 2000; 152(6):548–557.

36. Polednak, AP. Use of selected high fat foods by Hispanic adults in the northeastern U.S. Ethn Health 1997; 2(1–2):-71–76.

37. Frith-Terhune AL, Cogswell ME, Khan LK, Will JC, Ramakrishnan U. Iron deficiency anemia: high prevalence in Mexican American than in non-Hispanic white females in the third National Health and Nutrition Examination Survey, 1988–1994. Am J Clin Nutr 2000; 72(4):963–968.

38. Winkleby MA, Kraemer H, Ahn DK, Varady AN. Ethnic and socioecnomic differences in cardiovascular disease risk factors: findings for women from the Third National Health and Nutrition Examination Survey, 1988–1994. JAMA 1998; 280(4):356–362, 4(3):367–376.

39. Luepker R. Cardiovascular disease among Mexican Americans. JAMA 2001; 110(2):147–148.

40. Pandey KE, Labarthe DR, Goff, DC. Community-wide coronary heart disease mortality in Mexican Americans equals or exceeds that in non-Hispanic whites: the Corpus Christi Heart Project. Am J Med 2001; 110:81–87.

41. Goff DC, Ramsey VC. Mortality after hospitalization for myocardial infarction among Mexican Americans and non-Hispanic whites: the Corpus Christi Heart Project. Ethn Dis 1993; 3:55–63.

42. Goslar PW, Macera CA, Castellanos LG, Hussey JR, Sy FS, Sharpe PA. Blood pressure in Hispanic women: the role of diet, acculturation, and physical activity. Ethn Dis 1997; 7(20):106–113.

43. Harris MI, Flegal KM, Cowie C, et al. Prevalence of diabetes, impaired fasting glucose, and impaired glucose tolerance in U.S. adults: the Third National Health and Nutrition Examination Survey, 1988–1994. Diabetes Care 1998; 21(4):518–524.

44. Nurko AC, Aponte-Merced L, Bradley EL, Fox L. Dental caries prevalence and dental health care of Mexican American workers' children. J Dent Children 1998; 65:65–72.

45. Lo EY. Chinese Kitchen. New York, NY: William Morrow, 1999, 1–39, 105–110.

46. Satia JA, Patterson RE, Taylor VM, et al. Use of qualitative methods to study diet, acculturation, and health in Chinese-American women. J Am Diet Assoc 2000; 100(8):934–940.

47. Chau P, Lee H, Tseng R, Downes NJ. Dietary habits, health beliefs and food practices of elderly Chinese women. J Am Diet Assoc 1990; 90:579–580.

48. Wu Ha, Ziegler RG, Horn-Ross PL, et al. Tofu and risk of breast cancer in Asian Americans. Cancer Epidemiol Biomarkers Prev 1996; 5(11):901–906.

49. Sun WY, Wu JS. Comparison of dietary self-efficacy and behavior among American- born and foreign-born Chinese adolescents residing in New York City and Chinese adolescents in Guangzhou, China. J Am Coll Nutr 1997; 16(2):103–104.

50. Ziegler RG, Hoover RN, Nomure AM, et al. Relative weight, weight change, height, breast cancer risk in Asian-American women. J Natl Cancer Inst 1996; 88(10):650–660.

51. Lands EM, Hamazaki T, Yamazaki K, et al. Changing dietary patterns. Am J Clin Nutr 1990; 51:991–993.

52. Kudo Y, Falciglia GA, Couch SC. Evaluation of meal patterns and food choices of Japanese American females born in the United States. Eur J Clin Nutr 2000; 54(8):665–670.

53. Tsunehara CH, Neonetti DL, Fujimoto WY. Diet of second-generation Japanese American men with and without non-insulin dependent diabetes. Am J Clin Nutr 1990; 52:731–738.

54. Lauderdale DS, Jacobsen SJ, Furner SE, Levy PS, Brody JA, Goldberg J. Hip fracture incidence among elderly Asian American populations. Am J Epidemiol 1997; 146:502–509.

55. Marchand LL. Combined influence of genetic and dietary factors on colorectal cancer incidence in Japanese Americans. J Natl Cancer Inst 1999; 26(monograph):101–105.

56. Kamineni A, Williams MA, Schwartz SM, Cook LS, Weiss NS. The incidence of gastric carcinoma in Asian migrants to the U.S. and their descendants. Cancer Causes Control 1999; 10(1):77–83.

57. Fujimoto WY, Bergstrom RW, Boyko EJ, et al. Preventing diabetes: applying pathophysiological and epidemiological evidence. Br J Nutr 2000; 82(S2):S173–S176.

58. Hara H, Egusa G, Yamakido M. Incidence of non-insulin–dependent diabetes mellitus and its risk in Japanese-Americans. Diabetic Med 1996; 13(S6):S133–S142.

59. Alexander GR, Mor JM, Kogan MD, Leland MNL, Keiffer E. Pregnancy outcomes of U.S. born and foreign-born Japanese Americans. Am J Public Health 1996; 86(6):820–824.

60. Kim J, Chan M. Nutrition and health of Korean Americans: a review of the literature. Top Clin Nutr 2000; 16(1):59–70.

61. Lee S, Sobal J, Frongillo EA. Acculturation and health in Korean Americans. Soc Sci Med 2000; 51(2):159–173.

62. Kamath SK, Murillo G, Chatterton RT, et al. Breast cancer risk factors in two distinct ethnic groups: Indian and Pakistani vs American premenopausal women. Nutr Cancer 1999; 35(1):16–26.

63. Hughes, IO. Insulin, Indian origin and ischaemic heart disease. Intl J Card 1990; 26:1–4.

64. DiPasquale-Davis J, Hopkins S. Health behaviors of an elderly filipino group. Public Health Nurs 1997; 14(2):118–122.

65. Ikeda JP, Ceja DR, Glass RS, Harwood JO, Lucke KA, Sutherland JM. Food habits of Hmong living in central California. J Nutr Ed 1991; 23:168–175.

66. Newman V, Norcross W, McDonald R. Nutrient intake of low-income Southeast Asian pregnant women. J Am Diet Assoc 1991; 91:793–799.

67. Kremezi A. The foods of the Greek islands. New York, NY: Houghton Mifflin, 1995, 1–15, 147–142.

68. Pappas F, Gergen PJ, Carroll M. Hypertension prevalence and the status of awareness, treatment, control in the Hispanic Health and Nutrition Examination Survey, 1982–84. Am J Public Health 1990; 80(12): 1431–1436.

69. Bauer UE, Mayne ST. Do ethnic differences in dietary cation intake explain the ethnic differences in hypertension prevalence? Ann Epidemiol 1997; 7(7):479–485.

70. Gordon BM. Why we choose the foods we do. Nutr Today 1983; 3:17–24.

71. French S, Story M, Jeffrey R. Environmental influences on eating and physical activity. Ann Rev Public Health 2001; 22:309–315.

72. National Restaurant Association. (Website: http://www.restaurant.org/research/pocket/index.htm). Accessed 3/4/02.

73. Nestle M. Soft drink "pouring rights": marketing empty calories to children. Public Health Rep 2000; 115(4):308–319.

74. Wellman NS, Scarbrough FE, Ziegler RG, Lyle B. Do we facilitate the scientific process and the development of dietary guidance when findings from single studies are publicized? Am J Clin Nutr 1999; 70(5):802–805.

75. Worsley A. Perceived reliability of sources of health information. Health Ed Res 1989;367–376.

76. Rowe SB. Food for thought: an in-depth look at how the media report nutrition, food safety, and health. Am Med Writers Assoc J 2000; 15(4):5–9.
77. Ayoob K. Commentary on dietitian and the media: consumers want us and we need to be there. Topics Clin Nutr 2001; 16(2):1–7.
78. Davison K, Guan S. The quality of dietary information on the World Wide Web. J Can Dietetic Assoc 1996; 57(4):137–141.
79. Jaffrey M. Far Eastern cookery. New York, NY: Harper and Row, 1989; 22–25, 30-4411.
80. Roden, C. The new book of Middle Eastern Food. New York, NY: Alfred Knopf,2000; 3–53, 109–141, 365–400.

II SYNERGISTIC RELATIONSHIPS BETWEEN ORAL AND GENERAL HEALTH

5

Bidirectional Impact
of Oral Health and General Health

Angela R. Kamer, David A. Sirois,
and Maureen Huhmann

1. INTRODUCTION

Oral manifestations of systemic disease or its treatment have been the subject of an extensive body of biomedical literature; several textbooks cover the subject in great detail *(1,2)*. More recently, the impact of oral health on systemic health and disease has been the subject of intense investigation, leading to provocative ideas about oral risk factors for systemic disease and novel approaches to health promotion and disease prevention. This collective understanding of the reciprocal oral and systemic risks for disease will require, more than ever before, an expanded scope of dental, medical, and nutrition professional training to achieve competency in risk assessment and risk reduction. Translation into practice will require consultation among and collaboration between clinicians and should lead to innovative health care delivery systems that efficiently bring these caregivers and services to the patient.

The scope of the bidirectional impact of oral and general health is so extensive that only a survey of selected topics can be explored in this chapter. From the perspective of five oral conditions (periodontal disease, caries, mucosal disease, dysphagia, and chronic orofacial pain), this chapter reviews the bidirectional relationship between selected systemic illness and each oral condition. Table 1 summarizes a broader range of oral-systemic problems that have demonstrated bidirectional impact and should always prompt the primary-care provider to initiate evaluation by the dentist, registered dietitian, or physician. Several of these, and related topics, are discussed in other chapters of this book.

2. PERIODONTAL DISEASE

2.1. Systemic Disease Impact on Periodontal Disease

Periodontal diseases are a heterogeneous group of diseases that affect supporting structures of the teeth. Their diagnosis is based on specific signs and symptoms. In 1999, a new classification system was developed based on the current knowledge of the etiol-

From: *Nutrition and Oral Medicine*
Edited by: R. Touger-Decker, D. A. Sirois, and C. C. Mobley © Humana Press Inc., Totowa, NJ

Table 1

Selected Disorders or Events for Which a Clinical Pathway Including
Referral Between Dental, Medical, and Nutrition Clinicians is Recommended

Systemic

- Diabetes
- Pregnancy (for periodontal disease assessment and care)
- Elderly patients, especially those taking multiple medications
- Cardiac valvular disorders (risk for infective endocarditis)
- Systemic immunosuppressive therapy (organ transplant, primary immunologic disorders)
- Pathologic immunosuppression (HIV, AIDS, malignancy)
- Osteoporosis
- Autoimmune disorders (Sjogren's syndrome, lupus erythematosis, rheumatoid arthritis, pemphigus vulgaris, cicatricial pemphigoid)
- >10% unexplained weight changes in the past 6 mo
- Tobacco use
- Coagulation disorders
- Malabsorption
- Neurodegenerative disorders affecting physical ability
- Hemodialysis

Oral

- Dysphagia
- Chronic orofacial pain
- Oral or pharyngeal cancer (pre-, intra-, and posttherapy)
- Chronic or recurrent oral mucosal lesions
- High caries risk (three or more carious lesions in the past 12 mo)
- Xerostomia

ogy and pathogenesis of periodontal diseases. In this classification system, significant attention has been given to infectious periodontal disease caused by bacteria in the dental plaque such as dental plaque-induced gingival diseases, chronic periodontitis, aggressive periodontitis, and necrotizing periodontal diseases. Although periodontopathic bacteria are needed for initiation, maintenance, and progression of these infectious periodontal diseases, the response of the host to the bacterial challenge is just as important in determining the expression of the specific periodontal disease. An important corollary is that any systemic condition that is able to modulate the bacterial makeup or the host response to the bacterial challenge can constitute a risk factor for periodontal diseases. Identifying and addressing factors that significantly contribute to the development and progression of periodontal diseases is also important in the effective management of such patients. Some of the most frequent conditions identified as modifying the expression of periodontal diseases are smoking, diabetes mellitus, immunosuppression, and conditions related to hormonal changes.

To better understand the relationship between systemic conditions and the possible impact that they may have on periodontal diseases, one must appreciate the maintenance of a fine balance between two main factors, bacterial plaque and the host response to this bacterial challenge. Host response mechanisms encompass both the inflammatory and the immune responses. Although these mechanisms appear independently, they act in concert to resolve the bacterial challenge, inducing changes in vasculature and various inflammatory and immune cells *(2a,2b)*. These responses are coordinated by a multitude of mediators including interleukin (IL)-1 IL-6, and tumor necrosis factor (TNF)-α that eventually activate the effectors of periodontal inflammation and destruction such as proteinases and osteoclasts.

Under normal conditions, the balance between bacteria and host response is maintained, and a clinical healthy periodontal state is achieved. When this balance is disturbed by any factor affecting either arm of the balance, periodontal disease may occur. Several systemic conditions can modulate the expression of periodontal disease by affecting the host response, and these modulating factors can intervene at any level in the chain of pathogenesis of periodontal diseases.

2.1.1. PLAQUE-INDUCED GINGIVAL DISEASE

Plaque-induced gingival diseases are inflammatory conditions of the gingiva, called gingivitis, and they are characterized by the absence of clinical attachment loss. Clinical signs of gingivitis include erythema; edema of the gingiva; changes in contour, consistency, and texture; and bleeding on provocation. Plaque-induced gingivitis is a common occurrence in both children and adults *(3)*. However, several systemic conditions such as hormonal-associated physiological (pregnancy, menstrual cycle, puberty) or pathological conditions (e.g., diabetes mellitus), nutrition, blood disorders, and various medications have been found to significantly increase the risk of gingivitis.

2.1.2. PREGNANCY-ASSOCIATED GINGIVITIS

Pregnancy is associated with an increase in prevalence, severity, and extent of gingivitis. The prevalence of gingivitis in pregnant women can vary between 30 and 100% *(4,5)* and may be higher in woman with previous pregnancies *(4,5)*. During pregnancy, gingivitis increases in severity as early as the second month of pregnancy, increases further as the pregnancy advances, reaches a maximum around months 7 and 8, decreases in month 9 *(6,7)*, and returns to prepregnancy values in the postpartum period *(8,9)*. These changes are independent of plaque accumulation *(9)*, suggesting that the host factors are involved in its pathogenesis. The clinical signs of pregnancy gingivitis are similar to the signs of plaque-induced gingivitis. For example, there is a significant increase in inflammatory indexes such as gingival bleeding, pocket depth, and gingival crevicular fluid *(10)*. The percentage of bleeding sites may almost double in pregnant women compared to nonpregnant women *(9)*. The percentage of pregnant woman with pockets deeper than 4 mm may be twice that of nonpregnant women *(11)*. In a significant percentage of women, there may also be significant enlargement of the gingiva, particularly affecting areas of previous gingival inflammation.

2.1.3. MENSTRUAL CYCLE-ASSOCIATED GINGIVITIS

Changes in gingival appearance may also occur in relation to the menstrual cycle. These changes may be less obvious and may manifest themselves as increases in gingival crevicular fluid. It appears that this increase occurs particularly during the ovulation period and depends on the presence of bacterial plaque *(12,13)*.

2.1.4. Puberty-Associated Gingivitis

Puberty is a stage in the development of human beings characterized by sexual maturation. Studies suggest that the prevalence, severity, and extent of gingivitis increase in children reaches a peak around the age of 12–14 and decreasing thereafter, with significantly lower values by the age of 16–17 *(14)*. The increase in the severity and extent of gingivitis appear to parallel sexual maturation rather than plaque index, suggesting an enhanced response of gingival tissues to the presence of dental plaque and supporting the role of puberty in the pathogenesis of gingivitis *(15)*.

One of the most significant changes occurring during pregnancy, menstrual cycle, and puberty are major hormonal shifts, and these hormonal changes have been proposed as one of the mechanisms responsible for the increase in the expression of gingivitis during these physiological states *(10,16)*. During pregnancy, there is a significant increase in gonadotropins in the first trimester and progesterone and estrogens in the second and third trimesters. The menstrual cycle is also associated with significant surges in progesterone and estrogen, although these changes are less dramatic than those seen in pregnancy. During puberty, the changes in the hormonal makeup vary between girls and boys. In girls, there is a significant increase in estrogen and progesterone; in boys, testosterone reaches significantly high values. The main mechanisms by which sex hormones affect periodontal tissues are the effects on the elements of the host response such as increased blood vessel permeability, vasodilation, decreased epithelial keratinization, reduction in neutrophil chemotaxis, and changes in T cells and signal transduction molecules *(4,17)*. Studies have shown that the bacterial makeup changes during pregnancy and puberty, with a significant increase in the proportion of anaerobic to aerobic bacteria, particularly the periodontopathogen *Provotella intermidia*, probably because of the ability of these bacteria to use progesterone and estrogen as growth factors *(9)*.

2.1.5. Diabetes-Associated Gingivitis

The relationship between diabetes and periodontal disease is also discussed in Chapter 11; the topic is reviewed here in the context of diabetes risk factors for periodontal disease. Diabetes mellitus (DM) is an endocrine disorder with significant metabolic disturbances. Type 1 diabetes (T1DM) is characterized by destruction of the pancreatic β-cells through autoimmune mechanisms with consequent decrement or complete depletion of the insulin. Type 2 DM (T2DM) is characterized by the inability of insulin to exert its functions on target tissues because of deficiencies in its transduction system. T1DM constitutes 5–10% of all diagnosed diabetes, generally has its onset before the age of 21, and affects approx 1 in 400–500 children and adolescents. T2DM constitutes 90–95% of all diagnosed cases of diabetes and has its onset in adulthood, although it has become increasingly diagnosed in children and adolescents *(18)*.

Although gingivitis is prevalent in children, adolescents, and adults, DM adds an additional risk to its development *(3,19)*. In adults, the prevalence of people with diabetes having gingival inflammation is higher than in people without diabetes, whereas in children and adolescents with diabetes, the prevalence of gingivitis may almost double compared to healthy children and adolescents *(20,21)*. When evaluated in children, the severity and extent of gingivitis may also be significantly increased *(22–27)* and may depend on glycemic control *(25,28)*. Moderate to severe gingivitis is twice as extensive in subjects with diabetes compared to subjects without diabetes *(24)*.

2.1.6. Chronic Periodontitis: Diabetes Mellitus As a Risk Factor

Periodontitis is characterized by features similar to plaque-induced gingivitis but, in addition, there is clinical attachment loss and often bone loss. Approximately 35% of the dentate US adults between 30 and 90 yr of age have periodontal disease (29). Periodontal disease prevalence increases with age, reaching approx 50% among persons over the age of 55 yr (30). Diabetes is considered a risk factor for periodontal diseases. Unlike gingivitis, periodontitis is uncommon in children. Children with T1DM do not appear to be at an increased risk of developing periodontitis. In adolescents, however, T1DM may increase the susceptibility to periodontitis (23,31). For example, one study reported that nearly 10% of adolescents with T1DM had periodontitis compared to less than 2% of adolescents without T1DM (23). During adolescence, there may be an amplified inflammatory reaction of the gingiva to gingival plaque (32). It is therefore possible that the presence of diabetes adds an additional element to this already-modified host response, resulting in periodontal breakdown.

T2DM affects approx 15 million Americans (33). The prevalence of this condition among children younger than 10 yr of age, although historically low, is steadily increasing concurrent with the rise in childhood obesity (34,35). The prevalence and characteristics of periodontitis in children with T2DM has not received adequate study. To our knowledge, there is only one study evaluating periodontal disease in children under 10 yr of age (36), and unfortunately in that study, the data analysis aggregated periodontal findings for children, adolescents, and young adults. Therefore, any conclusions relating T2DM to periodontal disease in children cannot be drawn. Considering the low prevalence of this condition among children, however, acquiring more data would be challenging.

The status of periodontal disease in adolescents with T2DM is also poorly defined. Among studies investigating the relationship between T2DM and periodontal disease, only four included adolescents, and all subjects were Pima Indians. One study included only three subjects aged 15–19 yr (37), and the other three investigations combined persons aged 15–34 yr of age in the presentation of study findings (38,39). Nevertheless, the prevalence of periodontal disease among subjects with diabetes aged 15–34 was five to six times higher than the prevalence among subjects without diabetes (38,39), suggesting that younger people with T2DM are at particularly high risk of developing periodontal disease. Further conclusions about the relationship between T2DM and periodontal disease in adolescents would be premature.

T2DM in adolescents is considered to have reached epidemic proportions, and it is predicted that its incidence will continue to rise (40). There is a disproportionate increase in T2DM among children and adolescent minorities compared to whites (41), and these populations are also at an increased risk for complications of diabetes. Therefore, complications related to their diabetes, including periodontal disease, are expected to rise. Moreover, some of the characteristics of these populations such as race, obesity, and poor glycemic control of their diabetes (40,42,43) may add additional risk factors for periodontal breakdown (44–46), resulting in unusually aggressive periodontal diseases. Therefore, there is an imperative need to characterize the status of periodontal disease in adolescents with T2DM and to evaluate its magnitude as a health problem. Until additional studies are conducted, it is prudent, from a practical point of view, to assume that children and adolescents with T2DM are at an elevated (high) risk of developing periodontal diseases. As such, appropriate measures should be taken to diagnose and, if necessary, treat them.

In adults, considerable evidence exists suggesting that T1DM and T2DM increase the risk for periodontitis *(47)*. For example, the reported odds ratios for periodontal disease among subjects with T2DM ranged from 2 to 4, meaning that the odds of having periodontitis in patients with T2DM are two to four times the odds of having periodontitis in subjects without T2DM *(37,38,48,49)*. The presence of periodontitis in patients with diabetes appears to depend on factors such as metabolic control, duration of diabetes, and possibly the age of the patient. A number of studies showed that poor metabolic control increased the likelihood of periodontitis in persons with diabetes. Patients with poor metabolic-controlled T2DM may have two times more sites with attachment loss of more than 5 mm relative to subjects with good metabolic control *(50)*. In patients with T2DM, the odds of having severe periodontal disease in patients with fair-to-good glycemic control (HbA1c <9%) were approx 50% higher than among subjects without diabetes, whereas for subjects with poor glycemic control (HbA1c >9%), the odds of severe periodontal disease were 200% higher than those subjects without diabetes *(49)*. These findings suggest that there may be a dose–response relationship between periodontal disease risk and glycemic control. Some investigations suggest that patients who have had diabetes for more than 10 yr and those aged 30–50 yr and smokers may also be at higher risk of periodontal breakdown *(23,49,51)*. However, more clinical studies are needed to clarify the significance of these factors.

2.2. Periodontal Disease Impact on Cardiovascular Disease and Pregnancy

The host response to infection (production of inflammatory mediators) and the direct products of bacteria (endotoxin, lipopolysaccharides) appear to play a major role in the proposed relationship between periodontal disease and cardiovascular disease or premature birth. Several microbiological and immunological events associated with periodontal disease that can influence systemic health are reviewed below. In terms of the inflammatory events associated with periodontal disease, these same events can have variable effects on different organ systems (i.e., cardiovascular, genitourinary).

2.2.1. CARDIOVASCULAR DISEASES

Recent evidence suggests that periodontal disease could affect the expression of systemic diseases such as cardiovascular diseases and diabetes as well as cause adverse pregnancy outcomes *(52–56)*. As with other microorganisms, it is conceivable that periodontal bacteria could induce damage at sites distant from the location of initial colonization. This phenomenon, called focal infection, received considerable attention in the early literature but later fell out of favor. More recently, the concept of focal infection has been revisited as more and more evidence has accumulated to implicate periodontal disease in the pathogenesis of a variety of systemic diseases.

There are a number of plausible mechanisms by which periodontopathic bacteria could induce distant pathology. One such mechanism is via direct bacterial access to the systemic circulation and its subsequent metastasis to various anatomical sites. There is significant evidence for this mechanism in both the periodontal and general dental literature; for example, bacteremia induced by tissue manipulation may result in metastatic implantation of bacteria at damaged or prosthetic heart valves. Alternatively, bacterial products such as endotoxin may gain access to the circulation and affect various patho-logical processes at distant sites. Still another pathogenic mechanism involves the host response. Challenged with bacteria, the host produces a multitude of mediators including cytokines and other inflammatory proteins that again gain access to the circulatory sys-tem, with resulting systemic effects.

The term cardiovascular disease encompasses several pathological conditions involv-ing the heart and vascular system. The major cardiovascular diseases are coronary heart diseases, cerebrovascular diseases, and peripheral vascular diseases. The most common pathologic basis for these diseases is atherosclerosis. The major risk factors for athero-sclerosis and cardiovascular disease include dyslipidemia, hypertension, obesity, smok-ing, and diabetes, and together, these factors account for more than two-thirds of all myocardial infarctions (MI), the most common acute coronary syndrome *(57)*. However, acute coronary syndrome occurs in people without the "classical" risk factors, suggesting that other risk factors exist.

In addition to the traditionally recognized risk factors for cardiovascular disease, significant evidence now exists to suggest that inflammation is also an important risk factor. Several systemic markers defining the inflammatory status of an individual have been assessed in clinical studies to determine their role in predicting cardiovascular events. These systemic markers include proinflammatory cytokines (IL-6 and TNF-α), inflammatory-sensitive proteins (C-reactive protein [CRP], serum amyloid A [SAA], serum amyloid P, complement proteins, and fibrinogen) and adhesion molecules *(58–62)*. Other inflammatory-sensitive proteins found to be associated with an increased risk of cardiovascular events are fibrinogen *(63)* and SAA *(64)*. One study assessed the risk of MI in humans in relation to the level of five inflammatory-sensitive proteins. The subjects were grouped according to the presence of major cardiovascular risk factors (dyslipidemia, hypertension, smoking, and diabetes), with "low" risk being defined as having no major risk factors and "high" risk as having more than two risk factors. The results of this study revealed that in both the low- and high-risk groups, the risk of MI increased with the number of elevated inflammatory-sensitive proteins. In the low-risk group, subjects with at least three elevated inflammatory-sensitive proteins had more than three times the risk of MI relative to subjects without an elevated level of inflam-matory-sensitive proteins. This increase in risk was detectable only after 10 yr, suggest-ing that chronic inflammatory processes may have delayed effects on the pathogenesis of cardiovascular events. This study also suggested that elevations of inflammatory markers that may occur in periodontal disease could increase the risk of cardiovascular events even decades after exposure.

The role of the inflammatory process in the pathogenesis of cardiovascular disease is further suggested by studies demonstrating that anti-inflammatory agents, such as aspi-rin, and drugs with a serum CRP-lowering effects, such as statins, also lower the risk for cardiovascular events, again suggesting that CRP and perhaps other inflammatory mark-ers are in the pathogenic chain *(65,66)*. These inflammatory markers could be derived from the liver (CRP) or some other damaged tissues. Some of these inflammatory mark-ers such as IL-6 and TNF-α could be spilled into the plasma from diseased periodontal tissue and further stimulate the liver production of acute phase proteins (CRP). Thus, it appears that in addition to the "classical" risk factors, chronic inflammatory conditions such as periodontal disease may constitute risk factors for cardiovascular diseases. It is notable that Periostat (low-dosage doxycycline hyclate), a drug used to treat periodontal disease, has also been found to decrease CRP levels by 60%.

2.2.2. ATHEROSCLEROSIS

Atherosclerosis is a disease that affects the mid- and large-sized arteries, and its characteristic lesions are formed within the intimal layer of the vessels. Morphological characterization of atherosclerotic lesions clearly shows that they are inflammatory lesions. Moreover, the atheromatous lesions are particularly prone to complications in areas of significant inflammatory progression *(67)*. The molecular pathogenesis of atherosclerosis appears to recapitulate the molecular events of an evolving inflammatory process, with macrophages and lymphocytes playing a significant role. Endothelial dysfunction leading to the initiation of the atherosclerosis process may be caused by hemodynamic (hypertension), chemical (cholesterol, cigaret smoking, glycated proteins), immunologic (immune complexes), viral, bacterial, endocrine, paracrine factors (cytokines such as IL-1, IL-6 and TNF-α, angiotensin II), and inflammatory-sensitive proteins (e.g., CRP). Because atherosclerosis is an inflammatory process, modulating inflammatory processes may contribute not only to the initiation of the atherosclerotic lesion but may have significant effects in the progression and complication of these lesions and subsequent clinical events. Periodontal diseases are inflammatory conditions with the potential of influencing the atherosclerosis pathogenesis.

2.2.3. CLINICAL STUDIES EXPLORING THE ASSOCIATION BETWEEN PERIODONTAL AND CARDIOVASCULAR DISEASE

Both mechanistic and association clinical studies have been conducted to examine the possible involvement of periodontal diseases in the pathogenesis of cardiovascular diseases. Mechanistic studies have evaluated serological, pathological, and inflammatory marker data in order to assess the biological plausibility of a relationship between periodontal and cardiovascular disease. One seroepidemiological study from Finland found that the risk of having coronary heart disease in subjects with an antibody response to two periodontal pathogens (*Porphyromonas gingivalis* and *Actinobacillus actinomycetemcomitans*) was increased by 50% *(68)*, results consistent with studies showing that antibody levels to *P. gingivalis* are significantly higher in subjects with elevated CRP *(69)*. Another study showed that patients testing positive for *Bacteroides forsythus* in their periodontal pockets were three times more likely and subjects testing positive for *P. gingivalis* were 2.5 times more likely to have suffered a nonfatal MI. The evaluation of atheroma samples has demonstrated that periodontal pathogens are often present. In addition, the intimamedia wall thickness is considered a measure of subclinical atherosclerosis, and it is associated with cardiovascular events *(70)*. When subjects with and without periodontal disease were studied, it was found that those persons with severe periodontal disease were 30% more likely to have a thick carotid arterial wall *(71)*.

Several studies examining various populations reported an association between elevated levels of CRP and periodontal disease *(72–76)*, as well as degree of overweight or obesity as measured by body mass index (BMI). For example, data derived from the third National Health and Nutrition Examination Survey (NHANES III) showed that subjects with extensive periodontal disease had significantly higher CRP levels than subjects without periodontal disease *(75)* and that this difference was higher in subjects without other risk factors for elevated CRP. These results are supported by another study examining the Atherosclerosis Risk in Communities (ARIC) population *(77)*. The ARIC study was designed to investigate the etiology and natural history of atherosclerosis and clinical cardiovascular diseases in four US communities. In that investigation, subjects with periodontal disease were twice as likely to have elevated CRP levels among those persons with a low BMI but not among those with a high BMI, suggesting that if CRP production is stimulated by other causes, the stimulation coming from periodontal disease may be influenced by other factors and not add a further increment in its values *(77)*. At least one other study, however, failed to show increased CRP levels in subjects with periodontal diseases *(78)*, although methodological limitations may be responsible. Recent studies suggest that even modest elevations in CRP levels may increase the risk factors for cardiovascular diseases. Periodontal disease-induced increases in CRP levels may be just enough to constitute a risk for cardiovascular diseases. Since other inflammatory markers have been found to be associated with cardiovascular disease, these are also being investigated to determine a possible link between periodontal and cardiovascular diseases.

Numerous association studies have been conducted to examine the relationship between periodontal disease and cardiovascular events. Some of these investigations have suggested a clinically important relationship *(79,80)*; however, other studies have not found an association *(81–83)*, thus questioning the causal effect of periodontal disease in the pathogenesis of the cardiovascular diseases. These inconsistencies across studies may result from the fact that both study populations and methodological approaches varied by investigation. In addition, when the strength of the relationship is in the slight to moderate range, it is expected that some studies would not show any association. A recent meta-analysis of nine cohort studies found a relative risk of 1.19, a result consistent with a relatively weak relationship *(84)*. Interestingly, several studies including the meta-analysis found that in younger subjects the association between periodontal disease and cardiovascular disease was greatest in younger individuals *(83,85)*. These results are consistent with the suggestion that periodontal disease may be an important risk factor for cardiovascular disease in some but not all individuals.

Continued work is necessary to determine what factors in patients with periodontal disease additionally predict risk for cardiovascular disease as well as alternate explanations for the observed association between periodontal and cardiovascular disease *(86)*. Future studies should explore confounding factors (i.e., shared risk factors for periodontal and cardiovascular diseases) that could explain the observed associations between periodontal and cardiovascular diseases. Additional prospective, case-controlled studies are needed to clearly demonstrate that proposed associations are real and independent of common risk factors.

2.2.4. PREGNANCY AND PRETERM BIRTH

An estimated 10,000 babies are born each day in the United States. Of these babies, 800 are born at low birth weight and 150 at very low birth weight *(87,88)*; more than 50% will die, and a significant number will have permanent deficits. A growing body of evidence has revealed an increased risk for premature birth in women with varying degrees of periodontal disease *(89–92)*. As discussed in the preceding section on cardiovascular disease, the cytokines and other inflammatory mediators produced in gingivitis or periodontitis result in local tissue destruction and also enter the bloodstream, where they may reach significant levels and affect placental tissues. Numerous studies have demonstrated that genitourinary tract infection increases the risk for premature rupture of membranes and premature labor *(93,94)*. The bacteria found in periodontal disease include Gram-negative rods and anaerobes similar to those found in vaginal infection *(95,96)*. Even at a distant site such as the mouth, these bacteria can lead to the release of cell-wall components that trigger the maternal release of factors that can initiate labor or, by spreading to the upper genital tract, could lead to membrane rupture and premature labor similar to that seen vaginal infection. Several published reports have demonstrated vaginal infection with organisms that originate from oral (periodontal) sites *(97–99)*. Thus, periodontal disease may influence pregnancy and gestational development by direct infection of the genital tract as well as the release of inflammatory mediators that trigger from a distance hormonal events leading to premature labor and premature birth *(100)*.

One recent controlled clinical trial demonstrated a significant reduction of premature birth associated with prenatal periodontal therapy *(101)*, and several case-control studies have demonstrated increased risk for premature birth in women with periodontal disease compared to those without disease *(90,92,102)*, and risk varied with degree of periodontal disease. Although there remains considerable work ahead to understand the mechanisms and causal relationship, even at this stage public health recommendations are changing to emphasize dental and periodontal health as an important component of prenatal care.

3. CARIES

Dental caries is an infectious microbial disease that results in dissolution and destruction of calcified tooth structure. Caries and periodontal disease are probably the most common chronic infectious diseases in the world *(103)*. In industrialized nations, outstanding progress has been made over the past 50 yr in reducing the incidence and consequences of dental caries: by 1991, 50% of children aged 5–17 yr had no caries in their permanent dentition *(104)*, with 80% of the caries observed among only 25% of the children. This high-risk group represents children with primarily socioeconomic risk factors for disease. Over the past 25 yr, the percentage of adults with no caries increased from 15.7% to 19.6% in those aged 18–34 yr and from 12 to 13.5% in those aged 35–54 yr *(105,106)*. The trend in older adults has been worsening, with the percentage of teeth free of caries and restorations declining from 10.6 to 7.9% in those aged 55–64 yr and from 9.6 to 6.5% in those aged 65–74 yr *(105)*. In particular, there is increased risk for root caries in these older individuals who have experienced varying degrees of gingival recession because of periodontal disease *(107,108)*. Although fluoridation has had the single largest impact on the incidence of caries, improved oral hygiene, diet, education, and overall health have also played major roles *(109)*.

Although the most common risk factors for caries are lack of daily tooth brushing, frequency of carbohydrate intake, low income, low education, and lack of community fluoridation, any systemic or local disease that results in salivary hypofunction may dramatically increase the risk for and incidence of dental caries *(110,111)*. Impaired salivary gland neurosecretory action caused by pharmacologic blockade is a common side effect of many medication classes (particularly antihypertensive and antidepressant medications), and any person with three or more carious lesions in 1 ar and who is taking a new medication should be evaluated for possible drug side effects *(112)* *(see* Chapter 6). Several autoimmune disorders (most notable Sjogren's syndrome) can result in salivary gland injury, hyposalivation, and increased caries incidence *(see* Chapter 14). Radiation therapy for the treatment of malignancy in the head and neck regions, when the major salivary glands are included in the treatment field, can result in profound xerostomia and rampant caries *(113)* *(see* Chapter 12).

Dental caries can result in pain, loss of teeth, and limited ability to chew, thus potentially affecting short- and long-term ability to bite and chew foods, limiting food selection. Any patient with three or more carious lesions in the past 2 mo is considered at high risk for future caries and should be evaluated for underlying causes (diet, hygiene, xerostomia, and medications).

4. ORAL MUCOSAL DISEASE

Painful oral mucosal lesions can result in a number of local, systemic, and nutrition-related problems: impaired chewing ability because of pain, damaged epithelial integrity as a portal for infection, altered taste, and a variety of complications related to treatment of the disorder *(see* Chapters 6, 8, and 14). Representative oral mucosal disorders include local (oral cancer, aphthous stomatitis, reactive or traumatic lesions, recurrent [herpetic] viral lesions, candidiasis) and systemic disorders with oral manifestations (lichen planus, pemphigus vulgaris, benign mucous membrane pemphigoid, lupus erythematosis). The prevalence of these disorders and an assessment of the related public health need has recently been reviewed *(114)*. The first large-scale study of oral soft tissue lesions was published by Knapp in 1971 *(115)*. Of 181,388 young adult army inductees, 1.36% had oral soft tissue lesions. However, in a study of 14,749 adults over 35 yr of age, 10% had oral soft tissue lesions *(116)*. Axell *(117)* assessed the prevalence of oral mucosal diseases in 20,333 adults and found more than 60 different conditions. The prevalence of the more common lesions were as follows: herpes labialis, 17.38%; aphthous stomatitis, 17.7%; leukoplakia, 9.95%; snuff dippers' lesions, 8.04%; fibroepithelial polyp, 3.25%; denture stomatitis, 16.02%; angular cheilitis, 3.76%; benign migratory glossitis, 8.45%; and lichen planus, 1.89%. The original Health and Nutrition Examination Survey (HANES I) (1971–1974) study showed that 9.5% of 20,749 persons ages 1 to 74 yr had oral soft tissue lesions *(118)*. Bouquot et al. *(119,120)* found that 10.3% of the 23,616 who participated in a mass oral screening had at least one oral soft tissue lesion and of these, 25% had more than one lesion. Of the 10.3% with lesions, nearly 17% had oral leukoplakia, and 7% of these were carcinoma or severe dysplasia. In the HANES II study, Hand and Whitehill *(121)* reported that 23.1% of 629 Iowans over 65 yr of age had oral mucosal lesions. Studies performed by Kleinman et al. *(122)* have demonstrated that approx 10% of the population has oral soft tissue lesions at any one time. The more common lesions noted included recurrent aphthous stomatitis, 46%; recurrent herpetic infections, 17–38%; oral sores, 8.4%; leukoplakia, 5%; and lichen planus, 1%. The clinical significance of proper evaluation of these lesions cannot be underestimated. Sciubba et al. *(123)* reported in a nationwide survey that 12.3% of 945 epithelial lesions judged to be clinically suspicious by specialists in oral and maxillofacial pathology, oral and maxillofacial surgery, and oral medicine were dysplastic or malignant.

Table 2
Causes of Dysphagia

Neurogenic	Myogenic
• Stroke	• Muscular dystrophy
• Multiple sclerosis	• Myasthenia gravis
• ALS	• Aging
• Diabetic neuropathy	
• Cerebral palsy	Other
• Guillain-Barré	• Reumatologic disorders
	• Connective tissue disorders
Obstructive	• Vagotomy
• Candidiasis	• Gastrointestinal resection
• Head and neck cancer	

ALS, amyotrophic lateral sclerosis.

5. CHRONIC OROFACIAL PAIN

Persistent orofacial pain can lead to impaired ability to eat, reduced socializing, and depression. The painful conditions can result from local orofacial disorders or as regional manifestations of systemic illness. Pain is the most common reason for patients to seek health care. Chronic pain, both medical and dental, is a leading cause of disability, second only to respiratory infections for lost work days, and by far the leading reason for long-term disability. As detailed in the World Workshop on Oral Medicine in 1988, billions of dollars are expended annually for the diagnosis and treatment of pain, a significant portion of which is spent on inappropriate or ineffective diagnostic and treatment modalities for temporomandibular disorders (TMD) *(124)*. In a study of 45,711 US adults, Lipton et al. *(125)* demonstrated that approx 22% of the population, or 39 million persons, have orofacial pain. Nearly half of this pain is caused by toothache, but approx 10 million people have painful oral lesions, 4.3 million have TMD and related pain, 500,000 have face or cheek pain, and 300,000 complain of burning mouth symptoms. These findings were recently confirmed by Riley et al. *(126)*, who reported that of 5860 older adults interviewed (mean age, 73 ± 6.1 yr), 32% had painful oral sores, 50% had burning mouth, 56% reported jaw joint pain, 61% had facial pain, and 62% had toothache pain *(126)*. Oral discomfort has also been reported in 45–60% of menopausal women *(127)*. Additionally, patients are seen by dental providers with pain that can be diagnosed as vascular, neurologic, atypical facial pain, and other poorly understood head and neck pain syndromes. Cases of migraine have been documented to occur in 43 per 1000 persons, and neuralgia has been reported to occur in 2 per 1000 persons *(128)*. Oral burning might occur in up to 15% of adults *(129)*.

6. DYSPHAGIA

Swallowing dysfunction, better known as dysphagia, is common after acute stroke; it is also associated with traumatic brain injury, Parkinson's disease, aging, and the treatment and physiology of certain malignancies. Dysphagia can result in numerous complications including aspiration of food, chest infection, compromised nutritional status, increased mortality, increased length of stay, and overall disability (*see* Table 2) *(130,131)*.

Clinical characteristics of dysphagia include dysphonia, dysarthria, abnormal gag, abnormal volitional cough, cough and/or voice change after swallow, abnormal lip closure and tongue movement, lingual discoordination, delayed oral and pharyngeal transit, incomplete oral clearance, regurgitation, pharyngeal pooling, delayed or absent trigger of swallow, and dyspraxia *(132)*.

There are two main types of dysphagia: oropharyngeal and esophageal dysphagia. Oropharyngeal dysphagia can be related to neurogenic disorders, decreased salivation, oropharyngeal lesions, weakness of lips, decreased oral sensitivity, Sjogren's syndrome (dry mouth), or cognitive disorders. Esophageal dysphagia can be related to obstructive disorders, motility disorders, or motor dysfunction.

6.1. Complications of Dysphagia

Documented complications of dysphagia include increased length of stay, chest infections, disability/decreased functional status, decreased nutrition status, increased likelihood of discharge to institutionalized care, and increased mortality *(133–135)*. The "silent aspiration," or aspiration without a reflexive cough, is a serious concern with dysphagic individuals and is often the cause of several of the above-mentioned complications *(136)*. Silent aspiration accounts for 40 to 70% of aspiration in patients with dysphagia. Those patients who do silently aspirate often present with pneumonia and chest infections *(137)*. Smithard et al. in 1996, illustrated that patients with dysphagia secondary to acute stroke as assessed at the bedside had a 33% incidence of chest infections, double that of patients with a "safe swallow" *(133)*. Increased length of stay and risk of mortality are also higher in these subjects *(133–135)*.

6.2. Nutritional Implications of Dysphagia

Dysphagia usually results in insufficient food intake. In most incidences, this is because of the difficulty in consuming an adequate volume. Malnutrition occurs secondary to insufficient protein intake, as well as an overall lack of calories and micronutrients. Dietary intake may be affected for long periods of time *(132,134)*. Malnutrition significantly impedes the recovery process *(138)*. Nutrition status changes, as indicated by changes in skin-fold thickness and albumin, are apparent in patients who exhibit dysphagia *(133)*. Smithard found that deterioration of nutrition status began to improve 1 mo after appropriate diet and speech intervention *(133)*.

6.3. Dysphagia Screening

Dysphagia screening is defined as "a procedure designed to detect any clinical indication of potential neurological deglutition dysfunction" *(132)*. Early screening and treatment of dysphagia leads to more cost-effective treatment and improved quality of care and ensures optimal outcome *(134,139)*.

The Registered Dietitian Dysphagia Screening Tool, designed by Brody et al., utilizes medical record review, patient questioning, and observation of a meal (Table 3). Observation includes assessment of drooling of liquids and solids, cough during or after a swallow, facial or tongue weakness, difficulty with secretions, pocketing, change in voice quality, posture and head control, percentage of meal consumed, eating time, and presence of voluntary and dry cough *(140)*.

Table 3
Registered Dietitian (RD) Dysphagia Screening Tool (2003)

To be completed at the time of initial chart review by RD

Medical Record # _____   Date of Admission _____

Subject # _____

Gender _____   Date of Screen _____

I. INITIAL CHART REVIEW

MD/RN Documentation of:

Difficulty Swallowing: Fluids		Y	N
Choking During or After Meals		Y	N

If diagnosis and/or diet order meet screening criteria: patient appropriate for screening
AND/OR: If one or more of the above are yes: patient appropriate for screening

Screening to be completed		Y	N
Inappropriate for screening due to alternate mode of feeding		Y	N
Pt already referred or seen by SLP for Bedside Dysphagia		Y	N
Evaluation		Y	N

II. COGNITION

Is the patient alert and able to remain awake during the interview?		Y	N
Is the patient able to follow basic directions?			
Open your mouth		Y	N
Stick out your tongue		Y	N

If NO on either and patient is on an oral diet:

AT RISK—Refer to SLP for Bedside Dysphagia Evaluation.
Evaluate for nutrition support.
Complete Data Collection Form.

III. OBSERVE DURING A MEAL

Observe and ask patient if they exhibit or have a recent history
(within the last month) of any of the following:

		Observed		Self-Reported	
Drooling of:	liquids?	Y	N	Y	N
	solids?	Y	N	Y	N
Coughing:	during a swallow?	Y	N	Y	N
	after a swallow?	Y	N	Y	N
Facial or tongue weakness?		Y	N	Y	N
Difficulty managing own secretions?		Y	N	Y	N
Pocketing?		Y	N	Y	N
Change in voice quality (wet/gurgly)?		Y	N	Y	N
Poor head control or posture?		Y	N	Y	N
Failure to consume >50% of meal?		Y	N	Y	N
Prolonged eating time?		Y	N	Y	N

IV. CONDUCT

Voluntary Cough	Present?		Y	N
Dry Swallow	Present?		Y	N

Number of symptoms observed: _____

Number of symptoms self-reported: _____

Adapted with permission from Rebecca Brody, MS, RD, CNSD

Other screening methods for dysphagia include the Burke Dysphagia Screening Test, which incorporates the individual consuming 3 oz of water, the Standardized Swallowing Assessment; the Hinds and Wiles timed test; and the Smithard et al. Bedside Swallowing Assessment *(132)*. All of these tools look at the following similar clinical features and contain a component with or without the administration of water. These features include administration of water to assess for holding, leakage, coughing, choking, breathlessness, and quality of voice *(141,142)*. The literature reviewed indicates that a registered nurse, registered dietitian, physician, or speech–language pathologist (SLP) can perform these screenings in patients *(132,133,137–140,143–148)*.

6.4. Diagnosis of Dysphagia

Bedside dysphagia evaluations are performed by the SLP and help to identify patients at risk for dysphagia and increase timely and appropriate diet and dysphagia therapy *(130)*. The evaluation includes observation of a range of textures and consistencies, resulting in a detailed description of the clinical function of component phases of swallowing, usually accompanied by judgment of degree of dysfunction and aspiration risk *(132)*. It must be performed by a certified SLP. Clinical assessment focuses on oral–motor and oral–sensory function, protective reflexes, and respiratory status. Observations are made on level of arousal, cognitive–linguistic status, and perception *(149)*. Treatment including alteration in the consistencies of foods and the use of swallowing therapies improves swallowing function in these patients. This leads to improvements in nutritional status and overall health *(131)*.

6.5. Dysphagia Treatment

Once the presence of dysphagia is identified, treatment should commence. Goals for treatment may include the promotion of good nutrition status, weight maintenance, diminution of the risk of aspiration, promotion of eating independence, and enjoyment of mealtime *(150)*. The treatment of dysphagia typically includes oral motor exercises, swallowing techniques, positioning during feeding, and diet modification. Elmstahl et al. found in 1999 that the combination of these techniques reduced the degree of oral and pharyngeal dysfunction in acute stroke patients. This in turn led to improved nutrition status, as indicated by increases in albumin and total iron-binding capacity *(131)*.

6.6. Diet Management

Eating and drinking have important social, cultural, and emotional meaning in all societies *(151,152)*. Initiating safe oral nutrition and hydration is a priority for patients with dysphagia *(140)*. A diet order is recommended once the degree of dysphagia is assessed. Modifications in diet can include changes in food consistencies and/or liquid consistencies, or even elimination of intake by mouth and initiation of tube feeding. Liquid or pureed foods are sometimes the only consistency tolerated by patients with mechanical disorders that cause dysphagia but may not be the most appropriate choice for individuals with oropharyngeal dysphagia. Semisolid consistencies that are easy to chew are more often the best choices in this population *(153)*. Cohesive foods that are moist are easier to manage for most individuals with dysphagia *(150)*. Liquids often have to be thickened to decrease transit time and allow for protection of the airway *(150,153)*. The patient should take nothing by mouth if aspiration is present. Withholding oral intake

Table 4
Stages of National Dysphagia Diet

Stage	Description	Examples
Dysphagia puree	• Uniform • Pureed • Cohesive • "Pudding-like" texture	• Smooth hot cereals cooked to a "pudding" consistency • Mashed potatoes • Commercial slurried/pureed bread • Applesauce or pureed fruit • Pureed meat • Pureed pasta or rice • Pureed vegetable • Yogurt • Custard
Dysphagia mechanically altered	• Moist • Soft-textured • Easily forms a bolus	• Soft pancakes moistened with syrup • Cooked cereals • Dry cereals moistened with milk • Canned fruit (excluding pineapple) • Soft, moist cakes • Moist ground meat • Cottage cheese • Scrambled eggs • Tuna salad (no large chunks) • Potato salad • Well-cooked noodles in sauce/gravy • Well-cooked, diced vegetables
Dysphagia advanced	• Regular foods (with the exception of very hard, sticky, or crunchy foods)	• Moist breads (with butter, jelly, etc.) • Well-moistened cereals • Peeled soft fruits (peach, plum, kiwi) • Tender, thin-sliced meats • Eggs • Rice • Baked potato (without skin) • Tender, cooked vegetables • Shredded lettuce
Regular	• All foods	• No restrictions

of food and fluid reduces the volume of material aspirated and may reduce the severity of the pneumonia *(154)*.

In 2002, the American Dietetic Association published the National Dysphagia Diet Task Force's National Dysphagia Diet. The diet has four levels of consistencies: dysphagia puree, dysphagia mechanically altered, dysphagia advanced, and regular (Table 4). There are also four levels of National Dysphagia Diet liquid consistencies: thin liquids (low viscosity), nectar-like liquids (medium viscosity), honey-like liquids (viscosity of honey), and spoon-thick liquids (viscosity of pudding) *(155)*.

Compliance with the puree diet can be a problem for patients who previously consumed whole foods. Patients often find these foods unappetizing, especially if they are coming from a baby food jar. Several food service companies now provide individualized as well as bulk varieties of pureed foods for the hospitality industry. Unfortunately, these items are often very expensive, preventing their widespread use.

Patient positioning is also a very important part of feeding a patient with dysphagia. The patient must be sitting upright and should be supervised. Correct anatomical alignment is necessary for the passage of food through the pharynx and esophagus. Patients should be well supported whether they are in a chair or a bed.

7. SUMMARY

This chapter highlights bidirectional relationships between oral and systemic health and disease. What emerges are several themes of interaction that the clinician should be aware of: inflammation, infection, oral function, and salivation. Oral disease with an inflammatory component (primarily although not exclusively periodontal disease) can affect systemic immune and hormonal status, increasing risk for cardiovascular disease and pregnancy complications; this scope of influence will likely expand as this new area of investigation continues. Likewise, systemic inflammatory diseases (autoimmune and immune mediated) can have significant oral manifestations, including chronic mucosal ulceration and salivary gland hypofunction. Oral infection is common (caries and periodontal disease) and can be life threatening in patients with other systemic risk factors such as cardiac valve disorders (infective endocarditis) and immunsuppression caused by disease or medical therapy; oral infection is also the initiating event in the aforementioned inflammatory disorders. Oral function, including dysphagia, can be impaired whenever there is a painful condition (mucosal, periodontal, dental, musculoskeletal, or neuropathic) and affect oral intake of nutrients; these oral disorders may be primary or secondary to a number of neurological, rheumatological, and orthopedic problems. Saliva is essential for normal oral immune surveillance, mastication, swallowing, and digestion. Hyposalivation is a common complication of medical management of a wide variety of medical illnesses as well as radiation and chemotherapy for malignancy.

Physicians, dentists, and registered dietitians need improved cross training in oral–systemic–nutrition relationships. Greater awareness of the signs, symptoms, and management strategies for oral–systemic disease must be translated into clinical practice and include clinical pathways for referral and/or consultation for patients with high-risk findings or illnesses (*see* Table 1).

REFERENCES

1. Greenberg MS, Glick M, eds. Burket's Oral Medicine: Diagnosis and Treatment. 10th Ed. Hamilton, Ontario: BC Decker Inc., 2003
2. Little J, Falace D, Miller C, Rhodus N, eds. Dental management of the medically compromised patient. 6th Ed. St. Louis, MO: Mosby Inc., 2002
2a. Genco RJ. Host responses in periodontal diseases: current concepts. J Periodontol 1992; 63(4 Suppl.): 338–355.
2b. Kornman KS, Page RC, Tonetti MS. The host response to the microbial challenge in periodontitis: assembling the players. Periodontol 2000 1997; 14:33–53.
3. Jenkins WM, Papapanou PN. Epidemiology of periodontal disease in children and adolescents. Periodontol 2000 2001; 26:16–32.
4. Hugoson A. Gingival inflammation and female sex hormones: a clinical investigation of pregnant women and experimental studies in dogs. J Periodontal Res 1970; (Suppl. 5):1–18.
5. Loe H. Physiology of the gingival pocket. Acad Rev Calif Acad Periodontol 1965; 13(1):6–14.

6. Tilakaratne A, Soory M, Ranasinghe AW, Corea SM, Ekanayake SL, de Silva M. Periodontal disease status during pregnancy and 3 months post-partum, in a rural population of Sri-Lankan women. J Clin Periodontol 2000; 27(10):787–792.

7. Loe H. Periodontal disease in pregnancy. 3. Response to local treatment. Acta Odontol Scand 1966; 24(6):747–759, .

8. Cohen DW, Shapiro J, Friedman L, Kyle GC, Franklin S. A longitudinal investigation of the periodontal changes during pregnancy and fifteen months post-partum. 2. J Periodontol 1971; 42(10):653–657.

9. Kornman KS, Loesche WJ. The subgingival microbial flora during pregnancy. J Periodontal Res 1980; 15(2):111–122.

10. Mariotti A. Sex steroid hormones and cell dynamics in the periodontium. Crit Rev Oral Biol Med 1994; 5(1):27–53.

11. Miyazaki H, Yamashita Y, Shirahama R, et al. Periodontal condition of pregnant women assessed by CPITN. J Clin Periodontol 1991; 18(10):751–754.

12. Holm-Pedersen P, Loe H. Flow of gingival exudate as related to menstruation and pregnancy. J Periodontal Res 1967; 2(1):13–20.

13. Lindhe J, Attsfrom R. Gingival exudation during the menstrual cycle. J Periodontal Res 1967; 2(3):194–198.

14. Sutcliffe P. A longitudinal study of gingivitis and puberty. J Periodontal Res 1972; 7(1):52–58.

15. Mombelli A, Gusberti FA, van Oosten MA, Lang NP. Gingival health and gingivitis development during puberty: a 4-year longitudinal study. J Clin Periodontol 1989; 16(7):451–456.

16. Amar S, Chung KM. Influence of hormonal variation on the periodontium in women. Periodontol 2000 1994; 6:79–87.

17. Miyagi M, Aoyama H, Morishita M, Iwamoto Y. Effects of sex hormones on chemotaxis of human peripheral polymorphonuclear leukocytes and monocytes. J Periodontol 1992; 63(1):28–32.

18. National Diabetes Statistics 2000. Available at (Website: http://diabetes.niddk.nig.gov/dm/pubs/statistics/index/htm).

19. American Academy of Periodontology position paper 2003. Available at (Website: http://www.perio.org/resources-products/posppr2.html).

20. de Pommereau V, Pare C, Bordais P, Robert JJ. Insulin-dependent diabetes and periodontal disease in young patients. Ann Pediatr (Paris) 1992; 38(4):235–239.

21. Rylander H, Ramberg P, Blohme G, Lindhe J. Prevalence of periodontal diseases in young diabetics. J Clin Periodontal 1987; 14:38–43.

22. Bernick SM, Cohen DW, Baker L, Laster L. Dental disease in children with diabetes mellitus. J Periodontol 1975; 46(4):241–245.

23. Cianciola LJ, Park BH, Bruck E, Mosovich L, Genco RJ. Prevalence of periodontal disease in insulin-dependent diabetes mellitus (juvenile diabetes). J Am Dent Assoc 1982; 104(5):653–660.

24. de Pommereau V, Dargent-Pare C, Robert JJ, Brion M. Periodontal status in insulin-dependent diabetic adolescents. J Clin Periodontol 1992; 19(9 Pt 1):628–632.

25. Gislen G, Nilsson KO, Matsson L. Gingival inflammation in diabetic children related to degree of metabolic control. Acta Odontol Scand 1980; 38(4):241–246.

26. Novaes Junior AB, Pereira AL, de Moraes N, Novaes AB. Manifestations of insulin-dependent diabetes mellitus in the periodontium of young Brazilian patients. J Periodontol 1991; 62(2):116–122.

27. Pinson M, Hoffman WH, Garnick JJ, Litaker MS. Periodontal disease and type I diabetes mellitus in children and adolescents. J Clin Periodontol 1995; 22(2):118–123.

28. Karjalainen KM, Knuuttila ML. The onset of diabetes and poor metabolic control increases gingival bleeding in children and adolescents with insulin-dependent diabetes mellitus. J Clin Periodontol 1996; 23(12):1060–1067.

29. Albandar JM, Brunelle JA, Kingman A. Destructive periodontal disease in adults 30 years of age and older in the United States, 1988–1994. J Periodontol 1999; 70(1):13–29.

30. Albandar JM, Rams TE. Global epidemiology of periodontal diseases: an overview. Periodontol 2000 2002; 29:7–10.

31. Harrison R, Bowen WH. Periodontal health, dental caries, and metabolic control in insulin-dependent diabetic children and adolescents. Pediatr Dent 1987; 9(4):283–286.

32. Mariotti A. Dental plaque-induced gingival diseases. Ann Periodontol 1999; 4(1):7–19.

33. National Diabetes Statistics 2002. Available at (Website: http://diabetes.niddk.nig.gov/dm/pubs/statistics/index/htm).
34. Fagot-Campagna A. Emergence of type 2 diabetes mellitus in children: epidemiological evidence. J Pediatr Endocrinol Metab 2000; 13(Suppl. 6):1395–1402.
35. Fagot-Campagna A, Pettitt DJ, Engelgau MM, et al. Type 2 diabetes among North American children and adolescents: an epidemiologic review and a public health perspective. J Pediatr 2000; 136(5):664–672.
36. Shlossman M, Knowler WC, Pettitt DJ, Genco RJ. Type 2 diabetes mellitus and periodontal disease. J Am Dent Assoc 1990; 121(4):532–536.
37. Taylor GW, Burt BA, Becker MP, Genco RJ, Shlossman M. Glycemic control and alveolar bone loss progression in type 2 diabetes. Ann Periodontol 1998; 3(1):30–39.
38. Emrich LJ, Shlossman M, Genco RJ. Periodontal disease in non-insulin-dependent diabetes mellitus. J Periodontol 1991; 62(2):123–131.
39. Nelson RG, Shlossman M, Budding LM, et al. Periodontal disease and NIDDM in Pima Indians. Diabetes Care 1990; 13(8):836–840.
40. Rosenbloom AL, Joe JR, Young RS, Winter WE. Emerging epidemic of type 2 diabetes in youth. Diabetes Care 1999; 22(2):345–354.
41. Pinhas-Hamiel O, Dolan LM, Daniels SR, Standiford D, Khoury PR, Zeitler P. Increased incidence of non-insulin-dependent diabetes mellitus among adolescents. J Pediatr 1996; 128(5 Pt 1):608–615.
42. Auslander WF, Thompson S, Dreitzer D, White NH, Santiago JV. Disparity in glycemic control and adherence between African-American and Caucasian youths with diabetes: family and community contexts. Diabetes Care 1997; 20(10):1569–1575.
43. Neufeld ND, Raffel LJ, Landon C, Chen YD, Vadheim CM. Early presentation of type 2 diabetes in Mexican-American youth. Diabetes Care 1998; 21(1):80–86.
44. Albandar JM, Rams TE. Risk factors for periodontitis in children and young persons. Periodontol 2000 2002; 29:207–222.
45. Iacopino AM, Cutler CW. Pathophysiological relationships between periodontitis and systemic disease: recent concepts involving serum lipids. J Periodontol 2000; 71(8):1375–1384.
46. Wood N, Johnson RB, Streckfus CF. Comparison of body composition and periodontal disease using nutritional assessment techniques: Third National Health and Nutrition Examination Survey (NHANES III). J Clin Periodontol 2003; 30(4):321–327.
47. Ryan ME, Carnu O, Kamer AR. The influence of diabetes on the periodontal tissues. J Am Dent Assoc 2003; 134:34S–40S.
48. Persson RE, Hollender LG, MacEntee MI, Wyatt CC, Kiyak HA, Persson GR. Assessment of periodontal conditions and systemic disease in older subjects. J Clin Periodontol 2003; 30(3):207–213.
49. Tsai C, Hayes C, Taylor GW. Glycemic control of type 2 diabetes and severe periodontal disease in the U.S. adult population. Community Dent Oral Epidemiol 2002; 30(3):182–192.
50. Tervonen T, Oliver RC. Long-term control of diabetes mellitus and periodontitis. J Clin Periodontol 1993; 20(6):431–435.
51. Thorstensson H, Hugoson A. Periodontal disease experience in adult long-duration insulin-dependent diabetics. J Clin Periodontol 1993; 20(5):352–358.
52. Armitage GC. Periodontal infections and cardiovascular disease: how strong is the association? Oral Dis 2000; 6(6):335–350.
53. Genco RJ, Trevisan M, Wu T, Beck JD. Periodontal disease and risk of coronary heart disease. JAMA 2001 ; 285(1):40–41.
54. Madianos PN, Bobetsis GA, Kinane DF. Is periodontitis associated with an increased risk of coronary heart disease and preterm and/or low birth weight births? J Clin Periodontol 2002; 29(Suppl. 3):22–36; discussion 37–38.
55. Taylor GW. The effects of periodontal treatment on diabetes. J Am Dent Assn 2003; 134(Suppl.): 41S–48S.
56. American Academy Periodontology position paper 1998. Available at (Website: http://www.perio.org/resources-products/posppr2.html).
57. Stamler J, Stamler R, Neaton JD, et al. Low risk-factor profile and long-term cardiovascular and noncardiovascular mortality and life expectancy: findings for 5 large cohorts of young adult and middle-aged men and women. JAMA 1999; 282(21):2012–2018.

58. Mendall MA, Patel P, Asante M, et al. Relation of serum cytokine concentrations to cardiovascular risk factors and coronary heart disease. Heart 1997; 78(3):273–277.

59. Ridker PM, Rifai N, Pfeffer M, Sacks F, Lepage S, Braunwald E. Elevation of tumor necrosis factor-alpha and increased risk of recurrent coronary events after myocardial infarction. Circulation 2000; 101(18):2149–2153.

60. Ridker PM, Rifai N, Stampfer MJ, Hennekens CH. Plasma concentration of interleukin-6 and the risk of future myocardial infarction among apparently healthy men. Circulation 2000; 101(15): 1767–1772.

61. Ridker PM, Cushman M, Stampfer MJ, Tracy RP, Hennekens CH. Inflammation, aspirin, and the risk of cardiovascular disease in apparently healthy men. N Engl J Med 1997; 336(14):973–979.

62. Sakkinen P, Abbott RD, Curb JD, Rodriguez BL, Yano K, Tracy RP. C-reactive protein and myocardial infarction. J Clin Epidemiol 2002; 55(5):445–451.

63. Maresca G, Di Blasio A, Marchioli R, Di Minno G. Measuring plasma fibrinogen to predict stroke and myocardial infarction: an update. Arterioscler Thromb Vasc Biol 1999; 19(6):1368–1377.

64. Ridker PM. Novel risk factors and markers for coronary disease. Adv Intern Med 2000; 45:391–418.

65. Albert MA, Staggers J, Chew P, Ridker PM. The pravastatin inflammation CRP evaluation (PRINCE): rationale and design. Am Heart J 2001; 141(6):893–898.

66. Jialal I, Devaraj S. Inflammation and atherosclerosis: the value of the high-sensitivity C-reactive protein assay as a risk marker. Am J Clin Pathol 2001; 116(Suppl.):S108–S115.

67. van der Wal AC, Becker AE, van der Loos CM, Das PK. Site of intimal rupture or erosion of thrombosed coronary atherosclerotic plaques is characterized by an inflammatory process irrespective of the dominant plaque morphology. Circulation 1994; 89(1):36–44.

68. Pussinen PJ, Jousilahti P, Alfthan G, Palosuo T, Asikainen S, Salomaa V. Antibodies to periodontal pathogens are associated with coronary heart disease. Arterioscler Thromb Vasc Biol 2003; 23(7): 1250–1254.

69. Rahmati MA, Craig RG, Homel P, Kaysen GA, Levin NW. Serum markers of periodontal disease status and inflammation in hemodialysis patients. Am J Kidney Dis 2002; 40(5):983–989.

70. Chambless LE, Heiss G, Folsom AR, et al. Association of coronary heart disease incidence with carotid arterial wall thickness and major risk factors: the Atherosclerosis Risk in Communities (ARIC) Study, 1987–1993. Am J Epidemiol 1997; 146(6):483–494.

71. Beck JD, Elter JR, Heiss G, Couper D, Mauriello SM, Offenbacher S. Relationship of periodontal disease to carotid artery intima-media wall thickness: the atherosclerosis risk in communities (ARIC) study. Arterioscler Thromb Vasc Biol 2001; 21(11):1816–1822.

72. Craig RG, Yip JK, So MK, Boylan RJ, Socransky SS, Haffajee AD. Relationship of destructive periodontal disease to the acute-phase response. J Periodontol 2003; 74(7):1007–1016.

73. Ebersole JL, Machen RL, Steffen MJ, Willmann DE. Systemic acute-phase reactants, C-reactive protein and haptoglobin, in adult periodontitis. Clin Exp Immunol 1997; 107(2):347–352.

74. Noack B, Genco RJ, Trevisan M, Grossi S, Zambon JJ, De Nardin E. Periodontal infections contribute to elevated systemic C-reactive protein level. J Periodontol 2001; 72(9):1221–1227.

75. Slade GD, Offenbacher S, Beck JD, Heiss G, Pankow JS. Acute-phase inflammatory response to periodontal disease in the U.S. population. J Dent Res 2000; 79(1):49–57.

76. Wu T, Trevisan M, Genco RJ, Falkner KL, Dorn JP, Sempos CT. Examination of the relation between periodontal health status and cardiovascular risk factors: serum total and high density lipoprotein cholesterol, C-reactive protein, and plasma fibrinogen. Am J Epidemiol 2000; 151(3):273–282.

77. Slade GD, Ghezzi EM, Heiss G, Beck JD, Riche E, Offenbacher S. Relationship between periodontal disease and C-reactive protein among adults in the Atherosclerosis Risk in Communities study. Arch Intern Med 2003; 163(10):1172–1179.

78. Ide M, McPartlin D, Coward PY, Crook M, Lumb P, Wilson RF. Effect of treatment of chronic periodontitis on levels of serum markers of acute-phase inflammatory and vascular responses. J Clin Periodontol 2003; 30(4):334–340.

79. Arbes SJ Jr, Slade GD, Beck JD. Association between extent of periodontal attachment loss and self-reported history of heart attack: an analysis of NHANES III data. J Dent Res 1999; 78(12):1777–1782.

80. Beck J, Garcia R, Heiss G, Vokonas PS, Offenbacher S. Periodontal disease and cardiovascular disease. J Periodontol 1996; 67(10 Suppl.):1123–1137.

81. Hujoel PP, Drangsholt M, Spiekerman C, Derouen TA. Peridontal disease and coronary heart disease risk. JAMA 2002; 284:1406–1410.
82. Joshipura KJ, Rimm EB, Douglass CW, Trichopoulos D, Ascherio A, Willett WC. Poor oral health and coronary heart disease. J Dent Res 1996; 75(9):1631–1636.
83. Tuominen R, Reunanen A, Paunio M, Paunio I, Aromaa A. Oral health indicators poorly predict coronary heart disease deaths. J Dent Res 2003; 82(9):713–718.
84. Janket SJ, Baird AE, Chuang SK, Jones JA. Meta-analysis of periodontal disease and risk of coronary heart disease and stroke. Oral Surg Oral Med Oral Pathol Oral Radiol Endod 2003; 95(5):559–569.
85. DeStefano F, Anda RF, Kahn HS, Williamson DF, Russell CM. Dental disease and risk of coronary heart disease and mortality. Br Med J 1993; 306(6879):688–691.
86. Joshipura K, Ritchie C, Douglass C. Strength of evidence linking oral conditions and systemic disease. Compend Contin Educ Dent 2000; 21(Suppl.):12–23.
87. National Center for Health Statistics, 1998. Available at (Website: http://www.modimes.org. healthlibrary2/infanthealthstatistics/aveday2001.htm).
88. March of Dimes Perinatal Data Center. Final natality data, July 2000. Available at (Website: http://www.modimes.org.healthlibrary2/infanthaelthstatistics/preterm.htm).
89. Jeffcoat M, Geurs N, Reddy M, Glodenberg R, Hauth J. Current evidence regarding periodontal disease as a risk factor in preterm birth. Ann Periodontol 2001; 6:183–188.
90. Romero B, Chiquito C, Elejalde L, Bernardoni C. Relationship between periodontal disease in pregnant women and the nutritional condition of their newborns. J Periodontol 2002; 73:1177–1183.
91. Dasanayake A, Boyd D, Madianos P, Offenbacher S, Hills E. The association between *Porphyromonas gingivalis*-specific maternal serum IgG and low birth weight. J Periodontol 2001; 72(11):1491–1497.
92. Dasanayake A. Poor periodontal health of the pregnant woman as a risk factor for low birth weight. Ann Periodonal 1998; 3:206–212.
93. Hay PE, Lamont RF, Taylor-Robinson D, Morgan DJ, Ison C, Pearson J. Abnormal bacterial colonization of the genital tract and subsequent preterm delivery and late miscarriage. Br Med J 1994; 308:295–298.
94. Kempe A, Wishe B, Arkan SE, et al. Clinical determinants of racial disparity in very low birth weight. N Engl J Med 1992; 327:969–973.
95. Socransky SS, Haffajee AD. The bacterial etiology of destructive periodontal disease: current concepts. J Periodontol 1992; 63:322–331.
96. Zambon JJ. Periodontal diseases: microbial factors. 1996; 1:879–925.
97. Dixon NG, Ebright D, Defrancesco MA, Hawkins RE. Orogential contact: a cause of chorioamnionitis? Obstet Gynecol 1994; 84:654–655.
98. Wallace RJ. Capnocytophaga on the fetal surface of the placenta of a patient with ruptured membranes at 39 weeks gestation. Am J Obstet Gynecol 1986; 155:228–229.
99. Mercer LJ. Capnocytophaga isolated from the endometrium as a cause of neonatal sepsis: a case report. J Reprod Med 1985; 30:67–68.
100. Offenbacher S, Jared HL, O'Rielly PG, et al. Potential pathogenic mechanisms of periodontitis-associated pregnancy complications. Ann Periodontol 1998; 3:233–250.
101. Lopez N, Smith P, Gutierrez. Periodontal therapy may reduce the risk of preterm low birth weight in women with periodontal disease: a randomized controlled trial. J Periodontol 2002;73:911–924
102. Offenbacher S, Katz V, Fertik G et al. Periodontal infection as a possible risk factor for preterm low birth weight. J Periodontol 1996;67(Suppl.):1103–1113
103. Ettinger RL. Epidemiology of dental caries. Dent Clin N Amer 1999;43(4)679–694
104. Kaste LM, Selwitz RH, Oldakowski RJ, Brunelle JA, Winn DM, Brown LJ. Coronal caries in the primary and permanent dentition of children and adolescents 1–17 years of age. J Dent Res 1996;75:631–641
105. US Department of Health and Human Services. US Public Health Service. Oral health in America: a report of the surgeon general. Rockville, MD: National Institutes of Health, 2000.
106. Featherstone J. The science and practice of caries prevention. J Am Dent Assoc 2000; 131:887–899.
107. Steele JG, Sheiham A, Marcenas W, Fay N, Walls AW. Clinical and behavioral risk indicators for root caries in older people. Gerodontolgy 2001; 18(2):95–101.
108. Ship JA, Pillemer SR, Baum BJ. Xerostomia and the geriatric patient. J Amer Geriatr Soc 2002; 50(3):535–543.

109. Unell L, Soderfeldt B, Halling A, Birkhed D. Explanatory models for clinically determined and symp-tom-related caries indicators in an adult population. Acta Odontol Scand 1999; 57:132–138.
110. Guggenheimer J, Moore PA. Xerostomia: etiology, recognition, and treatment. J Am Dent Assoc 2003; 134:61–69.
111. Tenovuo J. Salivary parameters of relevance for assessing caries activity in individuals and populations. Community Dent Oral Epidemiol. 1997; 25(1):82–86.
112. Narhi TO, Meurman JH, Ainamo A. Xerostomia and hyposalivation: causes, consequences and treat-ment in the elderly. Drugs Aging 1999; 15:103–116.
113. D'Hondt E, Eisbruch A, Ship J. The influence of pre-radiation salivary flow rates and radiation dose on parotid salivary gland dysfunction in patients receiving radiotherapy for head and neck cancer. Spec Care Dent 1998; 18:102–108.
114. Miller CS, Epstein JB, Hall EH, Sirois DA. Changing oral care needs in the United States: the continuing need for oral medicine. Oral Surg Oral Med Oral Path Radiol Endo 2001; 91(1):34–44.
115. Knapp MJ. Oral disease in 181,338 consecutive oral examinations. J Am Dent Assoc 1971; 83:1288–1293.
116. Ross NM, Gross E. Oral findings based on an automated multiphasic health screening program. Bib-liographic links. J Oral Med 1971; 26:21–26.
117. Axell T. A prevalence study of oral mucosal lesions in an adult Swedish population. Odontol Rev 1976; 27:1–103.
118. National Health and Nutrition Examination Survey (NHANES I). Dental, ages 1–74 years (tape no. 4235). Hyattsville, MD: U.S. Dept of Health and Human Services, Public Health Service, Centers for Disease Control, National Center for Health Statistics, 1979.
119. Bouquot JE, Gundlach KK. Oral exophytic lesions in 23,616 white Americans over 35 years of age. Oral Surg Oral Med Oral Pathol 1986; 62:284–291.
120. Bouquot JE, Gorlin RJ. Leukoplakia, lichen planus, and other oral keratoses in 23,616 white Americans over the age of 35 years. Bibliographic links. Oral Surg Oral Med Oral Pathol 1986; 61:373–381.
121. Hand JS, Whitehill JM. The prevalence of oral mucosal lesions in an elderly population. J Am Dent Assoc 1986; 112:73–76.
122. Kleinman DV, Swango PA, Niessen LC. Epidemiologic studies of oral mucosal conditions: methodologic issues. Community Dent Oral Epidemiol 1991; 19:129–140.
123. Sciubba JJ, for the U.S. collaborative Oral CDX study group. Improving detection of precancerous and cancerous oral lesions. J Am Dent Assoc 1999; 130:1445–1457.
124. Millard HD, Mason DK, eds. World Workshop in Oral Medicine. Chicago, IL: Year Book Medical Publishers, 1989.
125. Lipton JA, Ship JA, Larach-Robinson D. Estimated prevalence and distribution of reported orofacial pain in the United States. J Am Dent Assoc 1993; 124:115–121.
126. Riley JL, Gilbert GH, Heft MW. Health care utilization by older adults in response to painful orofacial symptoms. Pain 1999; 81:67–75.
127. Ben Aryeh H, Gottlieb I, Ish-Shalom S, Szargel H, Laufer D. Oral complaints related to menopause. Maturitas 1996; 24:185–189.
128. Adams PF, Marano MA. National Health Interview Survey 1994. National Center for Health Statistics, Vital Health Statistics Series 10. Hyattsville, MD: U.S. Department of Health and Human Services, 1994.
129. Tammiala-Salonen T, Hiidenkari T, Parvinen T. Burning mouth in a Finnish adult population. Commu-nity Dent Oral Epidemiol 1993; 21:67–71.
130. Smithard DG, O'Neill PA, Park C, et al. Complications and outcome after acute stroke: does dysphagia matter? Stroke 1996; 27(7):1200–1204.
131. Elmstahl S, Bulow M, Ekberg O, Petersson M, Tegner H. Treatment of dysphagia improves nutritional conditions in stroke patients. Dysphagia 1999; 14:61–66.
132. Perry L, Love CP. Screening for dysphagia and aspiration in acute stroke: a systematic review. Dysph-agia. 2001; 16:7–18.
133. Smithard DG, O'Neill PA, Park C, et al. Complications and outcome after acute stroke: does dysphagia matter? Stroke 1996: 27(7):1200–1204.
134. Elmstahl S, Bulow M, Ekberg O, Petersson M, Tegner, H. Treatment of dysphagia improves nutritional conditions in stroke patients. Dysphagia 1999; 14:61–66.

135. Odderson IR, Keaton JC, McKenna BS. Swallow management in patients on an acute stroke pathway: quality is cost effective. Arch Phys Med Rehab 1995; 76:1130–1133.
136. Hammond CAS, Goldstein LB, Zajac DJ, Gray L, Davenport PW, Bolser DC. Assessment of aspiration risk in stroke patients with quantification of voluntary cough. Neurology 2001; 56:502–506.
137. Daniels SK, Ballo LA, Mahoney MC, Foundas AL. Clinical predictors of dysphagia and aspiration risk: outcome measures in acute stroke patients. Arch Phys Med Rehab 2000; 81:1030–1033.
138. Bending A. Meeting the challenges of managing dysphagia. Community Nurse 2001; 7(1):13–16.
139. Hinds NP, Wiles CM. Assessment of swallowing and referral to speech and language therapists in acute stroke. Q J Med 1998; 919(12):829–835.
140. Brody RA, Touger-Decker R, VonHagen S, O'Sullivan Maillet J. Role of registered dietitians in dysphagia screening. J Am Diet Assoc 2000; 100(9):1029–1037.
141. Wood P, Emick-Herring B. Dysphagia: a screening tool for stroke patients. J Neurosci Nurs 1997; 29(5): 325–329.
142. Perry L. Screening swallowing function of patients with acute stroke. 1. Identification, implementation, and initial evaluation of a screening tool for use by nurses. J Clin Nurs 2001; 10:463–473.
143. Perry L. Screening swallowing function of patients with acute stroke. 2. Detailed evaluation of the tool used by nurses. J Clin Nur 2001; 10:474–481.
144. Doggett DL, Tappe KA, Mitchell MD, Chapell D, Coates V, Turkelson CM. Prevention of pneumonia in elderly stroke patients by systematic diagnosis and treatment of dysphagia: an evidence-based comprehensive analysis of literature. Dysphagia 2001; 16:279–295.
145. DePippo KL, Holas MA, Reding MJ. The Burke Dysphagia Screening Test: validation of its use in patients with stroke. Arch Phys Med Rehab 1994; 75:1284–1286.
146. DePippo KL, Holas MA, Reding MJ. Validation of the 3-oz water swallow test for aspiration following stroke. Arch Neurol 1992; 49:1259–1261.
147. Davies S. Dysphagia in acute strokes. Nursing Standard 1999; 13(30):49–54.
148. Ellul J, Barer D. Intraobserver reliability of a standardized bedside swallowing assessment. Cerebrovasc Dis 1996; 6(Suppl. 2):152–153.
149. Davies S. Dysphagia in acute strokes. Nursing Standard 1999; 13(30):49–54.
150. Dorner B. Tough to swallow. Today's Dietitian 2002; 8:28–31.
151. Negus E. Stroke induced dysphagia in the hospital: the nutritional perspective. Br J Nur 1994; 3(6): 263–268.
152. Shaw C, Power J. Nutritional management of patients with dysphagia. Brit J Community Nurs 1999; 4(7):338–343.
153. Groher ME. Dysphagia: Diagnosis and Management. Boston, MA: Butterworth-Heinemann, 1997.
154. Kidd D, MacMahon J, Lawson J, Nesbitt R. The natural history and clinical consequences of aspiration in acute stroke. Q J Med 1995; 88(6):409–413.
155. National Dysphagia Diet Task Force. National Dysphagia Diet: Standardization for Optimal Care. Chicago, IL: American Dietetic Association, 2002.

6

Impacts and Interrelationships Between Medications, Nutrition, Diet, and Oral Health

Miriam R. Robbins

1. INTRODUCTION

Long-term medication therapy is common, allowing increasing numbers of people to control chronic illnesses and achieve improved quality of life. However, use of medications is rarely without side effect or risk, making prevention and management of medication complications more challenging. As patients with chronic illness age, it is more common to encounter multiple medications directed at multiple organ systems, compounding the challenge of managing the adverse effects of, and interactions among, multiple medications. Drug–nutrient interactions and nutritional deficiencies are a potential primary problem with many medications, which can also lead to secondary oral health complications. Likewise, medications can affect primarily the oral environment and have secondary nutritional and diet consequences. This chapter reviews common drug-induced nutrient deficits and their mechanisms, drug-induced adverse oral conditions, and selected interrelationships between medications and nutritional and oral health.

2. DRUGS AND NUTRITIONAL STATUS

Drug-induced nutritional deficiencies may develop through various mechanisms, occurring through different physiologic pathways. Drugs can interfere with synthesis of nutrients and alter the ability to transport, store, or metabolize nutrients. Nutrient depletion can result either by preventing nutrient absorption, enhancing nutrient elimination, or both. Drugs, even in therapeutic doses, can interfere with nutrient utilization, especially when the intake of nutrients is less than the demand or when nutrient stores are depleted *(1)*. Vitamin and mineral deficiencies can result from poor nutrient absorption caused by binding of nutrients to drugs, increased excretion, or impaired utilization. The inhibition of gastrointestinal (GI) absorption of vitamins by cholestyramine; the enhancement of potassium, magnesium, and zinc excretion by thiazide diuretics; and the acceleration of vitamin D metabolism and calcium depletion by anticonvulsants such as phenytoin and phenobarbital are well-documented examples *(2)*.

From: *Nutrition and Oral Medicine*
Edited by: R. Touger-Decker, D. A. Sirois, and C. C. Mobley © Humana Press Inc., Totowa, NJ

Drugs can produce damage to the exocrine pancreas, causing decreased production or release of pancreatic enzymes, which leads to decreased digestion of fat, protein, and starch. Some drugs decrease the absorption of macronutrients including sugars, fats, amino acids, vitamins, and minerals, causing nutritional deficiencies depending on the relative absorptive capacity of the small intestine *(3)*. Drugs can additionally have a direct depressant or stimulating effect on appetite and food intake.

Nutritional deficiencies and drug–nutrient reactions are more likely to occur among elderly patients taking multiple drugs for chronic illness who may also have other risks (economic, masticatory efficiency, access) for inadequate nutritional intake. Commonly prescribed drugs for chronic illness that disproportionately affect the elderly and can lead to significant health problems such as megaloblastic and iron-deficiency anemia, hyperkalemia, hyper- or hypocalcemia, osteomalacia, and osteoporosis, hip fractures, decreased wound healing, organic brain disease, and peripheral neuropathies include analgesics, anti-inflammatories, anticonvulsants, antidepressants and other psychotropics, antihypertensives, GI protectors, and hormone replacement therapy *(4)*. Drug-induced oral lesions, also prevalent among the elderly, can be a direct adverse effect of a drug or a result of drug-induced vitamin deficiencies *(5)*. Painful oral lesions can further impair the patient's ability to maintain adequate nutritional intake.

3. EFFECTS OF DRUGS ON NUTRIENT ABSORPTION AND METABOLISM

Most drugs taken orally are absorbed by the small intestine via transport across the mucosal membrane into the bloodstream. Once absorbed, the drug can be distributed in fat, muscle, or water, or bound to proteins, metabolized, and used by the body. Once metabolized, the drug is usually inactivated by the liver, which turns it into a form that can be readily eliminated by the kidneys. Chronic diseases or drug-induced cellular damage of intestinal mucosa can reduce drug absorption by damaging the transporters that carry drugs or nutrients into the bloodstream or interfering with the structural integrity of the villi. Decreased liver function can slow drug metabolism, especially in older adults, allowing more of the active form of a drug to be available for longer periods of time. A decline in renal function, especially caused by chronic diseases such as diabetes, can significantly decrease elimination of drugs *(6)*. Decreased absorption, increased elimination, or altered metabolism of drugs can contribute to drug-induced nutritional deficiencies, mostly in the form of vitamin or mineral deficiencies. Table 1 summarizes drugs that can result in nutritional deficits, and Table 2 summarizes foods that can alter drug absorption.

Primary malabsorption occurs when drugs depress uptake of nutrients from the small intestine without interfering with metabolism. Drugs can alter nutrient absorption in many ways: blocking transport systems, changing the pH of the stomach, inactivating intestinal enzymes, removing bile salts from the sites of absorption of fat-soluble vitamins, or reducing bacterial flora. Commonly used drugs that cause malabsorption include antacids, laxatives, tetracycline, neomycin, colchicine, and cholestyramine (used to lower serum cholesterol) *(7)*. Abuse of antacids can lead to phosphate depletion and osteomalacia (vitamin D deficiency). Antacids also affect the absorption of riboflavin (B_2), copper, and iron. Tetracycline reduces calcium absorption by binding to calcium and forming an insoluble complex that is excreted. Bile acid sequestrants' cholesterol-lowering agents can cause alterations in the absorption of B_{12}, folic acid, iron, and the fat-soluble vitamins. Chronic use of medications that decrease the gastric acid can cause B_{12} deficiency because an acidic pH is necessary to free B_{12} from its protein-bound state and be available to react with intrinsic factor. Iron also requires acidic gastric conditions for optimal absorption, and deficiency can result from reduced gastric acid production. Drugs, such as metoclopramide, that increase gastric emptying, can cause rapid emptying of food into the small intestine, which results in reduced nutrients absorption from inadequate time for gastric digestion or saturation of absorption systems. Mineral oil and overuse of laxatives can lead to fat-soluble vitamin deficiencies by increasing the rate of intestinal motility, speeding transit time, and decreasing the amount of time available for nutrient absorption (8). Increased intestinal motility can also result in inadequate time for potassium reabsorbtion by the large intestine and can lead to hypokalemia and abnormal heart rhythms.

Secondary malabsorption is caused by the interference of a drug with the absorption or metabolism of another nutrient (9). The primary example are drugs that alter the metabolism of vitamin D, which is responsible for stimulating calcium and phosphorus absorption to levels that support normal bone mineralization (1). Vitamin D deficiency leads to inadequate calcium absorption, decreased calcium plasma levels, and reabsorption of calcium to maintain plasma levels (10). Glucocorticosteroids can cause a lowered production of a biologically active vitamin D metabolite, which leads to a consequent decrease in calcium absorption. They also have a direct action on bone mineralization by causing mobilization of calcium from the skeleton (1). Demineralization and fractures can result in steroid-induced osteopenia and osteoporosis with prolonged use (11), especially in postmenopausal women. Vitamin D deficiency in patients on chronic anticonvulsant drugs such as phenobarbital and phenytoin is caused by acceleration at the site of hepatic conversion of the vitamin and its active metabolite (25-hydroxycholecalciferol) to an inactive form, causing decreased serum calcium levels. Osteomalacia may occur within months of the initiation of anticonvulsant therapy, especially in patients with inadequate calcium intakes (12). In both cases, supplemental calcium with vitamin D should be provided routinely to avoid such risks.

Once absorbed, a nutrient is usually metabolized through enzyme pathways, providing another opportunity for drugs to interact and affect nutrient metabolism. Drugs can function as antivitamins by combining with or inhibiting enzyme systems required for the conversion of vitamins to their coenzyme or active form (1). Often, this interference with the body's utilization of a specific nutrient is the desired therapeutic outcome. Folate is necessary for cells and tissues that rapidly divide, such as cancer cells. Methotrexate, by binding to dihydrofolate reductase enzyme, prevents the conversion of folic acid (from dihydrofolate) to its biologically active form (tetrahydrofolate) and inhibits the growth of these cells. Coumarin anticoagulants function as antagonists to vitamin K activity by causing the retention of the inactive form of vitamin K, thereby inhibiting the coagulation process (1). With some drugs, the effect on nutrient metabolism is recognized as an avoidable side effect. Isoniazid and L-dopa both inhibit the normal metabolism of vitamin B_6, often causing neuropathies that can be reversed with supplements. Anticonvulsants, especially phenytoin and phenobarbital, not only cause vitamin D and K deficiency, but with prolonged use also cause folic acid deficiency (9) by inducing the liver enzymes that metabolize these vitamins.

Table 1
Drugs That Can Result in Nutrient Deficits

Drug	Examples	Nutrient Deficit	Possible Clinical Signs
Alcohol		Folic acid, thiamine, vit. C, niacin, vit. B_2, vit. B_6, vit. B_{12}, Mg, zinc	Peripheral neuropathy, angular stomatitis, cheilitis, glossitis
Analgesics	Salicylates	Folate, vit. C	Anemia
Antacids	Aluminum hydroxide, sodium bicarbonate	Folic acid, Ca, Mg, Cu, Fe, phosphate, Zn, K	Osteomalacia
Antibacterial agents	General	All B vitamins, vit. C, and K	
	Trimethoprim	Folic acid	Anemia, glossitis, cheilitis
	Sulfa	Folic acid	Anemia, glossitis, cheilitis
	Tetracyclines	Vit. B_6, vit. B_{12}, Ca, Mg, Zn	Peripheral neuropathy, angular stomatitis, cheilitis, glossitis
	Aminoglycosides (Neomycin)	Vit. B_{12}, vit. A, vit. K; Ca, Fe, Mg, K^+	
Anticoagulants	Coumadin	Vit. K	Hemorrhage
Anticonvulsants	Phenobarbital, phenytoin, primidone	Folic acid, vit. B_{12}, vit. D, Ca	Osteomalacia
	Carbamazepine, Tegretol	Folic acid	Megaloblastic anemia, glossitis, cheilitis
Oral hypoglycemic agents	Sulfonylureas	Thiamine	Megaloblastic anemia
	Biguanides (metformin)	Vit. B_{12}	
Anti-inflammatory agents	Corticosteroids	Vit. D, Ca, Zn, K	Osteopenia, osteoporosis
	Prednisone	Ca	Osteopenia
	Gout medication (colchicine)	Vit. K, vit. B_{12}, vit. A, K, Na	
	Sulfasalazine	Folic acid	Anemia, glossitis, cheilitis
	Aspirin	Folic acid, vit. C, Fe, protein	Anemia, glossitis, cheilitis
	NSAIDs	Folic acid	Anemia, glossitis, cheilitis
Anti-Parkinson drugs	L-Dopa	Vit. B_6	Peripheral neuropathy, angular stomatitis, cheilitis, glossitis

Drug category	Drug	Nutrients affected	Effects
Antiretroviral agents	AZT, Retrovir, Ribavirn, Zidovudine	Cu, Zn	
Antituberculosis drugs	Isoniazid	Vit. B_6, vit. D, vit. E, Ca, Niacin	Pellagra, peripheral neuropathy, angular stomatitis, cheilitis, glossitis
	Para-amino salicylic acid	Folic acid, vit. B_{12}	Megaloblastic anemia
Antiulcer agents	H_2 receptor antagonists, cimetidine, ranitidine	Folic acid, vit. B_{12}, vit. D, Ca, Fe, Zn	Pernicious anemia, neuropathy, dsypnea, redness and burning of the tongue
	Proton pump inhibitors	Vit. B_{12}	Pernicious anemia, neuropathy, redness and burning of the tongue
Cardiovascular agent	Cardiac glycosides	Ca, Mg	Pernicious anemia, neuropathy, redness and burning of the tongue
	Potassium chloride	Vit. B_{12}	
Dihydrofolate reductase inhibitors	Methotrexate	Folic acid	
Diuretics/antihypertensives	Thiazides	Mg, Zn, K, Na	
	Potassium-sparing	Folic acid, Ca	Megaloblastic anemia, anorexia, glossitis, cheilitis
	Loop diuretics	Vit. B_1, vit. B_6, Mg, Zn, K	Peripheral neuropathy, angular stomatitis, cheilitis, glossitis
	Hydralazines	Vit. B_6, Mg	Peripheral neuropathy, angular cheilitis
	Triamterene	Folic acid	
Female hormones	Oral contraceptives	Vit. B_2, vit. B_6, vit. B_{12}, folic acid, vit. C, Mg, Zn	Peripheral neuropathy, angular stomatitis, cheilitis, glossitis
Hypocholesterolemic agents	HMG-CoA reductases	Folic acid	Anemia, glossitis, cheilitis
	Bile sequestrants	Folic acid, vit. B_{12}, vit. A, vit. D, vit. E, Fe, fat	Anemia, glossitis, cheilitis
Laxatives	Mineral oil	Vit. A, vit. D, vit. E, vit. K	Osteomalacia
	Phenolphthalein	Vit. D, K, Ca,	
Tranquilizers	Chlorpromazine	Vit. B_{12}	Anemia, glossitis, cheilitis

Table 2
Food-Altering Drug Absorption

Decreased

Acetaminophen	Doxycycline	Penicillin G and V
Alcohol	Erythromycin	Rifampin
Ampicillin	Erythromycin stearate	Sulfadiazine sodium
Aspirin	Hydrochlorothiazide	Tetracycline
Atenolol	Isoniazide	Theophylline
Captopril	Levodopa	Tolbutamide
Ciprofloxacin	Metronidazole	

Delayed

Acetaminophen	Digoxin	Nifedipine
Amoxicillin	Furosemide	Quinidine
Aspirin	Glipizide	Potassium ion
Cefaclor	Indoprofen	Sulfadiazine
Cephalexin	Indomethacin	Sufadimethoxine
Cephradine	Ketoprofen	Sulfanilamide
Cimetidine	Midazolam	Valproic acid
Diclofenac		

Increased

Chlorothiazide	Hydrazaline	Nitofurantoin
Diazepam	Labetalol	Propanolol
Erythromycin ethylsuccinate	Lithium	Riboflavin
Griseofulvin	Metoprolol	Spirolactone

Adapted from refs. *1* and *4*.

Alcohol affects nutrient metabolism primarily through its affect on the liver and other organs. Alcohol-induced abnormal pancreatic function leads to changes in vitamin absorption and utilization. Alcohol interferes with thiamine metabolism, resulting in deficiency that in its extreme form can cause Wernicke-Korsakoff syndrome, a chronic degenerative neurologic disorder. Alcoholics also can develop peripheral neuropathies secondary to thiamine and vitamin B_6 deficiency and pellagra, secondary to niacin deficiency *(13)*. Folate deficiency is also frequent in chronic alcoholics because of interference with absorption, storage, and conversion to its active form, as well as altered vitamin A metabolism.

Vitamins and minerals are necessary for a number of metabolic functions. Requirements vary with life stage (*see* Chapter 1). Some vitamins act as coenzymes for biochemical reactions, while others function as hormones. The family of B vitamins is composed of coenzymes and precursors of coenzymes that are essential for a large number of metabolic reactions. Therefore, inadequate intake of one often impairs utilization of others. For example, thiamine (vitamin B_1), riboflavin (vitamin B_2), niacin (vitamin B_3), biotin, and pantothenic acid are involved with energy-release mechanisms, including glycolysis and the tricarboxylic acid cycle. Thiamine pyrophosphate, the active form of thiamine (vitamin B_1) is the cofactor of an enzyme that catalyses the oxydative decarboxylation of pyruvate to acetyl coenzyme A for the Krebs cycle. Riboflavin (vitamin B_2) and niacin (vitamin B_3) are required for oxidoreduction reactions associated with the release of energy from carbohydrate, protein, or fat metabolism. Pyridoxine (vitamin B_6) is a coenzyme for reactions of protein metabolism, glycogen release from the liver and muscles, and the synthesis of the neurotransmitter γ-aminobutyric acid (GABA). Pantothenic acid and biotin are particularly important in fatty-acid synthesis and glucogenisis. Vitamin A is an essential hormone for maintaining the structural and functional integrity of the epithelial membranes. Vitamin K is necessary for the synthesis of blood-clotting factors II, VII, IX, and X by acting as a cofactor of the carboxylase that forms γ-carboxyglutamate in the precursor proteins of those clotting factors. Vitamin D is a steroid hormone that in its biologically active form, 1,25-dihydroxy vitamin D_3 [1,25-$(OH)_2D_3$, or calcitriol], functions primarily to regulate calcium and phosphorous homeostasis. Most vitamins cannot be synthesized in the body and must be absorbed from food sources, either in an active form or as precursors that are then transformed into active entities. Vitamin K, biotin, and small amounts of vitamin B_{12} are produced by intestinal tract flora; folate needs to be activated by intestinal enzymes. Vitamin D is synthesized from a precursor in the skin by sunlight and is found in enriched milk and cereal products.

Based on their solubility characteristics, vitamins are classified as fat or water soluble. The fat-soluble vitamins include A, D, E, and K, which circulate with lipoproteins in the blood before reaching their target tissues. Excess amounts of these vitamins can be stored in fat tissue and utilized when needed, compensating for short-term intake deficits. Since fat-soluble vitamins are readily absorbed and stored, doses in excess of the dietary reference intake (DRI) should be avoided because of the risk of toxicities, particularly with vitamin A. An exception may be vitamin E, which, when taken in large doses, has pharmacologic properties as an antioxidant. The B vitamins (B_1, B_2, B_6, B_{12}, niacin, panthothenic acid, biotin, and folic acid) and vitamin C are water soluble and are absorbed directly into the bloodstream. Frequent consumption of these vitamins is necessary to maintain necessary tissue levels because there is limited storage, and excesses are quickly eliminated by the kidneys. Trace elements and minerals, such as calcium and magnesium, are needed in large quantities by the body as essential building blocks, while iron, zinc, copper, iodine, and a number of other trace elements have limited but essential functions (14) and are needed in much smaller amounts.

Whether drug-induced nutritional deficits translate into frank nutrient deficiencies depends on several factors, including the overall nutrition status of the individual. Inadequate diet and subsequent low store of nutrients can increase the chance of nutritional drug depletion, causing clinical symptoms of nutrient deficits. For example, nursing-home patients on anticonvulsants who get little exposure to sunlight and marginal dietary intake of vitamin D have a higher incidence of developing osteomalacia and osteoporosis (15). The length of time that a drug is taken also has significant impact on depletion of nutrients. The incidence of vitamin D deficiency in patients on anticonvulsants increases the longer the drug is taken (15). Multiple drug regimens also may increase the risk of nutritional deficiency if the drugs affect the same absorption or metabolic pathway. Individuals with tuberculosis and concurrent malnutrition taking isoniazid and para-amino salicylic acid can develop B_6, B_{12}, and folic acid deficiency and subsequently develop pellagra (niacin deficiency) because B_6 is needed to convert tryptophan to niacin. Increased body fat, decreased muscle mass, or dehydration can also effect the distribution of lipophilic (such as benzodiazapines, digitoxin, and synthetic steroids [16]) or hydrophilic (as warfarin, procainamide, atenolol, quinidine, propanolol, theophylline, digoxin, and cimetidine *[17]*) drugs, causing increased drug concentrations that can lead to displacement of nutrients from plasma proteins or tissue-binding sites. This can lead to increased excretion of the affected nutrient, either free or in drug–nutrient complexes.

Drugs used to treat chronic diseases can also lead to increased nutrient requirements. For example, select drugs such as sulfasalzine (Azulfadine), INH, and methotrexate contribute to folic acid deficiencies in patients with inflammatory bowel disease, tuberculosis, and rheumatoid arthritis *(8)*. Individuals with end-stage renal disease may develop deficiencies in riboflavin, vitamin C, and folic acid if they are not given supplemental doses of these nutrients because of the nature of the disease and use of diuretics and dialysis. Patients with chronic renal disease also have impaired absorption of calcium secondary to decrease in renal production of 1,25-dihydrocholecalciferol.

Intestinal enzymes such as pepsinogen, amylase, and lipase, which help to digest food and bacteria are needed to help absorb vitamins B_1, B_2, B_6, B_{12}, and vitamin K. Malabsorption of these nutrients can be caused by drugs that kill off these bacteria, such as broad-spectrum antibiotics, or drugs that damage the lining of the intestines, thus reducing absorption and enzyme action *(1)*. Table 3 summarizes the clinical manifestations of specific vitamin deficiencies.

4. DRUGS AND FOOD INTAKE

Drugs can affect appetite as well as GI function, resulting in alterations in food intake. Drugs affecting appetite may have either a central or peripheral effect. Some drugs such as antidepressants and prednisone may increase appetite and cause weight gain, whereas others such as chemotherapeutic agents contribute to weight loss by causing anorexia, nausea, and vomiting. Many drugs (*see* Table 1) have oral side effects such as xerostomia or stomatitis that can affect food intake. A wide variety of drugs can cause changes in taste or smell alterations. Potassium iodide is secreted into the saliva, producing a constant unpleasant taste that is difficult to eradicate. Chlorpromazine and metronidazole cause a persistent metallic taste that inhibits food intake. Penicillamine causes zinc depletion, leading to loss of taste and loss of desire for food *(18)*. Digitalis, especially in patients with decreased renal function, can cause marked nausea and vomiting. Biguanides, used as oral hypoglycemic agents, cause impaired appetite and decreased food intake. Chemotherapy drugs, especially cisplatin, actinomycin D, adriamycin, dacarbazine, streptozocin, nitrosoureas, nitrogen mustard, and cyclophosphamide, and folic acid analogs *(19)* induce nausea, vomiting, anorexia, and subsequent weight loss. In patients who may have marginal intake of required nutrients, drugs causing anorexia can result in nutritional deficiencies.

5. FOOD AND DRUG INTERACTIONS

Absorption of drugs may be decreased or more infrequently increased by the presence of food, which changes the pH, osmolality, secretions and motility of the gastrointestinal tract (Table 2) *(9)*. Drug bioavailability may be affected by direct interactions between the drug and food, such the formation of drug–protein complexes or chelation with polyvalent metal ions *(20)*. For example, tetracycline forms an insoluble complex with calcium, rendering it ineffective when taken with dairy products *(9)*. Food may act as a

Table 3
Clinical Manifestations of Specific Vitamin Deficiencies

Deficiency	Manifestations
Fat-Soluble Vitamins	
Vitamin A	Night blindness, impaired protein utilization, impaired healing, impaired bone and tooth formation
Vitamin D	Bone loss, osteoporosis, low blood calcium, rickets/osteomalacia, muscle weakness, impaired tooth development
Vitamin E	Rare: anemia, lethargy, neuromuscular disease
Vitamin K	Impaired blood clotting, bleeding gums, bruising, bleeding after injury or surgery
Water-Soluble Vitamins	
Vitamin B_1 (thiamine)	Impaired gastric acid production, tingling and numbness in fingers and toes, stomatitis, beriberi (disorder of the nervous and cardiovascular system), and Wernicke-Kosakoff syndrome
Vitamin B_2 (riboflavin)	Impaired metabolism of carbohydrates, fats, and proteins; impaired cell growth; seborrheic dermatitis; angular cheilitis; "magenta" tongue; split tongue; burning of oral mucosa; aphthous ulcers
Niacin	Pellagralike symptoms of dermatitis, dementia, diarrhea, angular stomatitis, lesions of tongue and oral mucosa, raw erythematous tongue
Vitamin B_6 (pyroxidine)	Hypochromic anemia, decreased antibody formation, dermatitis of face and scalp, burning feet, peripheral neuropathy, carpal tunnel syndrome, angular stomatitis, cheilitis, glossitis
Vitamin B_{12} (cobalamine)	Pernicious anemia, hypotension, neuropathy, fatigue, dsypnea, redness and burning of the tongue
Folic acid	Megaloblastic anemia, anorexia, glossitis, cheilitis, problems with clotting and bruising, birth defects
Vitamin C (ascorbic acid)	Compromised immune system, impaired wound healing, petechiae, bleeding gums and loosening of teeth, damage to nerves, eyes and vascular system
Minerals	
Calcium	Osteopenia, osteoporosis, muscle cramps, joint aches, heart rhythm irregularities, numbness in arms and legs, rickets
Iron	Angular cheilitis, glossitis, dysphagia, mucosal thinning, ulcerations, anemia
Zinc	Hypogeusia, dysgeusia, delayed wound healing

mechanical barrier, preventing access to the epithelial surface of the GI tract, increase transit time, or indirectly inhibit drug absorption because of increased digestion by GI secretions. Drugs taken with food may remain in the stomach for extended periods and be broken down before they can be absorbed in the intestines. This is especially significant with drugs that are meant to be rapidly absorbed or have a short half-life *(4)*. Delayed gastric clearance of such drugs as erythromycin, capoten (Captopril), penicillin, digoxin, and levodopa would cause more of the drug to be metabolized in the stomach and less of the active drug available for absorption, causing a suboptimal clinical response *(21)*. Nutrients can bind to drugs and make them unavailable. Iron binds with tetracycline, ciprofloxacin (Cipro), ofloxacin (Floxin), and enoxacine (Penetrax), causing reduced absorption and blood levels *(21)*. Fluid intake may affect how well water-soluble drugs are absorbed. Excessive consumption of foods rich in vitamin K can alter prothrombin times in patients on coumadin. Patients taking coumadin do not have to avoid foods high in vitamin K, such as liver, broccoli, brussel sprouts, and green leafy vegetables (e.g., spinach, Swiss chard, coriander, collards, cabbage), but it is important that the patient keep his or her intake consistent so that the amount of vitamin K eaten remains the same.

Certain foods can affect the rate of drug metabolism or elimination. Grapefruit juice, even consumed 24 h before taking certain drugs, can inhibit an intestinal enzyme necessary for drug breakdown, resulting in a more potent drug effect. Examples of these drugs include carbamazepine (Tegretol), amiodizine (Norvasc), nifedepine (Procardia), felodipine (Plendil), cisapride (Propulsid) *(22)*, and atorvastatin (Lipitor). Foods can affect the rate of elimination of a drug by changing the pH of the urine. If the pH of the urine is modified, it is possible that there will be prolonged effects of a drug by increasing the un-ionized form in the urine (favoring reabsorption) or expedited elimination by promoting the excretion of the ionized form. If the urine has a low pH, weakly basic drugs such as amitriptyline and chloroquine are excreted, because they form water-soluble salts *(4)*. Foods that can cause acidification of the urine include meat, fish, chicken, seafood, eggs, cheese, peanut butter, and most processed carbohydrates such as breads and pasta. Conversely, the action of some drugs is prolonged if the pH of the urine is high because there is decreased ionization and therefore reduced elimination and increased absorption by the kidneys. Low protein diets, chronic antacid use, citrus fruits, milk products, and most vegetables can raise urine pH *(23)*. This alkalinizing effect of the diet leads to less of the ionized form of basic drugs (such as gentamicin, quinine, or procainamide) presented in the renal tubule, leading to more of the drug being reabsorbed. Similarly, the elimination half-life of ephedrine and fexofenadine (Allegra) is increased in the presence of an alkaline urine pH, possibly leading to increased level of the drug unless the dosing schedule is adjusted *(24)*.

Interactions between drugs and foods or alcohol can result in systemic reactions, some of which can be life threatening. Tyramine, an amine that appears in some plant and animal products that have been fermented or aged, is a potent pressor that can cause marked elevation in blood pressure and, in severe cases, hypertensive crisis. Monoamine oxides, found in the liver, GI tract, and adrenergic nerve endings, metabolize tyramine before it can reach systemic circulation *(25)*. Monoamine oxidase inhibitators (MAOIs) include drugs used to treat severe depression such as isocarboxazid (Marplan), phenelzine sulfate (Nardil) and tranylcypromine sulfate (Parnate), seligiline (Atapryl, Eldepryl, and Selpak) used to treat Parkinson's disease, and the antineoplastic drug procarbazine hydrochloride. If a patient taking these drugs eats foods containing tyramine, it is not metabolized and can cause a rapid increase in blood pressure and increased incidence of cerebrovascular accidents (CVAs). Examples of foods and beverages that contain tyramine include beer, ale, red wines including Chianti, vermouth, homemade breads, cheese, crackers (with cheese), sour cream, bananas, red plums, figs, raisins, avocados, fava beans, Italian broad beans, green bean pods, eggplant, pickled herring, chicken and beef liver, dry sausages, canned meats, salami, yogurt, soup cubes, commercial gravies, chocolate, and soy sauce *(26)*. All of these foods should be avoided by individuals taking MAOIs.

Alcohol is absorbed as a drug and is metabolized as both a nutrient and a drug. When consumed in excess, it causes malabsorption or decreased absorption of many nutrients, in particular intestinal absorption of the fat- and water-soluble vitamins *(27)*. In addition, there is malabsorption of folate, thiamin, vitamin B_{12}, calcium, magnesium, fatty acids, and protein in individuals with excess consumption *(27)*. Alcohol can cause hypoglycemic reactions in individuals taking oral hypoglycemic agents, which when combined with these agents can cause mental confusion, weakness, hypotension, and loss of consciousness. Tetraethylthiuram disulfide (Disulfiram or Antabuse) produces a "disulfiram" reaction (flushing, headache, nausea, vomiting, and chest and abdominal pain) *(28)* when even very small amounts of alcohol are consumed. A similar reaction is seen with alcohol and other drugs, including metronidazole, oral hypoglycemic agents such as the sulfonylureas, hydrochloride, chloramphenicol, and griseofulvin. Alcohol has an additive or synergistic central nervous system (CNS) depressant effect when combined with barbiturates. It increases the risk of phenytoin-induced folate deficiency and can cause hypotension when combined with coronary vasodilators, such as nitroglycerin *(28)*. Alcohol dissolves capsules and increases the rate of dissolution and absorption of drugs given in capsule form. It potentiates the adverse nutritional effects of other drugs that cause anorexia, malabsorption, vitamin antagonism, and mineral wasting *(29)*. Health care providers should be aware of the possibility of interactions with alcohol, both with the medications they prescribe and with other medications people may take, and advise patients accordingly.

6. DRUGS THAT AFFECT ORAL HEALTH AND NUTRITIONAL INTAKE

Many prescription and over-the-counter medications have the potential to cause adverse oral conditions. Drug-induced oral lesions or disorders occur frequently, especially among the elderly who take multiple medications to treat chronic diseases. Synergistic effects between medications can increase the incidence of such adverse events, either directly as an adverse effect of the drug or indirectly as the result of drug-induced vitamin deficiencies *(5)*. These effects can present as part of a general systemic effect, a specific oral adverse effect to the systemic use of a drug, or a local effect secondary to direct contact with the oral mucosa. The presence of these adverse drug effects can impair appetite and food intake and adversely affect the nutritional status of the patient. Table 4 *(30,31)* summarizes common drug-induced adverse oral conditions.

6.1. Xerostomia

Xerostomia is the perception of dry mouth and may or may not be associated with actual hyposalivation. Xerostomia is probably the most frequent, undesirable effect of drugs. Commonly used classes of medications such as anticholinergics, centrally acting antihypertensives, antihistamines, antipsychotics, narcotic analgesics, hypnotics, muscle relaxants, anticonvulsants, antineoplastics, antidepressants, and diuretics (Table 4) *(32)* can all cause a decrease of normal salivary secretion. Drug-induced xerostomia can cause alterations in taste and difficulty in chewing and swallowing, leading to decreased food intake, subclinical malnutrition, and reduced resistance to disease and stress, especially among the elderly *(33)*. Lack of lubrication can cause mucosal irritation, inflammation, and ulceration, and make it difficult for the patient to wear removable dental prostheses.

Table 4
Drug-Induced Adverse Oral Conditions

Category	Examples of drugs
Xerostomia	Anti-anxiety, anticonvulsants, anticholinergics, antidepressants (tricyclics and SSRIs), antihistamines/decongestants, HAART, protease inhibitors, antihypertensives, anti-Parkinson's, antipsychotics, antispasmodics, appetite suppressants, disopyramide, diuretics, hypnotics, muscle relaxants, narcotics, over-the-counter sleep aids, systemic bronchodilators, methyldopa, clonidine, reserpine, β-blocker
Soft-tissue reaction (erythema, fixed eruptions, glossitis, stomatitis, ulceration)	Ampicillin, anticoagulants, aspirin, captopril, barbiturates, sulfonamides, penicillamine, gold salts, chloroquine, isoniazid, nonsteroidal anti-inflammatory drugs, indomethacin, cytotoxic antineoplastic drugs, tetracycline, methyldopa
Movement disorders/dysphagia	Antipsychotics, lithium, levodopa, amoxapine, metoclopramide
Gingival overgrowth	Diltiazem, nifedipine, phenytoin, cyclosporin
Taste changes	Enalapril, captorpril, D-penicillamines, griseofulvin, metronidazole, chlorhexidine, carbenicillin, chloral hydrate, diltiazem, gold salts, guanethidine, iron, nifedipine, ethambutol, sulfasalazine, azathiprine, allopurinol, phenylbutazone, baclofen, levodopa, carbamazepine

Adapted from refs. *30* and *31*.

Xerostomia increases the development of candidal infections, often leading to complaints of pain, burning, and altered taste. Decreases in salivary flow leads to decreased enzymatic debridement of plaque, decreased buffering and neutralization of acid formed in the tooth decay process, and increased accumulation of food debris, resulting in increased caries and periodontal disease *(34)*.

6.2. Changes in Taste Sensations

Many drugs induce abnormalities of taste and smell. The alteration may be a decreased sensitivity in taste perception (hypogeusia), a total loss in the ability to taste (ageusia), or an unpleasant or altered taste sensation (dysgeusia) *(35)*. Although ageusia is rare, drugs can give rise to dysgeusia or hypogeusia by interfering in the chemical composition and amount of saliva, by directly affecting taste-receptor function or signal transduction (either stimulating or desensitizing), or by adversely affecting the renewal process of taste buds *(35)*. The effect of drugs on taste may also be mediated by their actions on trace metals such as copper, zinc, and nickel *(36)*. Reduction in salivary flow may concentrate electrolytes in the saliva, resulting in a salty or metallic taste. Alterations in taste can cause anorexia, food aversion, and weight loss.

Classifications of medications that can alter taste or smell include antihistamines, anticonvulsants, antidepressants, antihistamines, antihypertensives, anti-inflammatories, antimicrobials, antineoplastics, asthma medication, bronchodilators, lipid-lowering drugs, muscle relaxants, and vasodilators *(37)*. Griseofulvin, metronidazole (Flagyl), capoten (Captopril), penicillamine, and metformin (Glucophage) are frequently associated with altered taste. Up to 4% of patients treated with angiotensin-converting enzyme (ACE) inhibitors may have dysgeusia, although this adverse effect is self-limiting and reversible within a few months, even with continued therapy *(38)*. Therapies such as HAART, protease inhibitors, clarithromycin, and lansoprazole (Prevacid) therapy for *Heliobacter pylori* infection, terbinafine, pentamidine, and isotretinoin (Accutane) may cause some degree of loss of taste or altered taste. Taste disturbances tend to be self-limiting and often reversible in 2–3 mo following discontinuation of the medication. It may be feasible to contact the patient's physician to see whether there are substitute medications that can be used that have less effect on either salivary flow or taste. Possible approaches to relief from dysgeusia include increased use of flavoring agents during food preparation, substituting alternative protein sources if the patient is unable to tolerate meat, and use of artificial saliva as needed. Optimal oral hygiene is essential. Use of a "swish and spit" with iced lemon water can temporarily decrease dysgeusia and increase patient comfort and satisfaction with subsequent meals *(39)*. Patients should be reassured that, in most cases, taste will return to baseline. If the patient has persistent taste disturbances, a referral to an oral medicine specialist would be appropriate.

6.3. Stomatitis/Glossitis

Stomatitis (inflammation of the mucosal lining of the mouth) from medications can be caused by both local effects and systemically mediated responses. Pain from mucosal lesions can be severe and can interfere with eating. Some cases of drug-induced stomatitis have no clinical presentation other than erythema, whereas other cases can be categorized as allergic stomatitis, lichenoid drug eruptions, lupus erythematouslike eruptions, pemphiguslike drug reactions, and erythema multiforme *(40)*. Ulceration of the oral mucosa is a common side effect of a wide variety of antineoplastic agents, including methotrexate, 5-fluorouracil, doxorubicin, daunorubicin, bleomycin, and melphalen through inhibition of epithelial cell mitosis *(41)*. Allergic reactions can occur either locally from contact with the medication or from systemic administrations of the drug. Lichenoid drug eruptions have been linked to a number of medications, including antibiotics (tetracycline, penicillin, sulfonamides, nitrofurantoin, isoniazid, para-amino salicylic acid, streptomycin, ketoconazole, griseofulvin), oral hypoglycemics (sulfonylureas), antihypertensives (β-adrenergic blocking agents [methyldopa]); ACE inhibitors (captopril; reserpine), nonsteroidal anti-inflammatory agents (indomethacin, azulfidine, phenylbutazone, naproxen) *(42)*, and heavy metals (especially gold compounds) *(43)*. Secondary oral effects may be seen with drug-induced vitamin deficiencies (Table 2), including the B-complex vitamins, iron, vitamin C, and vitamin A. Thiamine deficiency (often the result of chronic alcoholism) may lead to painful mucosa and small vesicles on the buccal mucosa and tongue. Riboflavin (vitamin B_2) and pyridoxine (vitamin B_6) deficiency has been associated with angular cheilitis, atrophic glossitis, burning mouth, and mucosal ulcerations. Isoniazid, which inhibits the metabolism of B_6, can be associated with peripheral neuritis affecting the cranial nerves that supply the oral cavity. Acute deficiencies in niacin, folic acid, or vitamin B_{12} can cause the oral mucosa to become red, swollen, and tender to the touch. Pernicious anemia caused by vitamin B_{12} deficiency and folic acid deficiency can cause painful glossitis and gingivitis, as well as atrophy of the papillae of the tongue, resulting in a "bald" tongue. Long-term use of methotrexate, cholestyramine (Questran), colchicines, sodium aminosalicylate, ethanol, metformin (Glucophage), methyldopa, cimetidine (Tagamet), allopurinol (Zyloprim), and oral contraceptives have all been implicated in vitamin B_{12}

deficiency *(43)*. Niacin deficiency (pellagra) also causes an atrophic glossitis. Vitamin C deficiency causes red, spongy gingiva that bleeds easily and, in severe cases, can cause extensive destruction of the periodontium *(1)*. When prescribing drugs with a well-documented history of causing vitamin deficiencies, concomminant vitamin supplements should be prescribed. A good example of this would be the use of vitamin B_6 with isoniazid or prescribing folic acid supplements for patients taking medications known to cause folic acid deficiencies, such as anticonvulsant medications (e.g., dilantin, phenytoin, and primidone), oral hypoglycemic agents (metformin), anti-inflammatory agents (sulfasalazine, which is used to control inflammation associated with Crohn's disease and ulcerative colitis), diuretics (triamterene), and methotrexate *(44)*.

6.4. Dysphagia

Drugs that cause xerostomia can interfere with a patient's ability to swallow. Antipsychotic drugs can cause laryngeal dystonia early in treatment and tardive dyskinesias with chronic treatment that can cause dysphagia. Drug-induced esophageal injury can also cause difficulty in swallowing, usually as result of nonchewable tablets or capsules that get lodged within the esophagus, dissolve, and release their concentrated contents, causing direct mucosal damage *(45)*. An important warning sign is a dull, aching pain in the chest or shoulder after taking the drug. Almost 100 different drugs are known to cause esophageal damage *(46)* (*see* Table 5; *47,48*). Many factors influence the severity of drug-induced injury to the esophagus. Chemical and physical properties of the drug, such as its chemical formula, pH, concentration of medication, drug formulation, and size and shape of the tablet or capsule, play a role. Other factors include delay in transit time of the drug and duration of contact with esophageal mucosa. When gelatin capsules are administered with inadequate liquid, they may become sticky as they dissolve and delay transit time of the drug *(45)*. When a gelatin capsule becomes lodged in the esophagus, it may be difficult to dislodge with repeated swallows of water. Preexisting swallowing problems (esophageal dysmotility conditions, stroke) or anatomical abnormalities (esophageal strictures) may alter the passage of the drug to the stomach *(45)*.

Aspirin, tetracycline, quinidine, potassium chloride, vitamin C, and iron can all cause esophageal ulcers *(49)*. Alendronate (Fosamax) in particular can cause esophagitis, including severe ulcerations. Patients should take alendronate with at least 180 mL of water and remain in an upright position for at least 30 min before eating to prevent esophageal ulceration.

The best treatment for drug-induced esophageal damage is the discontinuation of the problematic drug. Patients should be instructed to swallow several sips of water to lubricate the throat before taking a tablet or capsule and then take the medication with at least 8 oz of liquid. Tablets or capsules should be swallowed while in an upright or sitting position, and the patient should not lie down immediately after taking a tablet or capsule to ensure that the solid dosage forms pass through the esophagus and into the stomach. Patients should also avoid irritating foods such as citrus juices and alcohol *(45)*.

6.5. Gingival Hyperplasia

Enlargement and overgrowth of the gingiva was originally recognized in patients using phenytoin and more recently in the calcium channel blocker class of cardiac drugs, cyclosporine, and the anticonvulsant valproate sodium. An inverse relationship appears

Table 5
Drugs Associated With Esophageal Damage

Acid-containing products	Clindamycin (Cleocin)
	Doxycycline (Vibramycin)
	Erythromycin (Ery-tabs, E-mycin)
	Minocycline (Minocin)
	Pentamidine (NebuPent)
	Tetracycline (Sumycin)
Antiarrhythmics	Quinidine (Quinaglute, Cardioquin)
Aspirin	Bayer Aspirin, others
Bisphosphonates	Alendronate (Fosamax)
	Tiludronate (Skelid)
Iron-containing products	FeoSol, Feratab, Slow FE, Fer-Iron, others
Methylxanthines	Theophylline (Theo-Dur, Unidur, Slo-Bid)
Nonsteroidal anti-inflammatory drugs	Ibuprofen (Advil, Motrin)
	Indomethacin (Indocin)
	Ketoprofen (Orudis)
	Naproxen (Aleve, Naprosyn)
Potassium chloride	K-Dur, K-Tabs, Klor-Con, Micro-K, Slow-K, others
Vitamin C (ascorbic acid) products	

Adapted from ref. *45, 47,* and *48.*

to exist between oral hygiene and the degree of gingival enlargement. In rare cases, the extent of the gingival hyperplasia is such that it impedes the patient's ability to eat, and excess tissue must be surgically removed.

7. CONCLUSION

The interactions between drugs and nutrition are becoming more important given the aging of the population and the increased usage of multiple medications on a chronic basis. Unwanted outcomes include reduction in the intended response to a therapeutic drug because of diet-induced changes in drug bioavailability or metabolism, drug-induced nutritional deficiencies, and drug–food/drug–nutrient incompatibility reactions *(50)*. Risk of drug–nutrient interactions and their outcomes depends on the patient's age, physiologic status including renal and hepatic function, number of drugs being taken, and the diet. Predictions of the risk of drug and nutrient interaction may be possible if the characteristics of prescribed drugs and diet are known. Diagnosis of a clinical problem as an adverse drug–nutrient interaction depends on recognizing that the problem appeared after the drug has been prescribed and/or a change in diet has occurred. Laboratory tests may be useful in clarifying the diagnosis, especially with drug-induced vitamin deficiencies. Avoidance of drug–nutrient interactions depends on knowledge of the risk as well as avoidance of drug–nutrient or drug–food intake that imposes a high-risk situation *(50)*. Careful monitoring of the oral cavity for signs of drug–nutrient vitamin deficiencies (such as atrophic glossitis) can allow intervention before a patient's nutritional status is further compromised. Use of sialagogues and topical fluorides can prevent damage of the oral mucosa and teeth as the result of drug-induced xerostomia. In summary, it is incumbent on the members of the health-care team to have a current knowledge of drug–nutrient interrelationships and to understand how adverse drug reactions can have a negative impact on a patient's nutritional status. Review and frequent update of all medications that a patient is taking, both prescribed and over the counter, and appropriate dietary evaluation with an eye to the patient's underlying medical condition are vital in order to anticipate and possibly prevent and appropriately treat unwanted interactions.

Guidelines for Practice

	Nutrition Professional	*Oral Health Professional*

Assessment
• Prolonged medication program/multiple medications/compromised patient (elderly, systemic disease)
	• Physical examination with attention to evidence of nutritional deficiency
	• Clinical signs of deficiencies
	  ◆ Altered taste
	  ◆ Angular chelitis
	  ◆ Bleeding
	  ◆ Glossitis
	  ◆ Stomatitis
	• Attention to adequacy of diet and need for supplements
	  ◆ Evaluation of daily diet with respect to nutritional adequacy
	    ▪ Elderly
	    ▪ Borderline or inadequate dietary habits
	    ▪ Chronically ill
	  ◆ Dietary alterations
	  ◆ Nutritional supplementation
	  ◆ Medication dose changes
	  ◆ Medication changes
		• Physical examination with attention to evidence of nutritional deficiency
		• Clinical signs of deficiencies
		  ◆ Altered taste
		  ◆ Angular chelitis
		  ◆ Bleeding
		  ◆ Glossitis
		  ◆ Stomatitis
		• Look for common drug-induced oral side effects

Prevention	• Awareness of possible nutritional effects of medication(s)
	• Awareness of various adverse effects
	• Awareness of incompatibilities associated with combination of medications
	• Update patient's medication history frequently
	  ◆ Prescription
	  ◆ Over-the-counter
		• Topical fluoride for patients on xerostomic drugs
		• Sialagogues
		• Medications taken with adequate water and in upright position
		• Periodic evaluations of daily diet and review of systems and physical exam

Intervention	• Appropriate supplements when indicated • Encourage adequate intake • With physician, adjustment of dosage up or down to accommodate for systemic disease	• Palliative relief of symptoms • Referral to registered dietitian as needed for diet intervention

REFERENCES

1. Roe DA. Drug-Induced Nutritional Deficiencies, 2nd Ed. Westport, CT: Avi Publishing, 1985.
2. Rikans LE. Drugs and nutrition in old age. Life Sci 1986; 39(12):1027–1036.
3. Branda R. Effects of drugs on cellular transport of nutrients. In Winick M, ed. Nutrition and Drugs. New York, NY: John Wiley, 1983, 13–29.
4. Lamy PP. Drug–nutrient interactions in the aged. In Watson RR, ed. Handbook of Nutrition in the Aged, 2nd Ed. Boca Raton, FL: CRC Press, 1994, 165–200.
5. Lamy ML. Drugs and oral health. The Maryland 1984; 60(7):125–135.
6. Blumberg J, Couris R. Pharmacology, nutrition and the elderly: interactions and implications. In Chernoff R, ed. Geriatric Nutrition: The Health Professionals Handbook. Gaithersburg, MD: Aspen Publishers, 1999L, 342–365.
7. Roe DA. Drugs, diet and nutrition. J Dent Children 1978; September–October:68–70.
8. Moseley V. Medications and malnutrition: cause and effect. J S C Med Assoc 1980; 76(7):339–342.
9. Zeman FJ. Drugs and Nutritional Care in Clinical Nutrition and Dietetics. Lexington, MA: D.C. Heath, 1983, 49–75.
10. Mohs ME. Assessment of nutritional status In Watson RR, ed. Handbook of Nutrition in the Aged, 2nd Ed. Boca Raton, FL: CRC Press, 1994, 145–164.
11. Roe DA. Drug-Induced Nutritional Deficiencies. In Roe DA, ed. Diet and Drug Interactions. Westport, CT: Avi Publishing, 1989, 83–103.
12. Dickerson JW. Some adverse effects of drugs on nutrition. Royal Soc Health J 1978; 98(6):261–265.
13. Zeman FJ Liver Disease and Alcoholism in Clinical Nutrition and Dietetics. Lexington, MA: D.C. Heath, 1983, 441–470.
14. Roe DA. Effects of drugs on nutrition. Life Sci 1974; 15(7):1219–1234.
15. Roe DA. Medications and nutrition in the elderly. Primary Care 1994; 21:135–147.
16. Eddington ND. Pharmacokinetics. In Roberts J, Snyder DL, Friedman E, ed. Handbook of Pharmacology of Aging. Boca Raton, FL: CRC Press, 1996, 1–22.
17. Bressler R. Adverse drug reactions. In Bressler R, Katz MD, ed. Geriatric Pharmacology. New York, NY: McGraw-Hill, 1993, 41–61.
18. Roe DA. Drug-induced malnutrition in geriatric patients. Compr Ther 1977; 3(10):24–28.
19. Casciato DA. Supportive care. In Casciato DA, and Lowitz BB, ed. Manual of Clinical Oncology, 3rd Ed. Boston, MA: Little, Brown, 1996, 61–63.
20. Viswanathan CT, Welling, PG. Food effects on drug absorption. In Roe DA, ed. Drugs and Nutrition in the Geriatric Patient. New York, NY: Churchill Livingstone, 1984, 47–70.
21. Kirk KJ. Significant drug–nutrient interactions. Am Fam Phys 1995; 51:1175–1182.
22. Dresser GK, Bailey DG. Grapefruit juice–drug interactions. Clin Pharmacol Ther 2000; 68:28–34.
23. Neuvonen PJ, Kivistoe KT. The clinical significance of food–drug interactions: a review. Med J Austral, 1989, 150:36–41.
24. Lambert ML. Drug and diet interactions. Am J Nurs 1975; 75(3):402–406.
25. Roe DA. Interactions between drugs and nutrients. Med Clin North Am 1979; 63:998.
26. Holt GA. Food & Drug Interaction. Chicago, IL: Precept Press, 1998, 319–326.
27. Roe DA. Alcohol and the Diet. Westport, CT: Avi Publishing, 1979.
28. Roe DA. Drug-Induced Reactions to Alcohol and Food in Diet and Drug Interactions. Westport, CT: Avi Publishing, 1989, 59–71.
29. Lieber CS. Alcohol, protein nutrition and liver injury. In Winik M, ed. Nutrition and Drugs. New York, NY: Wiley-Interscience, 1983, 49–71.
30. Lewis IK, Hanlen JT, Hobbens MJ, Beck JD. Use of medications with potential oral adverse drug reactions. Special Care Dent 1993; 12(4):171–176;
31. Abdhollahi M, Radfar M. A review of drug-induced oral reactions. J Contemp Dent Prac 2003; 1:10–31.
32. Lamy PP. Drugs, older adults and oral health. J Gerontol Nurs 1985; 11(10):36–37.
33. Soon JA. Effects of drug therapy on oral health of older adults. Can Dent Hygiene/Probe 1992; 3:(26):118–120.
34. Seymour RA. Oral and dental disorders. In Davies DM, Ferner RE, DeGlanville H, eds. Davies's Textbook of Adverse Drug Reactions, 5th Ed. London, UK: Chapman & Hall Medical, 1998, 234–250.

35. Porter SR, Scully C. Adverse drug reactions in the mouth. Clin Dermatol 2000; 18(5):525–532.
36. Guggenheimer J. Oral manifestations of drug therapy. Dent Clin North Am 2002; 46:857–868.
37. Shiffman SS. Taste and smell losses in normal aging and disease. JAMA 1997; 278(16):1257–1362.
38. Henkin RI. Drug-induced taste and smell disorders. Drug Safety 1994; 11:318–377.
39. Frankmann CB. Medical nutrition therapy for neoplastic disease. In Mahan K, Escott-Stump S, eds. Krause's Food, Nutrition and Diet Therapy, 10th Ed. Philadelphia, PA: WB Saunders, 2000, 867–888.
40. Wright JM. Oral manifestations of drug reactions. Dent Clin North Am 1984; 28(3):529–543.
41. Sonis ST. Oral complications of cancer therapy. In DeVita VT, Hellman S, Rosenberg SA, eds. Cancer: Principles and Practice of Oncology, 5th Ed. Philadelphia, PA: Lippincott-Raven, 1997, 2385–2393.
42. Korstanje MJ. Drug-induced mouth disorders. Clin Exp Dermatol 1995; 20(1):10–18.
43. Duxbury AJ. Systemic pharmacotherapy. In Jones JH, Mason DK, eds. Oral Manifestations of Systemic Disease, 2nd Ed. London, UK: Bailliere Tindall, 1990, 411–479.
44. Linker CA. Folic acid deficiency. In Tierney LM, et al., eds. Current Medical Diagnosis and Treatment 2002, 41st Ed. New York, NY: Lange Medical/McGraw-Hill, 2002, 524–525.
45. Boyce HW Jr . Drug-induced esophageal damage: diseases of medical progress. Gastrointest Endosc 1998; 47:547–550.
46. Kikendall JW. Pill-induced esophageal injury. In: Castell DO, Richter JE, eds. The Esophagus. Philadelphia, PA: Lippincott Williams & Wilkins, 1999.
47. Sliwa JA, Lis S. Drug-induced dysphagia. Arch Phys Med Rehabil. 1993; 74:445–447.
48. Balzer KM. Drug-induced dysphagia. Intl J MS Care 2000; 2(1):6.
49. U.S. Department of Health and Human Services. Harmful effects of medicines on the adult digestive system. NIH Publication No. 97-3421, September 1992.
50. Roe DA. Diet, nutrition and drug reactions. In Shils ME, Olson JA, Shike M, eds. Modern Nutrition in Health and Disease, 8th Ed. Philadelphia, PA: Lea and Febiger, 1994, 1399–1416.

III

RELATIONSHIP BETWEEN NUTRITION AND ORAL HEALTH

7 Oral Consequences of Compromised Nutritional Well-Being

Paula J. Moynihan and Peter Lingström

1. INTRODUCTION

Nutrition affects the development of the teeth and the development and maintenance of the oral tissues. Often, the very early signs of suboptimum nutritional status are first seen in the mouth, which has been described as a "mirror of nutritional status." Dental health professionals are therefore in a position to be the first to notice compromised nutrition, and a sound knowledge of the symptoms and signs will enable them to take the appropriate action. A role for dental health professionals in providing dietary advice is being encouraged, and therefore knowledge of the consequences of compromised nutritional status on the mouth is essential in order to fulfill this important role. The dental health professional should recognize when a patient needs to be referred to a dietitian, and, likewise, dietitians should recognize the oral symptoms of nutritional deficiencies.

In this chapter, compromised nutritional well-being encompasses general undernutrition such as protein energy malnutrition (PEM), deficiencies of specific nutrients, and diets that fall short of current recommendations for intakes of food types, such as a low intake of fruits and vegetables.

This chapter discusses each oral disease or disorder in turn, relating the condition to compromised nutrition. The conditions covered include enamel developmental defects, dental caries, impaired salivary gland function, disorders of the oral mucosa including noma and oral cancer, and periodontal disease.

2. COMPROMISED NUTRITIONAL STATUS AND ENAMEL DEVELOPMENTAL DEFECTS

Calcification of enamel of deciduous incisors begins at 14 wk *in utero* and continues until about 4 mo after birth. Lesions to the enamel of the deciduous incisors are therefore most likely to be caused by perinatal or neonatal insults. Simultaneously with calcification of the deciduous dentition, the tooth germs for the permanent teeth develop. Mineralization of the permanent dentition starts with the first molars around birth, and all teeth (with the exception of the third molars) have normally started to mineralize before 3 yr of age. The crowns are complete at 5 to 7 yr of age, and root formation is complete

From: *Nutrition and Oral Medicine*
Edited by: R. Touger-Decker, D. A. Sirois, and C. C. Mobley © Humana Press Inc., Totowa, NJ

between 10 and 15 yr of age. A full description of the development of the dentition is provided by Rugg-Gunn 1993 *(1)*.

Developmental defects may be broadly classified into opacities (white or yellow areas of opaque enamel) that are caused largely by excess fluoride ingestion, or "hypoplasia," a term that describes surface defects of enamel (pits, fissures, or larger areas of missing enamel). There are many causes of enamel developmental defects including congenital defects, effects of drugs, trauma, infection, and metabolic disturbances *(2)*; compromised nutritional status is just one cause. Most attention has focused on excess ingestion of fluoride as a cause of opacities and disturbances of calcium and phosphorus metabolism and deficiencies of vitamins A and D and protein as nutritional causes of hypoplasia. Damage to the teeth during the development is permanent damage that affects the aesthetics of the teeth and the susceptibility to dental diseases.

2.1. Protein Energy Malnutrition and Enamel Developmental Defects

The most common enamel abnormality in severely malnourished children is linear enamel hypoplasia (LEH) *(3,4)*, characterized by a horizontal groove on the labial surface that stains posteruption. In developing countries, hypoplasia is common and linked to malnutrition in children. Both malnutrition in early childhood and impaired maternal nutritional status can result in hypoplasia. Enwonwu *(5)* reported the prevalence of hypoplasia to be approx 21% in 4-yr-old Nigerian children from low socioeconomic backgrounds compared with 0% in affluent areas. Almost 75% of the defects were caused by prenatal damage. Sweeney *(4)* reported a prevalence of LEH of 73% in children with third-degree malnutrition compared with 24% in children with lesser malnutrition. The reason why malnourished children were more susceptible to hypoplasia was unclear until Nikiforuk and Fraser found, in a study of subjects with disturbances of calcium and/or phosphate metabolism, that hypocalcemia was associated with hypoplasia *(6)*. In chronic undernutrition, hypocalcemia develops as a result of diarrhea and thus may explain the association between PEM and defective enamel development. Acute diarrheal disease may also lead to low serum levels of vitamin A, which may contribute to the development of hypoplasia.

Opacities are largely caused by excessive fluoride ingestion; however, PEM has also been shown to exacerbate the effect of excessive fluoride ingestion, causing more severe enamel opacities *(7)*.

2.2. Deficiencies of Vitamins A and D and Enamel Hypoplasia

Vitamin A is important in maintaining normal epithelial tissue integrity and histodifferentiation of the tooth. Vitamin A functions in the normal differentiation of the enamel organ, which is an essential prerequisite for tooth development to occur normally. Numerous animal studies have shown that a deficiency of vitamin A impairs histo-differentiation of the tooth *(8)*. Vitamin D is intricately involved in mineralization processes, and, therefore, a deficiency of this vitamin will impair normal mineralization.

The early half of the 20th century was an exciting time in the discovery of the vitamins, and during this period Lady May Mellanby conducted extensive studies on the effects of the vitamins on the development of the teeth and their resistance to disease *(9– 12)*. In 1918 *(9)*, she reported that dogs reared on a diet deficient in vitamin D had delayed development of teeth that were poorly aligned with deficient calcification of enamel. Mellanby noticed the high prevalence of hypoplasia in the primary dentition of British children and suggested that this was caused by vitamin deficiencies, especially vitamins A and D *(10)*. She attributed the improvements in British children's teeth between 1929 and 1943 to the improved diet of the wartime food policy, which provided cheap milk; free cod liver oil to pregnant mothers, infants, and young children; fortification of white flour with calcium carbonate; and the addition of vitamins A and D to margarine *(11)*.

Mellanby examined teeth of children in England and in India and found that gross hypoplasia was slightly more prevalent in India; however, the prevalence of mild hypoplasia was similar in the two countries. She attributed the higher gross hypoplasia in India to the poor diet and greater diarrheal disease and the lower-than-expected mild hypoplasia to the high exposure to sunlight and resulting good status of vitamin D *(12)*. In support of these observations, Cockburn et al. *(13)* found that supplementation with vitamin D during pregnancy resulted in raised cord-blood vitamin D levels and reduced incidence of enamel defects in deciduous teeth in the offspring.

2.3. Association Between Hypoplasia of Enamel and Dental Caries

In addition to the aesthetic disadvantages of enamel defects, there is evidence that hypoplasia is associated with an increased risk of caries *(14–17)*. Mellanby *(14)* studied more than 300 teeth from at least 200 British children aged 2–13 yr. Nearly all teeth with hypoplasia were carious, whereas only 25% of teeth without hypoplasia were carious. In Guatemalan children aged 2–6 yr, 48% of children without hypoplasia were caries free but only 31% of children with hypoplasia were caries free *(15)*. In a study of Chinese children, Li et al. *(16)* found that almost 25% of children aged 3–5 yr had hypoplasia, and only 7% of these children were caries free compared with 21% of children without hypoplasia. Matee et al. *(17)* found a higher incidence of nursing-bottle caries in young children with hypoplasia.

3. THE EFFECT OF COMPROMISED NUTRITIONAL STATUS ON DENTAL CARIES

3.1. PEM

The worldwide distribution of severity of dental caries has changed markedly since the late 1970s, with a marked decrease in prevalence in developed countries but an increase in many developing countries that parallels an increase in sugars consumption. Where sugars are available in developing countries, the level of caries observed is higher than expected from observations in industrialized countries, and this has led to the hypothesis that malnutrition enhances the cariogenic effects of sugars *(5,18)*. This has been demonstrated in animal experiments, which have shown increased caries in rat pups whose dams received a protein-deficient diet during pregnancy and lactation *(19)*. However, the milk quantity as well as quality would be affected in such an experiment, making if difficult to separate the effect of deficient calories from deficient protein. Further research showed that addition of protein alone was able to restore the low level of caries observed in the well-fed rats.

There are three potential mechanisms to explain how deficiency of protein, energy, or both increase caries susceptibility. First, malnutrition results in defectively formed enamel that is poorly calcified (see the discussion of hypoplasia above) and therefore susceptible to dental decay. Second, undernutrition causes delayed eruption of the dentition, and this affects the caries prevalence at any given age *(5, 20–22)*. Enwonwu found that malnourished children aged 7–24 mo had 2.5 fewer erupted teeth compared with well-nourished children of a similar age. Alvarez and colleagues *(20–22)* conducted a series of investigations into nutritional status and eruption and exfoliation of dentition in Peruvian children from a poor area of Lima. Occurrence of caries as a function of time was shifted to the right and occurred 15 mo later in malnourished children compared with well-nourished children. This suggested that one reason for a higher level of caries in malnourished children at age 6 was the delay in exfoliation of the primary dentition. When the study was expanded to look at the permanent dentition *(21)*, eruption of the permanent dentition occurred 2.5 yr later, and hence caries prevalence at age 12 was lower because many of the secondary teeth had not erupted. The third mechanism by which PEM increases caries susceptibility is through its effects on salivary gland function and saliva quality. The effects of compromised nutritional status on salivary gland function are considered in a later section.

3.2. Vitamin Deficiencies and Dental Caries

3.2.1. VITAMIN D

Mellanby postulated that vitamin D deficiency was the cause of dental caries in British schoolchildren because deficiency of this vitamin resulted in hypoplasia that rendered the teeth susceptible to dental decay. She tested her vitamin-deficiency theory in intervention studies and found that initiation and spread of caries was lower and hardening of precarious lesions was higher in children receiving dietary supplements *(23)*. Children supplemented with cod liver oil developed fewer caries lesions in erupting permanent teeth (but not erupted teeth) compared with a control group receiving olive oil. Many investigators did not accept the vitamin theory and rightly claimed that the effect of dietary sugars was of greater significance. Mellanby modified her view to say that vitamin D was *a* factor during the development of teeth rather than *the* factor responsible for caries.

Vitamin D deficiency is rare nowadays except in countries with limited natural sunlight. However, a modern intervention study in which full-spectrum lighting was installed into classrooms in Alberta, Canada, found that fewer caries developed in the schoolchildren compared with children from classrooms with conventional lighting *(24)*. In some religions, females fully veil themselves and receive little vitamin D through the action of sunlight on the skin. This renders them susceptible to deficiency of vitamin D and may result in increased caries susceptibility in their offspring. An intervention study conducted in Scotland in which pregnant mothers received a vitamin D supplement from the 12th wk of pregnancy resulted in fewer caries in the children at age 3 yr compared with the children of a control group who did not receive a vitamin D supplement *(13)*. Deficiency of vitamin D during the development of the teeth is likely to cause defects in the enamel that render the tooth more susceptible to dental caries.

3.2.2. VITAMIN A

Animal experiments have shown that deficiency of vitamin A causes gross structural changes in teeth, and this increases risk of dental caries *(25–27)*. Vitamin A deficiency is often associated with diarrhea and PEM and may increase susceptibility to dental caries by causing hypoplasia and also by affecting normal salivary function.

In conclusion, PEM and deficiencies of specific nutrients per se will not cause dental caries in the absence of dietary sugars. Even in severely malnourished communities, dental caries is rare when intake of sugar is below 10 kg/yr. Likewise, optimum nutritional status will not protect against dental caries if the frequency and amount of intake of dietary free sugars is too high.

4. THE EFFECT OF COMPROMISED NUTRITIONAL STATUS ON SALIVARY SECRETION AND COMPOSITION

Saliva is a complex liquid consisting of secretions from the major and minor salivary glands where a number of physiological factors influence the composition of whole saliva. About 99% of saliva is water, whereas the remainder consists mainly of proteins and electrolytes. One of its major functions is to protect the soft tissues of the oral cavity. Other important functions are to clear the oral cavity of food residues, buffer the detrimental effects of strong acids and bases, provide ions to enhance the degree of remineralization of the teeth, and be involved in the preparation of food for digestion, as well as functioning in both taste and speech. Thus, there is an overwhelming risk that factors that compromise salivary gland function may also alter oral host defense and impact on oral health.

Nutritional deficiencies have been found to affect both salivary gland formation and function as well as saliva composition. Research into saliva covers a broad spectrum of factors that influence saliva, including the degree of malnutrition, timing of the deficiency, consistency of diet, salivary gland function, and the source of saliva. In relation to gland function, it is particularly important to determine the period when malnutrition takes place—for example, *in utero* and during lactation, in young age or in older age. Much of the research on nutrition and saliva has been conducted on animals.

4.1. Protein Deficiency

Both moderate and severe protein malnutrition result in alterations to salivary gland growth and function *(28–30)*. The results reported have varied depending on the point in the life cycle at which malnutrition occurred. When protein deficiency takes place at an early stage, the size of the submandibular gland has been found to be irreversibly reduced *(31)*. The effects that take place during these early stages of development may not be completely reversed when a diet adequate in protein is subsequently provided. Protein malnutrition induced in young adult rats resulted in increased parotid gland weight and a decreased β-adrenoceptor density, whereas submandibular gland weight and β-cell density were both reduced *(29)*. However, several studies have shown no effect on gland weight when protein malnutrition is induced in aged animals *(32)*.

Johnson et al. *(30)* evaluated the effect on parotid gland growth and secretory function of animals fed diets with different protein concentrations (20% or 7%) and different consistencies (powdered or solid). A reduced parotid gland weight was found in the rats fed the low protein (7%) diet. This reduced gland weight was observed for the low-protein diet when it was fed as either a solid or powdered form. However, the parotid gland weight observed in the animals fed the low-protein diets was similar to the animals fed a normal protein diet (20%) in a powdered form. The composition of the parotid gland saliva was higher in proline-rich proteins in both groups of animals on the low-protein diets. The flow rate of parotid saliva was significantly reduced by both the diet consistency and the dietary protein concentration. Although protein deficiency has a marked effect on salivary gland growth and function, diet texture, which affects the requirement for mastication, was also found to be a significant factor. This is supported by other researchers where a change in saliva volume *(33)*, gland weight *(34)*, and salivary composition *(32–34)* has been found during protein malnutrition. The majority of the work has been conducted on animals. However, although somewhat difficult to extrapolate the results to humans, one might expect someone with protein malnutrition to have a reduced gland function.

4.2. Vitamin and Mineral Deficiencies

Essential vitamins and minerals must be readily available for optimal gland function. It has been shown that when fed low-calcium diets, rats may develop a salivary secretion dysfunction *(35)*. Vitamin A has also been found to affect the morphology and function of salivary glands in animals *(36,37)*, and it has been observed that vitamin D deficiency reduces parotid gland secretion *(38)*. Different explanations have been suggested, but a function disorder in the salivary gland has been postulated to be the most likely explanation. For vitamin D, it has been proposed that the vitamin is necessary for the synthesis of proteins, which in turn is essential for the utilization of extracellular calcium in the secretion process *(38)*. Other effects of specific nutrient deficiencies on saliva cited in the literature include a reduction in acidic proline-rich proteins in parotid saliva of zinc-deficient rats *(39)* and reduced saliva secretion rate and impaired peroxidase protection in iron-deprived rats *(40)*. It is possible that reduced saliva calcium content may reduce the capacity for the hard tissues to remineralize.

4.3. Effects of Childhood Malnutrition on Saliva

In 8- to 12-yr-old Indian children with moderate to severe PEM, extensive analyses of their salivary production and composition revealed the following findings: (a) a decreased stimulated secretion rate that was related to the severity of PEM, but no difference in unstimulted secretion rate; (b) a lower content of calcium and chloride ions and total protein secretion in stimulated saliva; and (c) impaired immunological and agglutinating defense factors in unstimulated saliva *(41)*. The magnitude of decrease in salivary protein concentration and arginase activity increased with increased severity of PEM, which has led to the suggestion that protein content of saliva and its arginase activity may be used as an index of PEM in the early stages of the disease *(42)*.

4.4. Effects of Adult Moderate Malnutrition on Saliva

In one of the few studies carried out on human adults where a low energy (300 kcal/d) liquid diet was given for 7 d, a reduction in stimulated salivary secretion rate, phosphate, and calcium ion concentrations were found *(43)*. This occurred even when absence of chewing was compensated for. In a previous study by the same investigators, a significant decrease in secretion rate, phosphate, and sialic acid concentration of stimulated whole saliva was observed *(44)*.

5. COMPROMISED NUTRITIONAL WELL-BEING
AND DISORDERS OF THE ORAL MUCOSA

The oral tissues are composed of cells with a rapid turnover and so require a regular adequate supply of nutrients to maintain their integrity. Nutritional deficiencies lead to atrophy of the oral mucosa and can lead to thinning, inflammation, and ulceration of the oral mucosa and loss of filiform papillae on the lingual mucosa, resulting in glossitis (inflammation of the tongue). Nutritional deficiencies also cause atrophy, inflammation, and fissures to the labial mucosa of the lips, and a common feature of compromised nutritional well-being is angular chelitis (sores at the corners of the mouth), largely because of the high turnover of cells in the labial commissures. A suboptimum nutritional status will also increase the susceptibility to oral infections, including candidiasis, and secondary staphylococcal infections to damaged, inflamed tissues. The effects of specific nutritional deficiencies on the oral mucosal tissues are summarized in Table 1.

A deficiency of vitamin B_{12} causes reversible dysplasic changes to the oral mucosa and recurrent ulcers *(45,46)*. A deficiency of thiamine causes burning-mouth syndrome *(47)*, as do deficiencies of riboflavin and B_6 *(48)*. B_{12} deficiency has been associated with stomatitis (inflammation of the oral mucosa), which is common in patients with pernicious anemia.

PEM is associated with a smooth, red glossitis affecting in particular the anterior margins of the tongue. This condition is often referred to as "scarlet tongue." A deficiency of vitamin B_{12} also causes atrophy of the lingual papillae, but the condition responds well to vitamin therapy and is reversed within 3 wk. Glossitis is common in patients with iron deficiency anemia. However, glossitis is an early symptom of iron deficiency appearing prior to anemia. The severity of glossitis in iron deficiency is not as severe as that observed in deficiencies of vitamin B_{12} or folate. Cheilosis, or inflammation of the lips is a common sign of deficiency of the B vitamin complex, being associated with deficiencies of riboflavin, folate, and pyridoxine (Fig. 1).

5.1. Noma

Noma (also known as cancrum oris) is a gangrenous lesion of early childhood in which the perioral flesh is destroyed. The disease is exclusive to malnourished and poor communities and occurs most commonly in Africa, where the prevalence is 1–7 per 1000 population. Cases of noma have also been reported in Asian and Pacific countries *(49)*.

Details of the pathogenesis have been reported elsewhere *(50)*. In brief, compromised nutritional status and/or viral or other infections result in impaired immune function. Next, oral ulcers appear, such as acute ulcerative gingivitis, and these are exacerbated by malnutrition and/or viral infections. The ulcerated tissue provides a site of entry for organisms, including *Fusobacterium necrophorum* and *Prevotella intermedia*, that cause the gangrenous lesion *(51)*. Mortality from noma is very high (70–90%) *(52)*. The after effects are severe aesthetic and functional lesions. The prevention of this disfiguring disease relies on prevention of malnutrition in poor countries.

5.2. Oral Cancer

Cancers of the mouth and pharynx are the fifth most common cancers in the world and the seventh most common causes of death from cancer *(53)*. This is further detailed in

Table 1
The Role of Some Vitamins and Minerals in the Oral Tissues and the Oral Signs of Deficiency

Nutrient	Dietary source	Function	Oral sign of deficiency
Vitamin A	Carotenoids (found in dark-green and yellow fruits and vegetables (not citrus). Preformed vitamin found in oily fish, liver, eggs, and fortified margarine	Epithelial differentiation	Mucosal keratinization and leukoplakia; Cheilitis; Hypoplasia if deficiency occurs during mineralization of the enamel
Thiamin (B$_1$)	Fortified wheat flour and breakfast cereals, milk, eggs, yeast extract	Coenzyme thiamine pyrophosphate functions in energy metabolism	Oral sensitivity; Burning mouth syndrome; Reduced taste perception
Riboflavin (B$_2$)	Dairy products and eggs, fortified breakfast cereals, liver, kidney, and whole grains	Flavoproteins: coenzymes involved in energy metabolism	Angular cheilitis; Glossitis; Recurrent aphthae
Niacin (B$_3$)	Dairy products, liver, meat, eggs, yeast extract, pulses	Nucleotide coenzyme involved in energy metabolism	Mucosal atrophy and stomatitis; Glossitis; Angular cheilitis
Vitamin B$_6$	Liver, meat, fish, whole grains, milk, and peanuts	Coenzyme involved in amino acid metabolism	Glossitis; Cheilitis; Burning mouth syndrome; Ulceration; Lip fissures
Folate	Liver, kidney, green leafy vegetables, oranges, pulses, and fortified breakfast cereals (fortified flour in the United States and Canada)	Purine and pyrimidine synthesis	Glossitis; Stomatosis; Recurrent aphthae; Angular cheilitis; Candidosis
Vitamin B$_{12}$	Meat, fish, eggs, dairy products, fortified breakfast cereals	Purine and pyrimidine synthesis	Atrophic glossitis; Stomatitis; Recurrent aphthae; Dysplasia: Angular cheilitis; Candidosis
Vitamin C	Citrus fruits, berries, potatoes, green vegetables, bell peppers, parsley	Antioxidant involved in redox reactions	Recurrent aphthae; Angular cheilitis; Gingivitis/periodontitis
Vitamin D	Oily fish, fortified margarine, eggs, sunlight	Calcium homeostasis	Hypoplasia if deficiency occurs during tooth mineralization
Vitamin E	Vegetable oils, sunflower seeds, whole grains, eggs	An antioxidant	None
Vitamin K	Vegetables, pulses, liver	Formation of clotting factors	Gingival bleeding; Post extraction hemorrhage
Iron	Meat, fish, dark-green vegetables, pulses, cocoa, fortified breakfast cereals	Hemoglobin and myoglobin formation; enzyme component	Glossitis; Angular cheilitis; Mucosal atrophy (increases susceptibility to carcinoma); Candidosis
Zinc	Shellfish, fish, meat, poultry, dairy products, pulses	A component of >70 enzymes	Taste disturbances
Selenium	Richest source is animal products	Enzyme component in glutathione peroxidase; protects from oxidative damage	May be protective against oral cancer (high levels promote caries)

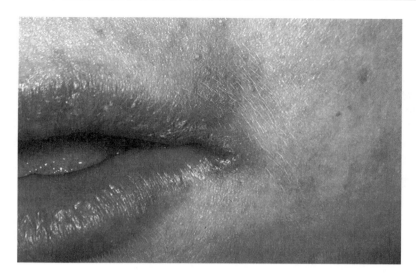

Fig. 1. Angular Cheilitis: vertical fissuring of lips as a consequence of B-vitamin deficiency.

Chapter 12. Oral cancer includes cancer of the tongue, gums, floor of the mouth and other mucosal surfaces, lips, and salivary glands. Oral cancer has a relatively high incidence in developing countries, and recent trends show an increase in Europe, Japan, and Australia. The incidence is generally higher in men than in women. Tobacco use and alcohol are the main etiological factors, causing damage to cells that results in compensatory hyperproliferation and increases the likelihood of unrepaired DNA damage. This damage, across generations of cells, results in an abnormal clone or precancerous lesion (leucoplakia). Leucoplakia is reversible, but further damage will ultimately result in carcinoma.

There has been much research into the associations between diet and oral cancer, including individual micronutrients, food types, and dietary supplementation. Arens *(54)* stated that regional variations in the intake of some micronutrients may be implicated in the geographical distribution of oral cancer in the United Kingdom, and, as early as 1933, Orr *(55)* suggested that the level of fruit and vegetable consumption determined differences in the risk of oral cancer in India.

5.2.1. MINERAL DEFICIENCY AND ORAL CANCER

There is some evidence for an association between deficiency of iron and oral cancer. In Sweden, a fall in the incidence of sideropenic anemia coincided with a fall in the incidence of oral cancer *(56)*. A higher susceptibility to oral cancer is associated with iron-deficiency states *(57)*. Case-control studies are few and show conflicting results: Rich and Radden *(58)* showed that elderly women with oral cancer had lower serum iron status compared with controls. However, Chyou et al. *(59)* found no association between iron status and cancer of the mouth. The evidence is therefore sparse, and the World Cancer Research Fund report "Food Nutrition and the Prevention of Cancer" stated that there was insufficient evidence to draw conclusions regarding iron status and oral cancer.

A few studies have investigated possible associations between selenium status and oral-cancer risk. Rogers found that low selenium concentration of toenails (as an index of status over the past year) was related to increased risk of oral cancer. This relationship was not observed for other minerals, including zinc and calcium *(60)*. Other studies have found low red blood cell concentrations of selenium and higher plasma concentrations of selenium in patients with oral cancer compared with control subjects without cancer *(61)*. In a cohort of US adults, studied between 1974 and 1990, high serum selenium concentrations were associated with increased risk of oral cancer *(62)*. On the basis of the limited number of studies, firm conclusions about the role of selenium in relation to oral cancer risk cannot be drawn.

5.2.2. VITAMIN STATUS AND RISK OF ORAL CANCER

The associations between diet and cancer have been researched for decades; however, most recent interest has focused on a potentially protective role of the antioxidant vitamins A, C, and E and the carotenoids, in particular β-carotene. The antioxidant vitamins scavenge potentially mutagenic free radicals from damaged cells.

Convincing evidence exists largely from case-control studies for a protective role of vitamin C. Overall, studies indicate that vitamin C intakes in the uppermost quartile are associated with half the risk of cancers of the oral tissues *(63–67)*. A low serum concentration of vitamin C has also been found in patients with precancerous oral lesions. Tobacco and alcohol abuse both result in a lower status of vitamin C.

Evidence for an association between vitamin E status and oral cancer is limited. Some studies have found lower serum vitamin E concentrations in patients with oral cancers compared with controls *(68)*, whereas others report no association *(69)*. A limited number of intervention studies show long-term supplementation with vitamin E to reduce risk *(68,70)*.

Case-control studies investigating the association between retinol status and oral cancer and leucoplakia have also produced conflicting results. Some studies found that retinol intakes were positively associated with increased risk *(65,71)*, and others have found low retinol status to be associated with increased risk of oral cancer *(69,72)*.

Precursors of vitamin A can modulate differentiation of the oral mucosa, and retinoids can suppress oral leukoplakia *(73)*. A low intake of carotenoids has been associated with increased risk of oral cancer in a small number of studies in humans *(66)*. A higher incidence of leukoplakia has been reported in subjects with a low carotenoid status *(74,69)*, and intervention studies have shown carotenoids to reduce the occurrence of leukoplakia in humans *(75,76)*. However, intervention with carotenoids in experimental animals has produced mixed results.

A meta-analysis by MacFarlane *(77)*, in which data from several studies were statistically combined to provide an analysis with greater power than any one individual study, looked at the effects of tobacco, alcohol, fruits and vegetables, macronutrients, vitamin C, and nonstarch polysaccharide (dietary fiber) on oral cancer. Dietary fiber and vitamin C status were inversely related to disease risk across study populations, and the greatest reduction in risk from vitamin C occurred in heavy smokers.

5.2.3 LOW INTAKE OF FRUIT AND VEGETABLES AND RISK OF ORAL CANCER

Overall intervention with individual vitamins has produced inconsistent results that suggest that the individual vitamins per se may not be the sole bioactive component and could serve as a marker for other bioactive substances found in the same food sources. This view is supported by the convincing evidence that diets high in fruits and vegetables offer protection against oral cancer, and therefore low intake of fruits and vegetables increases risk for the disease. Some research has investigated the protective role of different types of individual fruits or vegetables.

The protective effect of fruits and vegetables remains after adjusting for tobacco use and alcohol consumption. The majority of studies that have investigated fruits and vegetables as a broad category have found a protective association (64,67,78–80). Likewise, the majority of studies that have specifically looked at fruit have found significant associations between level of intake and oral cancer risk, daily consumption halving the risk compared with less than daily consumption (65,67,80–84). McLaughlin (65) investigated the protective role of a number of fruits and vegetables and found that the strongest protection was offered by fruits.

Considering individual vegetables and fruits, the evidence is most consistent for carrots, citrus fruits, and green vegetables (67,80,82). However, evidence of a protective effect of cruciferous vegetables is not as convincing, with the majority of studies not finding an association (67,84). Francheschi (80) reported a protective effect of green peppers, and Hirayama (85) found a reduced risk of oral cancer with an increased intake of yellow and green vegetables in Japan. In an ecological study of 59 countries that used food intake data from food balance sheets and mortality data from oral cancer, a protective association was found between cabbage consumption and oral cancer. Case-control studies have found conflicting evidence for a protective effect of legume intake on oral cancer (64,67,84). In conclusion, evidence from case-control studies strongly indicates a protective role of fruits and vegetables; however, well-designed dietary intervention studies that prospectively investigate the association between fruit and vegetable intake and risk of oral cancer are required.

6. NUTRITIONAL DEFICIENCIES AND PERIODONTAL DISEASE

Periodontal disease includes the gingival inflammation and the further development of loss of soft-tissue attachment to the tooth and resorption of the alveolar bone, ultimately leading to tooth loss. The disease is found primarily among adults with increased numbers in older age but can also be found in younger individuals (86,87).

Although convincing scientific evidence supports the fact that the pathogenesis of periodontitis involves anaerobic oral bacteria and that tissue damage occurs as a result of the complex interaction between pathogenic bacteria and the host's response to infection, several local and systemic factors are known to be associated with the risk or the severity of the periodontal disease (88,89). Nutrition is known to be important for maintaining periodontal health, and different dietary aspects have been put forward as possible aggravating factors.

The two potential mechanisms in the relation of diet to gingival and periodontal health are diet in relation to plaque formation and the effect of different nutritional deficiencies on the periodontal tissues. Research into the local effect of diet on plaque has focused largely on the effect of an abrasive diet in reducing plaque formation. Although animal studies have shown a relationship between diet and plaque formation (90,91), the significance to humans is questionable because of differences in tooth morphology. It is also unclear whether, in addition to the influence of diet on amount of plaque present, this relationship extends further to influence the development of gingivitis and periodontitis. A more important influence of diet on periodontal health is the relationship between suboptimal nutritional status and periodontal disease, where detrimental metabolic changes associated with compromised nutritional status increase susceptibility to periodontal problems. Attention has been drawn mainly to the role of vitamin C, calcium, vitamin D, and antioxidants in different chronic stages of disease.

6.1. History of Vitamin C and Scurvy

Vitamin C (ascorbic acid) is one of the most well-documented nutrients in relation to periodontal disease, and severe vitamin C deficiency is known to lead to scorbutic gingivitis (scurvy), characterized by ulcerative gingivitis and rapid periodontal pocket development with tooth exfoliation (92). During vitamin C deficiency, a lack of collagen formation and an increase in the permeability of endotoxin from the oral mucosa have been observed in histological studies (93). Studies have demonstrated that vitamin C enhances motility of polymorphonuclear leukocytes, and deficiency therefore decreases host immune responses (94,95). A rapid reduction in bleeding on probing after supplementation with vitamin C has been found, suggesting that the shifts in gingival indices are related to vascular changes or early inflammatory pathways (96). This implies that vitamin C status may influence early stages of gingival inflammation, particularly crevicular bleeding. Another suggested mechanism by which vitamin C depletion influences periodontal health is by decreasing bactericidal activity against *Actinimyces viscosus* (97).

Studies in animals have shown that a diet low in vitamin C increases susceptibility of the periodontium to chronic inflammation (98), and acute vitamin C deficiency increases the permeability of the gingival sulcular epithelium. These are changes that occur prior to development of scorbutic gingivitis (99). The periodontal effects of vitamin C deficiency in humans show contradictory results. Although some epidemiological and experimental evidence has failed to demonstrate any significant etiological relationship between vitamin C deficiency and the periodontal disease (100,101), others have reported a direct relationship between gingival inflammation and vitamin C status (96,102). When the effects of vitamin C depletion and supplementation on periodontal health were studied in experimental conditions in healthy nonsmoking men aged 19–28 yr, it was found that vitamin C deficiency influenced the early stages of inflammation, while no mucosal pathoses or changes in plaque accumulation or probing depths were noted during any of the periods of depletion or supplementation (96). The number of healthy sites observed after supplementation with 600 mg/d of ascorbic acid was reduced during the following period of depletion to 5 mg/d. These results are supported by Leggott et al. (102), who found a significant increase in gingival bleeding after a period with vitamin C depletion, while no significant changes in plaque accumulation, probing pocket depth, or attachment level during the study were found.

6.2. Relevance of Vitamin C Deficiency Today

Acute scurvy is a rare occurrence in industrialized societies; however, studies on vitamin C and its effect on the extracellular matrix and on immunologic and inflammatory responses provide a rationale for hypothesizing that vitamin C is a risk factor for periodontal disease. Epidemiological studies that have examined the relationship between vitamin C and periodontal disease show contradictory results, and there is great controversy concerning the amount of vitamin C necessary for health. The levels of vitamin C required to prevent or cure scurvy could conceivably be quite different from those necessary for the optimal beneficial effects of vitamin C.

The role of dietary vitamin C as a contributing risk factor for periodontal disease has been investigated using data from the Third National Health and Nutrition Examination Survey (NHANES III), and the results have been compared between smokers and non-smokers *(92)*. The periodontal health of 12,419 adults aged 20 or older was compared to their dietary vitamin C intake. The dietary intake of vitamin C showed a statistically significant relationship to periodontal disease in current and former smokers as measured by clinical attachment. It was concluded that those with the lowest intake of vitamin C, and who also smoke, are likely to show the greatest clinical effect on the periodontal tissues. Thus, a weak but significant dose–response increase of risk for periodontal disease in lower vitamin C intake groups was found.

The effect of megadoses of vitamin C on nondeficient individuals has received little attention. A relationship between low levels of vitamin C and impaired wound healing has been demonstrated, and it has been suggested that gingival tissues undergoing healing could benefit from increased levels of vitamin C. In healthy young adult males, classified according to periodontal status, one single intravenous dose of 500 mg of ascorbic acid resulted in statistically significant correlations between gingival status and ascorbic acid levels in whole blood and urine *(103)*. This is in contrast to a more recent study by Woolfe et al. *(104)*, who evaluated the relationship of vitamin C supplementation to gingival clinical parameters. An intake of 1 g vitamin C per day for 6 wk in normal human subjects did not have an effect on the gingival response to initial therapy, and identical gingival responses to periodontal therapy were found in control and vitamin C–supplemented patients. Final blood vitamin C levels appeared to have increased minimally, suggesting that excesses of the vitamin were excreted in the urine. On the basis of the best available evidence, there are no benefits to the periodontal patient of taking vitamin C supplements and the dietary reference intake (DRI) may be easily met through consumption of a healthy, balanced diet.

6.3. Dietary Calcium and Periodontal Disease

Dietary calcium has long been considered a candidate to modulate periodontal disease, and deficiency has been associated with changes in collagen synthesis and structure in oral connective tissue *(105)*. Both animal and human studies have indicated a relationship between calcium intake, bone mineral density (BMD), and tooth loss *(106)*. Calcium deficiency has, in animal studies, been associated with osteopenia or resorption of the alveolar bone *(105,107,108)*. Because calcium intake affects alveolar BMD, it is possible that it also affects periodontal disease, but to what extent has not been elucidated.

Human studies have not been conclusive in establishing a link between periodontal disease and dietary calcium. In a double-blind study, calcium supplementation (1 g) for 180 d without any subsequent periodontal treatment did not influence the periodontal status of patients with moderate to advanced periodontal disease *(109)*. The periodontal status of patients with a low calcium intake did not differ from those receiving adequate calcium. Other studies have reported positive associations between calcium supplementation and periodontal conditions *(110,111)*. Periodontal disease has, in humans, been found to be reversed when the patients were given 1 g calcium per day for 180 d *(111)*.

In a study of more than 12,000 adults, Nishida et al. *(106)* found a statistically significant association between lower dietary calcium intake and periodontal disease in young males and females and for older males. For the females with the lowest level of dietary calcium intake, there was a 54% greater risk of periodontal disease.

6.4. Other Nutrients and Periodontal Disease

A recent study of older adults reported that an intake of calcium and vitamin D, maintained at the US DRI values (in order to prevent osteoporosis) had a beneficial effect on tooth loss *(112)*. However, the number of teeth lost depended on self-reports, and the authors conclude that these findings need to be confirmed in an intervention trial. Although many human studies have evaluated the effect of both calcium and vitamin D deficiency, only a limited number of studies have looked at vitamin D separately. In one of the few studies, young rats were fed diets deficient in calcium, calcium plus vitamin D, or vitamin D *(113)*. Whereas the first two diets resulted in obvious effects on the periodontal tissues, the rats were found to be insensitive to vitamin D deficiency as long as an adequate supply of calcium was available. In one of the few studies evaluating the intake of a wide range of nutrients, dietary protein and vitamin A together with calcium were found to correlate to periodontal disease *(114)*.

6.5. Antioxidant Nutrients and Periodontal Disease

In response to periodontal pathogens, neuthrophils release oxidants, proteinases, and other destructive factors *(115)*. Different antioxidants, present in all body fluids and tissues, may protect against tissue-destructive effects of oxidants. These include, for example, ascorbic acid (vitamin C), α-tocopherol (vitamin E), and β-carotene found in extracellular fluid and dietary-derived components such as uric acid, nonprotein thiols, and glutathione *(116)*. In relation to periodontal disease, it has been found that *P. gingivalis* triggers the release of cytokines, resulting in increased activity of polymorphonucleocytes (PMN) and that increased oxidative damage to gingival tissue, periodontal ligament, and alveolar bone may occur *(116)*. A similar increase in PMN cells has been found after only 3 d plaque accumulation during experimental gingivitis *(117)*.

Data considering antioxidant status and periodontal disease are rare, but a reduced salivary antioxidant activity in patients suffering from periodontal disease has been reported *(116)*. In another study of only 28 healthy and 7 diseased subjects, no difference in salivary antioxidant capacity between diseased and healthy patients was found *(118)*. It has been suggested that an improved understanding of the role that antioxidants play in periodontal health and disease and the influence of diet and nutrition on antioxidant status may lead to a possible nutritional strategy for the treatment of periodontal disease *(116)*. However, there is no evidence to support supplementation with megadoses of antioxidant vitamins; once again, an adequate intake may be obtained by consumption of a healthy, balanced diet.

6.6. Nutrition and Diet in Relation to Dental Plaque

It is important to bear in mind the overall pathogenesis of periodontal disease and that the changes seen may vary both inter- and intraindividually in relation to the presence of dental plaque. Good dietary practices and optimal nutritional status are important in reducing the severity of inflammatory periodontal lesions but are likely to be of limited value if the stimuli from dental plaque are not removed. There is still little knowledge about the interaction between the presence or absence of plaque and coexisitance of nutritional deficiencies. Further studies are needed to clarify the role of nutrition in periodontal disease and to determine the extent to which adequate dietary intake will affect the initiation, progression, or treatment of periodontal disease.

7. SUMMARY OF THE RELEVANCE TO CURRENT-DAY DENTISTRY

Although severe nutritional deficiencies are rare in the Western world, they are commonly found in developing countries. In the latter, oral diseases are not the main target for health authorities where general health aspects take priority. However, it is generally believed that malnutrition impairs innate and adaptive defenses of the host and that the severity of oral infections can be intensified, leading to their development into life-threatening diseases such as noma *(50)*. As one tool in the combat against the different oral diseases discussed in this chapter, an optimal dietary intake of nutrients should be taken care of. Generally optimal oral health, including reduced levels of dental caries and periodontitis, is considered essential in order to retain a high number of teeth into older age and thereby have the ability to consume a healthy, varied diet. There is evidence that loss of teeth may be associated with suboptimal intake of nutrients *(119–121)*.

The primary oral infectious diseases, dental caries and periodontitis, can today be kept at a low level by different preventive tools such as adequate exposure to fluoride, restricted free sugars consumption (with respect to dental caries), and oral hygiene and different antimicrobial agents (with respect to periodontal disease). One may speculate whether the nutritional status is of lesser importance during high preventive measures. Unfortunately, there is still a lack of knowledge to which extent different nutrients interfere with the initiation and progression of certain oral diseases. Little is also known about how this differs among individuals and in relation to variation in a general health perspective. This is of particular interest for the increased number of older persons seen worldwide.

Today, many nutritional aspects are well understood but seldom considered in formulating and executing a treatment plan. Patients may not be aware of the effects of diet and/ or nutritional status on the development and maintenance of a healthy mouth, including teeth free from caries and signs of periodontal disease. It is important that all dental care providers look for potential signs of nutritional deficiencies or nutrition-related problems in all patients, but particularly for those with chronic diseases. The link between nutrition and oral health may vary from subtle to overt.

8. CONCLUSIONS AND RECOMMENDATIONS

An important consideration is that many of the oral consequences of compromised nutritional status discussed in this chapter may themselves directly or indirectly result in an aggravation of the malnutrition. This applies not only to developing low-income countries, because a clear example is the housebound older adult living in industrialized nations. One example is that a poor diet in earlier life results in tooth loss in later life. Tooth loss then limits the diet and compromises nutritional status, which may then predispose to other oral conditions and impaired general health. A second example is a reduced salivary secretion (which is common in older age) that results in sore gingiva and

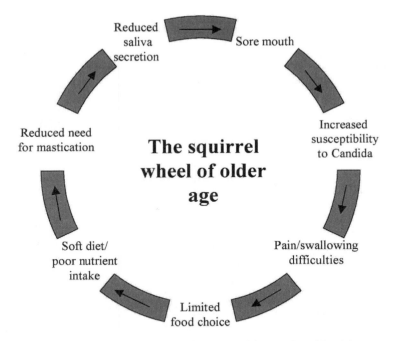

Fig. 2. The squirrel wheel of poor nutrition and oral health.

tongue, which then increases the susceptibility to infections such as candida. This subsequently results in swallowing difficulties and thereby limits dietary intake, further compounding poor nutrition. A reduced food intake of soft character will result in less activity for the salivary glands and a further decrease in saliva flow—the result is a downward spiral, a squirrel-wheel from which it is hard to escape (Fig. 2). Basically, any of the variables listed in the figure can start the wheel to turn.

To summarize the main issues addressed in this chapter:

1. Dental structures are influenced by nutritional status only during the period of tooth formation. Thereafter, deficient nutrition has no direct influence on tooth structure (but may influence the supporting structures of the teeth and the oral mucosa).

2. Adequate early feeding programs in developing countries are important in avoiding enamel defects and compromised salivary secretion, both of which may increase susceptibility to dental caries, the latter having more widespread oral consequences.

3. The early signs of nutritional deficiencies are seen in the oral soft tissues and include thinning, inflammation, and ulceration. Malnutrition also impairs immune responses and may predispose to life-threatening diseases of the oral soft tissues such as noma.

4. Oral cancer is the fifth most common cancer worldwide, and there is good evidence that vitamin C is protective, but evidence for other vitamins is less consistent. However, vitamin C may serve as a proxy for other bioactive components in fruits and vegetables; there is an increasing body of evidence that suggests that diets high in fruits and some vegetables protect against oral cancer.

5. An optimal nutritional status is important in reducing the origin and severity of periodontal disease but is likely to be of limited value if the stimuli from dental plaque are not

removed. Further research is needed in order to identify to what extent dietary modification and/or supplementation will modulate periodontal disease and tooth loss.

6. Nutritional status and oral health are reciprocally related, and each one affects the other—a downturn in nutrition impairs oral function, and this in turn compromises nutritional well-being.

REFERENCES

1. Rugg-Gunn A. Nutrition and Dental Health. Oxford, UK:Oxford University Press, 1993, 15–35.
2. Pindbord J J. Aetiology of developmental enamel defects not related to fluorosis. Int Dent J 1982; 32:123–134.
3. Infante PF, Gillespie GM. An epidemiological study of linear enamel hypoplasia of deciduous anterior teeth in Guatemalan children. Arch Oral Biol 1974; 19:1055–1061.
4. Sweeney EA, Saffir AJ, Leon R. Linear hypoplasia of deciduous incisor teeth in malnourished children. Am J Clin Nutr 1971; 24:29–31.
5. Enwonwu CO. Influence of socio-economic conditions on dental development in Nigerian children. Arch Oral Biol 1973; 18:95–107.
6. Nikiforuk G, Fraser D. The aetiology of enamel hypoplasia: a unifying concept. J Ped 1981; 98:888–893.
7. Rugg-Gunn AJ, Al-Mohammadi SM, Butler TJ. Malnutrition and developmental defects of enamel in 2- to 6- year-old Saudi boys. Caries Res 1998; 32:181–192.
8. Jontell K, Linde A. Nutritional aspects of tooth formation. World Rev NutrDiet 1986; 48:114–136.
9. Mellanby M. An experimental study of the influence of diet on teeth formation. Lancet 1918; 2:767–770.
10. Mellanby M. The role of nutrition as a factor in resistance to dental caries. Br Dent J 1937; 62: 241–252.
11. Mellanby M, Coumoulos H. The improved dentition of 5-year-old London schoolchildren. Br Med J 1944; 1:837–840.
12. Mellanby M, Martin WJ. Dental structure and disease in some 5-year-old Indian school children compared with the same age group in London. Arch Oral Biol 1962; 7:733–750.
13. Cockburn F, Belton NR, Purvis RJ, Giles MM. Maternal vitamin D intake and mineral metabolism in mothers and their newborn infants. Br Med J 1980; 2:11–14.
14. Mellanby M. The relation of caries to the structure of teeth. Br Dent J 1923; 44:1–13.
15. Infante PF, Gillespie GM. Enamel hypoplasia in relation to caries in Guatemalan children. J Dent Res 1977; 56:493–498.
16. Li Y, Navia JB, Bian JY. Caries experience in deciduous dentition of rural Chinese children aged 3–5 years old in relation to the presence or absence of enamel hypoplasia. Caries Res 1996; 30:8–15.
17. Matee MIN, van't Hof MA, Maselle SY, Mitx FHM. Nursing caries, linear hypoplasia and nursing and weaning habits in Tanzanian infants. Comm Dent Oral Epidemiol 1994; 22:289–293.
18. Alvarez JO, Navia JM. Nutritional status, tooth eruption and dental caries: a review. Am J Clin Nutr 1989; 49:417–426.
19. Navia JM, DiOrio LP, Menaker L, Miller J. Effect of undernutrition during the perinatal period on caries development in the rat. J Dent Res 1970; 49:1091–1098.
20. Alvarez JO, Lewis CA, Saman C, et al. Chronic malnutrition, dental caries, and tooth exfoliation in Peruvian children aged 3–9 years. Am J Clin Nutr 1988; 48:368–372.
21. Alvarez JO, Eguren JC, Caceda J, Navia JM. The effect of nutritional status on the age distribution of dental caries in the primary teeth. J Dent Res 1990; 69:1564–1566.
22. Alvarez JO, Dieguez-Marino B, Caceda J, Navia JM. A longitudinal study of infant malnutrition and dental caries. J Dent Res 1991; 70:339, abstr 590.
23. Mellanby M, Pattinson CL. The action of vitamin D in preventing the spread and promoting the arrest of caries in children. Br Med J 1928; 2:1079–1082.
24. Hargreaves JA, Thompson GW. Ultra-violet light and dental caries in children. Caries Res 1989; 23:389–392.
25. Wolbach SB, Howe PR. The incisor teeth of albino rats and guinea pigs in vitamin A deficiency and repair. Am J Pathol 1933; 9:275–294.
26. Salley JJ, Bryson WF, Eshleman JR. The effect of chronic vitamin A deficiency on dental caries in Syrian hamsters. J Dent 1959; 38:1038–1043.

27. Harris SS, Navia JM. Vitamin A deficiency and caries susceptibility of rat molars. Arch Oral Biol 1980; 25:415–421.
28. Johansson I, Alm P. Effect of moderate protein-deficiency on ultrastructure in parotid and submandibular acinar cells in the adult rat. Scand J Dent Res 1989; 97:505–510.
29. Johansson I, Ryberg M. The effects of moderate protein deficiency on β-adrenoceptor density in rat parotid and submandibular salivary glands. Arch Oral Biol 1991; 36:591–594.
30. Johnson DA, Lopez H, Navia JM. Effects of protein deficiency and diet consistency on the parotid gland and parotid saliva of rats. J Dent Res 1995; 74:1444–1452.
31. Menaker L, Navia JM. Effect of undernutrition during the perinatal period on caries development in the rat. 5. Changes in the whole saliva volume and protein content. J Dent Res 1974; 53:592–597.
32. Naini A, Morgan B, Mandel ID. Effect of protein malnutrition on the composition of submandibular glands of aged rats. Arch Oral Biol 1989; 34:985–988.
33. Johansson I, Ericson T. Saliva composition and caries development during protein deficiency and β-receptor stimulation or inhibition. J Oral Pathol 1987; 16:145–149.
34. Anderson LC. Effects of diabetes and dietary manipulation on rat parotid gland secretory response to sympathetic nerve stimulation. Comp Biochem Physiol 1991; 98:363–366.
35. Wang P-L, Shirasu S, Shinohara M, et al. Salivary amylase activity of rats fed a low calcium diet. Jpn J Pharmacol 1998; 78:279–283.
36. Trowbridge HO. Salivary gland changes in vitamin A deficient rats. Arch Oral Biol 1969; 14:891–900.
37. Anzano MA, Lamb AJ, Olsen JA. Impaired salivary gland secretory function following the induction of rapid, synchronous vitamin A deficiency in rats. J Nutr 1981; 111:496–504.
38. Glijer B, Peterfy C, Tenenhouse A. The effect of vitamin D deficiency on secretion of saliva by rat parotid gland in vivo. J Physiol 1985; 363:323–334.
39. Johnson DA, Alvares OF. Zinc deficiency–induced changes in rat parotid salivary proteins. J Nutr 1984; 114:1955–1964.
40. Johansson I, Fagernäs C. Effect of iron-deficiency anaemia on saliva secretion rate and composition in the rat. Arch Oral Biol 1994; 39:51–56.
41. Johansson I, Lenander-Lumikari M, Saellström A-K. Saliva composition in Indian children with chronic protein-energy malnutrition. J Dent Res 1994; 73:11–19.
42. Agarwal PK, Agarwal KN, Agarwal DK. Biochemical changes in saliva of malnourished children. Am J Clin Nutr 1984; 39:181–184.
43. Johansson I, Ericson T. Effect of chewing on the secretion of salivary components during fasting. Caries Res 1986; 20:141–147.
44. Johansson I, Ericson T, Steen L. Studies of the effect of diet on saliva secretion and caries development: the effect of fasting on saliva composition of female subjects. J Nutr 1984; 114:2010–2020.
45. Wray D, Fergason MM, Mason DK, Hutcheon AW, Dagg JH. Recurrent aphthae: treatment with vitamin B$_{12}$, folic acid and iron. Br Med J 1975; 2:490–493.
46. Theaker H, Porter SR. Vitamin B$_{12}$ deficiency and dysplasia of the oral mucosa. Oral Surg Oral Med 1989; 67:81–83.
47. Foy H, Kondi A, Mbaya V. Serum vitamin B$_{12}$ and folate levels in normal and riboflavin deficient baboons. Br J Haematol 1966; 12:239–245.
48. Lamey P, Hammond A, Allan BF, McIntosh WB. Vitamin status of patients with burning mouth syndrome and the response to replacement therapy. Br Dent J 1986; 160:81–83.
49. Bourgeois DM, Leclercq MH. The World Health Organization initiative on noma. Oral Dis 1999; 5:172–174.
50. Enwonwu CO, Phillips RS, Falkler WA Jr. Nutrition and oral infectious diseases: state of the science. Compend Contin Educ Dent 2002; 23:431–448.
51. Costini B, Larroque G, Duboscq JC, Montandon D. Noma or cancrum oris: etiopathogenic and nosologic aspects. Med Trop 1995; 55:263–273.
52. Bourgeois DM, Diallo B, Frieh C, Leclercq MH. Epidemiology of the incidence of orofacial noma: a study of cases in Kakar, Senegal, 1981–1993. Am J Trop Med 1999; 61:909–913.
53. World Cancer Research Fund/American Institute for Cancer. Food, Nutrition and the Prevention of Cancer: A Global Perspective, 1997.

54. Arens U. Oral health, diet and other factors. The Report of the British Nutrition Foundation Task Force. British Nutrition Foundation, 1999.
55. Orr IM. Oral cancer in betel nut chewers in Travancore. Lancet 1933; 2:575–580.
56. Larsson LG, Sandstrom A, Westling P. Relationship of Plummer-Vinson disease to cancer of the upper alimentary tract in Sweden. Cancer Res 1975; 35:3308–3316.
57. Warnakuylasuriya KAAS, Prabhu SR. Anaemia in the tropics. In Prabju SR, Wilson DS, Daftary DK, Johnson NW, eds., Oral Disease in the Tropics. Oxford, UK:Oxford University Press, 1992, 325–339.
58. Rich AM, Radden BG. Squamous cell carcinoma of the oral mucosa: a review of 244 cases in Australia. J Oral Path 1984; 13:459–471.
59. Chyou P, Nomura AM, Stemmermann GN. Diet, alcohol, smoking and cancer or the upper aerodigestive tract: a prospective study among Hawaii Japanese men. Int J Cancer 1995; 60:616–621.
60. Rogers MAM, Thomas DB, Davies S, Weiss NS, Vaughan TL, Nevissi AE. A case-control study of oral cancer and pre-diagnostic concentrations of selenium and zinc in nail tissue. Int J Cancer 1991; 48:182–188.
61. Goodwin W J, Lane H W, Bradford K, et al. Selenium and glutathione peroxidase levels in patients with epidermoid carcinoma of the oral cavity and oropharynx. Cancer 1983; 51:110–115.
62. Zheng W, Blot WH, Diamond EL, et el. Serum, micronutrients and the subsequent risk of oral and pharyngeal cancer. Cancer Res 1993; 53:795–798.
63. Marshall J, Graham S, Mettlin C, Shedd D, Swanson M. Diet in the epidemiology of oral cancer. Nutr Cancer 1983; 5:96–106.
64. Notani PN, Jayant K. Role of diet in upper aerodigestive tracts cancers. Nutr Cancer 1987; 10:103–113.
65. McLaughlin JK, Grindley G, Block G, et al. Dietary factors in oral and pharyngeal cancer. J Natl Cancer Inst 1988; 80:1237–1243.
66. Rossing MA, Baughan TL, McNight B. Diet and pharyngeal cancer. Int J Cancer 1989; 44:593–597.
67. Grindley G, McLaughlin JK, Block G. Diet and oral and pharyngeal cancer among blacks. Nutr Cancer 1990; 14:219–225.
68. Knekt P, Aromaa A, Maatela J, et al. Vitamin E and cancer prevention. Am J Clin Nutr 1991; 53:283S–286S.
69. Ramaswamy G, Rao VR, Kumaraswamy SV, Anatha N. Serum vitamins status in oral leucoplakias: a preliminary study oral oncology. Eur J Cancer 1996; 32B:120–122.
70. Barone J, Taioli E, Herbert JR, Wynder EL. Vitamin supplement use for oral and oesophageal cancer. Nutr Cancer 1992; 18:31–41.
71. Grindley G, McLaughlin JK, Block G, Blot WJ, Gluch M, Fraumeni JF Jr. Vitamin supplement use and reduced risk of oral and pharyngeal cancer. Am J Epidemiol 1992; 135:1083–1092.
72. Middleton B, Byers T, Marshall J, Graham S. Dietary vitamin A and cancer: multisite case control study. Nutr Cancer 1986; 8:106–115.
73. Scully C, Boyle P. Vitamin A related compounds in the chemoprevention of potentially malignant oral lesions and carcinoma. Eur J Cancer 1992; 28B:87–90.
74. Prasad MPR, Krishna TP, Pasricha S, Qureshi MA, Krishnaswamy K. Diet and oral cancer: a case control study. Nutr Cancer 1992; 18:85–93.
75. Stich HF, Rosin MP, Hornby AP, Mathew B, Sankaranarayanan R, Nair MK. Remission of oral leukoplakias and micronuclei in tobacco quid chewers treated with beta-carotene and with beta-carotene plus vitamin A. Int J Cancer 1988; 42:195–199.
76. Garewal HS. Emerging role of beta-carotene and other antioxidant nutrients in prevention or oral cancer. Arch Otolaryn Head Neck Surg 1995; 121:141–144.
77. Macfarlane GJ. The Epidemiology of Oral Cancer. Thesis. Bristol, UK: University of Bristol, 1993.
78. Jafarey NA, Mahmood Z, Savidi SH. Habits and dietary pattern of cases of carcinoma of the oral cavity and oropharynx. J Pak Med Assoc 1977; 27:340–343.
79. Oreggia E, De Stefani E, Correa P, Fierro L. Risk factors for cancer of the tongue in Uruguay. Cancer 1991; 67:180–183.
80. Franceschi S, Barro S, La Vecchia C, Bidoli E, Negri E, Talamini R. Risk factors for cancer of the tongue and mouth a case control study from Northern Italy. Cancer 1992; 70:2227–2233.
81. Winn DM, Zieger RG, Pickle LW, Gridley G, Blot WJ, Hoover RN. Diet in the etiology of oral and opharyngeal cancer among women from southern United States. Cancer Res 1984; 44:1216–1222.

82. Franco EL, Kowalski LP, Oliveira AV, et al. Risk factors for oral cancer in Brazil: a case control study. Int J Cancer 1989; 43:992–1000.
83. La Vecchia C, Negri E, D'Avanzo B, Boyle P, Francheschi S. Dietary indicators of oral and pharyngeal cancer. Int J Epidemiol 1991; 20:39–44.
84. Zheng W, Blot WJ, Shu XV, et al. Risk factors for oral and pharyngeal cancer in Shanghai with emphasis on diet. Cancer Epidemiol Biomarkers Prev 1992: 1:441–448.
85. Hirayama T. A large scale cohort study on cancer risks by diet with special reference to the risk reducing effect of green yellow vegetable consumption. Intl Symp Princess Takamatsu Cancer Res Fund 1985; 16:41–53.
86. Albandar JM, Rams TE. Global epidemiology of periodontal diseases: an overview. Periodontology 2000 2002;29:7–10.
87. Albandar JM, Tinoco EMB. Global epidemiology of periodontal diseases in children and young persons. Periodontology 2002; 29:153–176.
88. Genco RJ. Current view of risk factors for periodontal disease. J Periodontol 1996; 67(Suppl.):1041–1049.
89. Kornman KS, Löe H. The role of local factors in the etiology of periodontal diseases. Periodontology 1993; 2:83–97.
90. Jensen L, Logan E, Finney O, et al. Reduction in accumulation of plaque, stain and calculus in dogs by dietary means. J Vet Dent 1995; 12:161–163.
91. Logan EI, Finney O, Hefferren JJ. Effects of a dental food on plaque accumulation and gingival health in dogs. J Vet Dent 2002; 19:15–18.
92. Nishida M, Grossi SG, Dunford RG, Ho AW, Trevisan M, Genco RJ. Dietary vitamin C and the risk for periodontal disease. J Peridontol 2000; 71:1215–1223.
93. Alfano MC, Miller SA, Drummond JF. Effect of ascorbic acid deficiency on the permeability and collagen biosynthesis of oral mucosal epithelium. Ann NY Acad Sci 1975; 258:253–263.
94. Goetzl EJ, Wasserman SI, Gigli I, Austen KF. Enhancement of random migration and chemotactic response of human leukocytes by ascorbic acid. J Clin Invest 1974; 53:813–818.
95. Sandler JA, Gallin JI, Vaughan M. Effects of serotonin, carbamylchlorine and ascorbic acid on leukocyte cyclic GM and chemotaxis. J Cell Biol 1975; 67:480–484.
96. Leggott PJ, Robertson PB, Rothman DL, Murray PA, Jacob RA. The effect of controlled ascorbic acid depletion and supplementation on periodontal health. J Periodontol 1986; 57:480–485.
97. Goldschmidt MC, Masin WJ, Brown LR, Wyde PR. The effect of ascorbic acid deficiency on leukocyte phagocytisis and killing of *Actinimyces viscous*. Int J Vitam Nutr Res 1988; 58:326–334.
98. Alvares O, Altman LC, Springmeyer S, Ensign W, Jacobson K. The effect of subclinical ascorbate deficiency on periodontal health in nonhuman primates. J Periodontol Res 1981; 16:628–636.
99. Alvares O, Siegel I. Permeability of gingival sulcular epithelium in the development of scorbutic gingivitis. J Oral Pathol 1981; 10:40–48.
100. Ismail AI, Burt BA, Eklund SA. Relation between ascorbic acid intake and periodontal disease in the United States. J Am Dent Assoc 1983; 107:927–931.
101. Vogel RI, Lamster IB, Wechsler SA, Macedo B, Hartley LJ, Macedo JA. The effects of megadoses of ascorbic acid on PMN chemotaxis and experimental gingivitis. J Periodontol 1986; 57:472–479.
102. Leggott PJ, Robertson PB, Jacob RA, Zambon JJ, Walsh M, Armitage GC. Effects of ascorbic acid depletion and supplementation on periodontal health and subgingival microflora in humans. J Dent Res 1991; 70:1531–1536.
103. Shannon IL, Gibson WA. Intravenous ascorbic acid loading in subjects classified as to periodontal status. J Dent Res 1965; 44:355–361.
104. Woolfe SN, Kenney EB, Hume WR, Carranza FA Jr. Relationship of ascorbic acid levels of blood and gingival tissue with response to periodontal therapy. J Clin Periodontol 1984; 11:159–165.
105. Oliver WM, Leaver AG, Scott PG. The effect of deficiencies of calcium or of calcium and vitamin D on the rate of oral collagen synthesis in the rat. J Period Res 1972; 7:29–34.
106. Nishida M, Grossi SG, Dunford RG, Ho AW, Trevisan M, Genco RJ. Calcium and the risk for periodontal disease. J Periodontol 2000; 71:1057–1066.
107. Henrikson PA. Periodontal disease and calcium deficiency: an experimental study in the dog. Acta Odontol Scand 1968; 26(Suppl. 50):1–132.

108. Lundgren S, Rosenquist JB. Short term bone healing in calcium deficiency osteopenia and disuse osteopenia: experimental studies in adult rats. Scand J Dent Res 1992; 100:337–339.

109. Uhrbom E, Jacobson L. Calcium and periodontitis: clinical effect of calcium medication. J Clin Periodontol 1984; 11:230–241.

110. Spiller WF Jr . A clinical evaluation of calcium therapy for periodontal disease. Dent Digest 1971; 77:522–526.

111. Krook L, Lutwak L, Whalen JP, Henrikson P, Lesser GV, Uris R. Human periodontal disease: morphology and response to calcium therapy. Cornell Vet 1972; 62:32–53.

112. Krall EA, Wehler C, Garcia RI, Harris SS, Dawson-Hughes B. Calcium and vitamin D supplements reduce tooth loss in the elderly. Am J Med 2001; 111:452–456.

113. Oliver WM. The effect of deficiencies of calcium, vitamin D or calcium and vitamin and of variations in the source of dietary protein on the supporting tissues of the rat molar. J Peridont 1969; 4:56–59.

114. Freeland JH, Cousins RJ, Schwartz R. Relationship of mineral status and intake to periodontal disease. Am J Clin Nutr 1976; 29:745–749.

115. Enwonwu CO. Interface of malnutrition and periodontal diseases. Am J Clin Nutr1995; 61(Suppl.): 430S–436S.

116. Sculley DV, Langley-Evans SC. Salivary antioxidants and periodontal disease status. Proc Nutr Soc 2002; 61:137–143.

117. Zhang J, Kashket S, Lingström P. Evidence of the early onset of gingival inflammation following short-term plaque accumulation. J Clin Peridontal 2002; 29:1082–1085, 2003; 30:278.

118. Moore S, Calder KAC, Millar NJ, Rice-Evans CA. Antioxidant activity of saliva and periodontal disease. Free Radic Res 1994; 21:417–425.

119. Carlos JP, Wolfe MD. Methodological and nutritional issues in assessing the oral health of aged subjects. Am J Clin Nutr 1989; 50(Suppl.):1210–1218, 1231–1235.

120. Steele JG, Sheiham A, Marcenes W, Walls AWG. National diet and nutrition survey: people aged 65 and over. 2. Report of the oral health survey. London, UK: The Stationary Office, 1998.

121. Moynihan PJ, Butler T J, Thomason J M, Jepson NJA. Nutrient intake in partially dentate patients: the effect of prosthetic rehabilitation. J Dent 2000; 28:557–563.

8

Nutritional Consequences of Oral Conditions and Diseases

A. Ross Kerr and Riva Touger-Decker

1. INTRODUCTION

Oral health status is influenced by numerous oral diseases and conditions, including loss of teeth and supporting dental alveolar bone, xerostomia, loss of taste and smell, orofacial pain, oral movement disorders, and others. Other major factors include general health, socioeconomic status (SES), nutritional well-being, and dietary habits *(1)*. Diseases of the oral cavity, both local and systemic, can have a significant impact on ability to consume an adequate diet and consequently maintain optimal nutrition status. The impact of tooth loss, edentulism, and removable prostheses on dietary habits, diet adequacy, masticatory function, olfaction, and gastrointestinal (GI) disorders has been documented *(2–11)*. Inadequate intake of fruits, vegetables, and whole grains is common in edentulous individuals or those individuals with maxillary and mandibular complete dentures, resulting in an inadequate intake of dietary fiber and vitamins A and C *(5,9,10)*. Disorders of taste and smell can affect appetite and salivary flow and compromise dietary intake. Orofacial pain, salivary disorders, and oral movement disorders can also have a negative impact on appetite and impair normal oral function and eating ability. The relationship between oral disease and nutrition is synergistic. Oral diseases, along with acute, chronic, and terminal systemic diseases with oral manifestations, impact functional ability to eat as well as nutritional well-being *(11)*.

1.1. Nutrition Consequence Following Physical Loss of Masticatory Apparatus

1.1.1. TOOTH AND ALVEOLAR BONE LOSS AND THE EFFECTS OF DENTAL REHABILITATION

Data from the third National Health and Nutrition Examination Survey (NHANES III) conducted from 1988 to 1991 showed that approx 60% of US adults were missing at least one tooth, and 10% were edentulous *(12)*. Rates of edentulism correlated strongly with age, with the average number of teeth and a rate of edentulism in the over-75 age group estimated to be nine teeth per person and 44%, respectively. Despite the increasing number of senior citizens, the rate of tooth loss and edentulism has been declining and

From: *Nutrition and Oral Medicine*
Edited by: R. Touger-Decker, D. A. Sirois, and C. C. Mobley © Humana Press Inc., Totowa, NJ

is estimated to drop by approx 50% over the next 30 yr *(13)*. Nevertheless, a significant number of adults, particularly the elderly, have tooth loss in the United States today, and it is natural to hypothesize that this group is at nutritional risk *(11)*. Moynihan demonstrated that edentulous patients have about one-fifth the chewing ability of their dentate counterparts *(8)*. Many consume increasing amounts of medications (including laxatives and anti-reflux agents) for GI disorders *(14)*.

Many studies have clearly established that masticatory function is reduced following tooth loss *(2,3,9,10,15)*. Masticatory function is measured experimentally by assessing the particle-size distribution of food when chewed for a given number of strokes, often to the point before swallowing (masticatory performance), by counting the number of strokes to reduce a food to a given particle size (masticatory efficiency), or by the force exerted during chewing (masticatory force). Using the Swallowing Threshold Test Index to measure masticatory performance of a test food in four dentition status groups of all ages (intact [14–16 teeth bilaterally], partially compromised [10–13 teeth on one side and 14–16 teeth on the other], compromised [10–13 teeth bilaterally], and a complete denture group), there was a graded reduction in masticatory function with progressive loss of dentition, with denture wearers showing the poorest performance *(2)*. Persons with intact dentitions, followed closely by persons with partially compromised dentitions (with or without removable partial dentures), on average demonstrated a superior level of masticatory performance (>80%), compared to persons with compromised dentition or complete denture wearers, who demonstrated significantly lower and inadequate performance (<80%) *(3)*. A study employing two different methodologies to measure masticatory function yielded similar findings *(9)*, although it was observed that some persons with complete dentures had a high degree of function, comparable to persons with intact dentitions. This wide variation in masticatory performance was demonstrated in 367 subjects with complete dentures. Approximately half of these subjects demonstrated inadequate performance, primarily because of lack of satisfaction secondary to poor denture stability *(10)*.

In the clinical setting, however, masticatory function is not measured. It is incumbent on the practitioner to ask the patient simple questions about his or her eating ability *(16)*. Such questions (*see* Chapter 17) are as follow:

- Do you have any difficulty biting, chewing, swallowing foods?
     If yes, specify biting, chewing, swallowing (which one[s])?
     If yes, what specific foods are difficult?
- If you wear dentures, do you keep them in your mouth for eating?
     Which ones do you remove and why?

In patients with complete dentures, masticatory function is increased following replacement by implant-borne prostheses or by functionally corrected new dentures *(17)*, although it does not return to the performance levels seen in patients with an intact dentition. Allen and McMillan *(18)* compared individuals receiving implant-supported dentures, fixed bridges, and complete conventional dentures. Although individuals who received implant-supported dentures showed improved ability to chew as compared to the other two groups, food selection habits did not increase significantly in this group as compared to the other groups. These findings confirm those of others *(19,20)* that improvement in chewing ability does not necessarily mean improved dietary habits; individualized diet counseling may be needed in order to improve food choices.

Masticatory ability is subjective and relates to both the individual's self-assessed biting or chewing function and associated food preferences. Masticatory ability is correlated with masticatory function. Using surveys to assess perceived chewing difficulty and food acceptance (taste, texture, and frequency of ingestion) of 13 test foods with differing chewing hardness, it was demonstrated that both perception of chewing ability (2) and food acceptance (3) are correlated with masticatory function, with the greatest effect seen in edentulous persons. Younger patients (under 50 yr old) with compromised dentitions demonstrated increased perceived chewing difficulty compared to older patients, indicating adaptation over time (20). In a study (20) exploring diet adequacy and nutrition risk status before and after denture insertion in individuals getting new complete dentures, diet adequacy was assessed using a 3-d food diary, and nutrition risk status was determined using the Nutrition Screening Initiative (21) DETERMINE Checklist. Three months after denture insertion, 45% of the patients were at moderate nutrition risk; the three most common risk factors were eating alone (63%), living alone (45.6%), and continued tooth or mouth problems making eating difficult (40.4%). Diet adequacy compared to the food guide pyramid was poor; intake of all food groups with the exception of fats, sweets, and oils was below the recommended number of servings for all groups. Mean values for calcium, zinc, and vitamin B_6 was below the recommended daily allowances (RDA). Despite new dentures, 40% of subjects continued to experience perceived difficulty biting and chewing. This study demonstrated that although new dentures may improve functional chewing ability, they do not necessarily yield improved patient perception of chewing ability or improved diet quality.

Given that many foods with high nutrient value, such as fruits and vegetables, are more difficult to chew, the hypothesis that reduced masticatory function and ability can have a deleterious impact on nutritional intake seems strong, yet these relationships have been difficult to prove, and the conclusions of numerous studies remain equivocal. The field of dietary analysis is evolving, and many of the early studies assessing nutritional status in subjects with tooth loss are methodologically flawed, including cross-sectionally rather than longitudinally designed studies, lack of power because of small sample size, inadequate or inconsistent nutritional data collection or analysis, and failure to control or adjust for numerous potential confounding factors (such as age, gender, SES, caloric intake, medical status and medications, smoking, alcohol intake, salivary flow, anthropometric data). It is also difficult to compare results from studies because of a wide variation in both population composition (independent or free-living vs institutionalized, elderly vs adult, low vs high SES, and a myriad of populations categorized by discrete vs continuous variables of dentition or masticatory functional status) and nutritional assessment (single nutrient vs dietary pattern methods of measuring nutritional intake, comparison to control groups or RDA values, and inclusion vs exclusion of various objective measures of overall nutritional status). Furthermore, nutritional status is itself a risk factor for tooth loss, and the impact of poor dietary habits preceding tooth loss may perpetuate following tooth loss and replacement.

Shinkai et al. used the Interactive Healthy Eating Index as a measurement of diet quality in assessing dentition and nutrition status; results showed that diet quality did not differ by dentition status in a heterogeneous group of 731 independently living subjects (22). Oral function was not a predictor of overall diet quality in this study. Several studies have found significant changes in nutritional intakes in subjects with compromised dentitions (21–24). The design of the first NHANES, a large cross-sectional study of 13,479 adults aged 18–74 yr, included a 24-h dietary recall and collected information about tooth loss. Controlling for multiple variables, results indicated edentulous adults had significantly lower intakes of vitamin C, protein, and iron, and a lower consumption of fruits and vegetables compared to adults with teeth (23).

The Health Professionals Follow-Up Study collected information from 49,501 subjects to assess the nutritional consequences of tooth loss (25). Data collected included demographic and behavioral traits, number of teeth, medical history, and the estimated intake frequency of 131 food items over a 1-yr period. This approach was validated by collecting detailed 2-wk recalls from 127 subjects and showed Pearson correlation coefficients ranging from $r = 0.64$–0.77 for various nutrients. The nature of the population facilitated valid data and, in addition, the investigators adjusted for total calorie intake and other potential confounders. Edentulous subjects consumed, on average, significantly less dietary fiber, carotene, vegetables, fresh apples, pears, and carrots, and consumed more saturated fat and cholesterol compared to subjects with 25 or more teeth. The actual differences in intake between these two groups were relatively small, ranging from 2 to 13%, although, because of the higher SES and access to dental care of the patient population studied, the differences in the general population are likely to be higher. Papas et al. (26) studied nutrition and dentition status in 691 subjects in New England. All were over 60 yr old and the population was 95% white. Individuals who reported difficulty biting, chewing, and swallowing were more likely (80 vs 60% in males, 75 vs 66% in females) to wear dentures. Denture wearers had lower intakes of calories, protein, and folate than nonwearers.

In a cohort of 490 British seniors, the nutrient intake was associated with dental status (27). Nutritional intake was measured by 4-d recall and hematologic and biochemical measurement of various nutrients. Confounding factors were controlled by multivariate analysis. Edentulous independently living subjects consumed fewer calories, protein, intrinsic and milk sugars, fiber, calcium, nonheme iron, niacin, and vitamin C compared to dentate subjects. Only plasma nutrient levels of vitamin C and retinol were significantly reduced in the edentulous group. Fiber and sugar intake was significantly associated with both the number of teeth and occluding pairs of posterior teeth.

The health-related consequences of the nutritional differences in intake because of dentition status in the previously cited studies suggest that edentulous persons may be at higher risk for cardiovascular or GI diseases and cancer, along with increased associated morbidity and mortality. Persons with deficient masticatory function were shown to be more likely to have GI disorders, as concluded in a study of 367 elderly noninstitutionalized people, linking poor masticatory performance to a significantly increased prevalence in the use of medications to treat GI disorders (10). In a study evaluating the relationships between a functional measure of dental status, a nutritional intake profile, and mortality in a cohort of 1189 elderly community subjects in Italy, the authors concluded that dental status is among the major nutritional predictors of long-term mortality (28).

Although eating ability may impact food choices, the reported relationships between dentition status and nutrition status and diet adequacy has been variable for many reasons. A primary consideration not often cited is behavior patterns relative to food choices, which are difficult to change (18). Individuals with compromised dentition adjust their eating habits over time; once new dentures are placed, despite instructions, they may rely on previous eating habits, food preferences, and patterns because it has been typical behavior for an extended time period. In some instances, individuals may be afraid to try to eat a greater variety of foods that are perceived to be difficult to chew. The duration for all of the studies cited has been short; a longitudinal study of individuals with compromised dentition would more accurately characterize the impact of compromised dentition on morbidity, mortality, and disease risk. Despite the lack of adequate longitudinal data, the impact of compromised dentition on food habits is well documented. It is imperative for dietitians and dental practitioners to address dietary habits in the office setting. It is of vital importance to question all patients regarding perceived ability to bite, chew, and swallow foods, changes in eating habits secondary to oral dysfunction, and reasons why their eating habits have changed (*see* Chapter 17). Following insertion of permanent or removable prostheses, dental practitioners should instruct patients on a balanced diet and discuss how their ability to bite, chew, and swallow has been modified (*see* Chapter 3). Follow-up visits should include questions on changes in eating habits and reasons why or why not eating ability has or has not changed. Early intervention and frequent follow-up can help promote adjustment to a varied, balanced diet for individuals of all ages. Dietetics practitioners should question patients about use of removable prostheses, examine the dentition to note presence and degree of edentulism, and counsel patients accordingly as well as refer patients as needed to dentists.

1.2. Loss of Jaw or Soft Tissues (Tongue/Palate/Floor of Mouth/ Oropharynx)

Loss of jaw or soft tissues may occur congenitally, the most common example being cleft lip or palate, or following surgical resection of head and neck tumors. The nutritional impact of cleft lip or palate can be severe if a newborn is unable to feed, particularly because these babies have a low birthweight. The combined use of a palatal obturator and lactation education has been shown to reduce feeding time, increase volume intake, decrease infant fatigue, and result in favorable growth (29). Alternatively, when bottle feeding is preferred, successful feeding has been obtained using either a standard glass baby bottle with a crosscut nipple (30,31) or a squeezable cleft palate nurser (31) and feeding the infant in the sitting position and burping frequently.

A team approach to management is critical for optimal systemic, oral, and nutritional well-being. Dental, medical, and dietetics professionals along with the caregiver can plan strategies to achieve optimal dietary intake during all phases of rehabilitation.

Approximately 30,000 Americans are diagnosed with oropharyngeal cancer annually. Treatment involves a number of modalities including surgical resection, radiotherapy, and, in some cases, chemotherapy. More than 60% of patients with oropharyngeal cancer have advanced disease at the time of diagnosis (32) and up to 30–50% of this population are malnourished (33), presumably because of the increased metabolic requirements and the impact of tumor growth on the masticatory apparatus. Diet and nutrition issues of cancers of the head, neck, and oral cavity are addressed in Chapter 12.

1.3. Nutrition Consequence of Oral Pain

1.3.1. Odontogenic Pain

Odontogenic pain may arise as a result of disease or injury to the dental pulp or the periodontal apparatus. Patients with early pulpal disease, known as reversible pulpitis, have symptoms of a fleeting sharp pain elicited by exposure to a stimulus such as cold or sweet. Chronic and untreated pulpal disease progresses to an irreversible pulpitis, a condition resulting in pulpal death. This produces symptoms of poorly localized lingering pain described as boring or gnawing. It is aggravated by eating or exposure to a cold stimulus, as well as by lying down (i.e., many patients awake from their sleep with pulpitis pain). Pulpitis progression produces even more pain, frequently severe in nature, aggravated by heat, and often relieved by application of cold. Occasionally, chronic pulpitis results in the spontaneous development of pain. Pulpal death and necrosis can lead to an acute apical periodontitis and an acute apical abscess, both of which may cause a severe throbbing pain localized to the tooth involved, and regional lymphadenopathy. Ultimately, the abscess can disseminate into a cellulitis and fascial space infection, which will cause facial swelling, pain in the regional lymph nodes, fever, malaise, difficulty eating or opening the mouth, and dysphagia. In extreme cases, the infection and affiliated inflammatory products can become life threatening if vital structures become involved (e.g., dyspnea caused by compromised airway, infection of mediastinum, cavernous sinus). Periodontal pain is usually associated with an acute periodontal abscess, which can also result in serious sequelae.

Because odontogenic pain is generally acute in nature, prompt and effective treatment by tooth restoration, root-canal therapy, extraction, or periodontal curettage will result in the resolution of pain. As such, the nutritional impact is generally short-lived unless the treatment for the pain results in loss of teeth and associated sequelae (*see* Section 1.1.1.). However, in patients who are at risk for or have malnutrition and/or lack access to emergency care, the inability to chew may have a pronounced nutritional impact. Appetite and eating may be compromised by frequent use of analgesics, which may impact GI function and/or narcotics used for severe pain, which may diminish appetite (*see* Chapter 6).

1.3.2. CHRONIC OROFACIAL PAIN

In chronic pain disorders such as myofascial pain (MFP), eating ability may be hampered by pain. In studies of individuals with MFP, masticatory muscle function may fatigue more quickly than in individuals without MFP and raise pain scores *(34,35)*. Raphael et al. *(35)* studied patients with MFP; of 61 participants, 88.5% indicated difficulty chewing, 86.9% indicated difficulty eating hard foods, and 24.6% indicated difficulty eating soft foods. A trend, although not significant, was found for individuals who reported eating difficulty for hard foods; these subjects consumed a greater percentage of calories from protein. Those who experienced difficulty eating soft foods when compared to those who did not report this difficulty had a reduced intake of total calories (although not significant). Although comparison of the macro- and micronutrient intake of MFP patients to the US population revealed no significant difference in nutrient intake per se, when multiple linear regression was used, a significant difference in dietary fiber intake was noted for individuals with higher pain levels. There was a significant negative relationship between pain severity and dietary fiber intake ($p < 0.01$). The results of this study supported the concept that intake of high-fiber foods is more difficult for individuals with MFP. Dietary recommendations for patients with MFP should include high-fiber foods that do not require extensive masticatory function.

1.3.3. MUCOSAL PAIN

Oral or pharyngeal mucosal pain can result from a number of different disorders and can be categorized as acute or chronic. Mucosal pain generally occurs following the erosion or ulceration of the epithelium, leading to the exposure of the underlying mucosal nociceptors and, depending on the etiology, a variable release of mediators of inflammation that further sensitize the exposed nociceptors. Common causes for acute mucosal pain in otherwise well-nourished immunocompetent patients include traumatic ulcerations secondary to ill-fitting dentures, faulty restorations, or sharp teeth; minor recurrent aphthous stomatitis (also known as canker sores); mucosal burning secondary to xerostomia or candidiasis; and herpes virus infections, of which intraoral herpes simplex (HSV) or varicella zoster virus (VZV) infections are the most common. Many of these conditions are short-lived (7–10 d), self-limiting, or easily treated, and have minimal nutritional impact.

However, nutritional consequences are far more likely in mucosal disorders that take longer than 2 wk to resolve, recur frequently, are not self-limiting without treatment, are so severe that eating and swallowing solid food is impossible, or, if they occur in patients who are predisposed to malnutrition such as the elderly or other immunocompetent patients. Recurrent aphthous stomatitis can result in delayed healing, particularly if the ulcers are large, occur in crops, or recur frequently.

Erosive lichen planus, oral mucous membrane pemphigoid, pemphigus vulgaris, and a number of other rare immune-mediated disorders can involve multiple sites on the oropharyngeal mucosa, and, unless they are treated successfully, mastication and swallowing can be severely compromised. Infectious diseases, normally self-limiting in the immunocompetent patient, can become widespread and may lead to severe oral mucosal pain. Examples include viral infections such as HSV, VZV, and cytomegalovirus; fungal infections such as candidiasis and deep fungal infections; and bacterial infections such as necrotizing ulcerative gingival or periodontal infections. Disorders related to human immunodeficiency virus (HIV) are addressed in Chapter 13; lesions associated with autoimmune diseases are discussed in Chapter 14.

In all of these disorders, diet management should be individualized on the basis of the location and extent of the lesion(s). Use of a straw may be helpful to avoid contact of liquids with lesions. Common themes in diet management for individuals with mucosal lesions are as follows:

- try foods at room temperature or cool; avoid extremes in temperature, hot or cold;
- avoid citrus and acidic juices and fruits including oranges, grapefruit, lemon, lime, tomato, and pineapple;
- use herbs instead of spices and hot sauces for seasoning;
- keep foods easy to chew, limiting rough textured foods such as bread crusts, bagels, pretzels, crackers, chips, nuts, fruit skins, and salads;
- try fruit smoothies: frozen fruit (berries, bananas, melon) and milk or yogurt in the blender;
- try mild gravies;
- cut all food well prior to eating; and
- keep a water bottle handy at all times; drink with and between meals and snacks.

Clinical features and their associated oral findings and disorders, along with nutritional considerations, are addressed in Table 1.

Table 1
Abnormal Oral Findings: Associated Local and Systemic Diseases

Clinical feature	Associated finding	Associated disorders	Nutritional considerations
Xerostomia	Excessive dental caries, candidiasis, dysphagia, dysgeusia, burning mouth or tongue	Drug-induced xerostomia, head and neck irradiation, Sjögren's syndrome, diabetes	Increase fluids, minimize cariogenic foods, modify food consistency and flavoring, evaluate glucose control in diabetes
Burning mouth or tongue	May be associated with mucosal erythema or atrophy, glossitis	Anemia, diabetes, candidiasis	Determine etiology of anemia (iron, folate, B_{12}), modify food consistency and flavoring, evaluate glucose control
Angular cheilitis	Dry, cracked, fissured corner of the mouth	Dehydration, anemia, ill-fitting dentures (drooling)	Determine etiology
Candidiasis	White and/or red removable patches on the oral mucosa	Immunodeficiency, diabetes	Determine etiology
Difficulty chewing	Partial or complete edentulism, poor occlusion, ill-fitting dentures	Cranial nerve disorders (*see* Appendix D)	Determine etiology, referral for medical nutrition therapy

136

1.4. Nutritional Consequences of Oral Movement Disorders (e.g., Parkinson's)

Patients with oral movement disorders may be at risk for nutritional consequences. Many oral movement disorders are associated with pathologic alterations in the basal ganglia or their neuronal interconnections, although some are less clearly understood. Movement disorders are characterized either by an excess of movement (hyperkinesia or dyskinesia) or by a paucity of movement (hypokinesia or bradykinesia). Different neurological diseases may be characterized clearly by one type of dyskinesia (e.g., tics associated with Tourette's syndrome) or by a combination of overlapping movement disorders (e.g., dystonia, resting tremor, and bradykinesia associated with Parkinson's disease [PD]). In descending order of prevalence, the most common movement disorder is essential tremor, followed by PD, dystonia, and drug-induced dyskinesias.

Of the little research carried out in this area, most has focused on PD, a slowly progressive and debilitating degenerative disease caused by destruction in the dopaminergic neurons in the substantia nigra of the brain. Patients with PD have muscular rigidity (leading to difficulty in cutting up and moving food into their mouths, and chewing), difficulty swallowing (characterized by increased transit time and impaired tongue coordination), and diminished smell, and eventually they develop dementia. Furthermore, the medications they take, especially levodopa, can lead to xerostomia and GI sequelae such as nausea, vomiting, or constipation. All of these are risk factors for malnutrition, and these patients are often underweight and or malnourished.

Damage to the developing central nervous system may result in significant impairment in oral–motor function and can potentially contribute to feeding difficulty in disabled children and result in nutritional impairment. Early recognition, assessment, and treatment of an infant with neurological impairment that is compromising the normal feeding process is crucial. The elderly may be at risk for age-related diminution of oral–motor function *(36)*.

1.5. Nutritional Consequences of Xerostomia

Salivary hypofunction is estimated to affect approx 5% of the US population *(37)*, primarily the elderly, and has multiple causes including medical problems, medications (including antidepressants, anticholinergics, antispasmodics, antihistamines, antihypertensives, sedatives, and others), head and neck radiotherapy, and Sjögren's syndrome. Healthy saliva production is essential to the protection of the oral mucosae and teeth and for taste perception, food bolus formation, swallowing, speech, and early digestion. Hyposecretion of saliva exemplifies the importance of salivary flow: it causes food to stick to oral structures and compromises a person's ability to swallow food; predisposes persons to dental caries, which can result in dental pain and infection; causes hypogeusia or dysgeusia; and puts persons at risk for candidiasis, which can cause mucosal burning. Quality of life and nutritional intake can be affected by xerostomia. Although salivary function remains intact in healthy elderly persons *(38)*, the elderly population has a higher prevalence of the risk factors for xerostomia, and most of the research linking xerostomia to nutritional consequences is focused on this population, particularly in the institutionalized elderly. Sjögren's syndrome is an autoimmune exocrinopathy that is in part characterized by severe salivary hypofunction caused by infiltration of lymphocytes into the salivary gland parenchyma (*see* Chapter 14).

This disease serves as a good model for xerostomia. Elderly patients (>65) with this disease were shown to have significantly lower nutritional intake compared to nonxerostomic controls *(39)*. In a study of 28 free-living patients diagnosed with Sjögren's syndrome and abnormal unstimulated and stimulated salivary flow rates were matched (for age, medical conditions, and medication usage, and anthropometric data) with 24 control subjects with salivary flow rates greater than 0.5 ml/min; subjects, however, were not matched for other potentially important confounding factors such as masticatory function. A 5-d dietary record and patient interview was conducted. Not only did the xerostomia group show a significant reduction in intake of all 12 nutrients evaluated (in particular, fiber, potassium, zinc, and vitamin B_6) compared to the control group, but their intakes were also below RDA levels.

Xerostomia is potential major contributing etiological factor for nutritional deficiencies in the elderly *(40)*. Dietary intake of 43 elderly institutionalized subjects from an extended-care facility (21 subjects with sialometry-proven xerostomia and 22 closely matched control subjects without xerostomia) was analyzed based on a 5-d food diary. All meals were identical, and a videotape was taken to ensure documentation of all dietary intakes. Additional data collected by interview included food preferences, taste perception, self-perception of health, medication usage, and a number of anthropometric measurements used to assess nutritional status (height, weight, body composition, and body mass index [BMI]). There was a markedly greater proportion of subjects in the xerostomia group who had diets deficient in nutrients. Furthermore, in contrast to the control group in which no subject complained about the food, all of the xerostomic institutionalized subjects perceived the taste and quality of the food to be poor. Anthropomorphic measures revealed a significantly lower BMI in the xerostomic subjects compared to the control group, and abnormal serum albumin levels (an index of protein nutriture) were below normal in more than 50% of the xerostomic patients compared to only one subject from the control group. Because nutritional deficits are not uncommon in the free-living elderly population, the investigators also performed a nutritional assessment and interviews on 24 xerostomic free-living seniors and found that this group had a similar prevalence of nutritional deficits in their diets. It is, however, important to distinguish between dietary nutrient deficits and frank nutritional deficiencies. Recognition of dietary nutrient deficits early can prevent the development of frank nutrient deficiencies.

Sialometry-proven xerostomia was a significant risk factor for malnutrition in a cohort of 99 Swiss elderly, nonpsychiatric, hospitalized patients with a variety of medical conditions *(41)*. There was a significant association between symptoms of oral dryness in 51% of the cohort (e.g., dry mouth during the day, difficulty speaking, frequent water intake, and problems with denture wear) and abnormal unstimulated flow (<0.1 mL/min) in 17% and stimulated flow (<0.5 mL/min) in 26% of the cohort, respectively. The subjects with reduced flow rates demonstrated a significant reduction in anthropometric measures of nutrition status (BMI, triceps skin thickness, and arm circumference) and serum albumin levels compared to the subjects in the cohort with normal salivary flow tests.

Diet management guidelines for xerostomia may be found in the appendix. Of central importance is the need for individuals to keep a water bottle around at all times and practice good oral hygiene. Frequent rinsing with plain water will prevent accumulation of food remnants, particularly fermentable carbohydrates in the oral cavity, which could lead to increased caries risk. Dental and dietetics practitioners should provide patients with guidelines and refer to each other as needed to maximize patient care.

1.6. Nutritional Consequences of Diminished Taste and Smell

Adjusted national estimates of the 1994 Disability Supplement to the National Health Interview Survey reported prevalence rates of 1.4 and 0.6% for olfactory and gustatory problems, respectively, that these rates increase exponentially with age *(42)*, and that olfactory function may decline with age more than taste. Risk factors for diminished taste and smell include nervous system disorders, chronic renal and liver disease, endocrine disorders, medication use, and a multitude of disorders affecting the nasal and oropharyngeal regions *(43)*. Our capacity to taste and smell allows us to distinguish the flavor and aroma of foods or drinks, whether pleasant or unpleasant. Indeed, alterations in these senses significantly impact our quality of life *(44)*.

The clinical assessment of olfaction begins with threshold and suprathreshold testing, usually with phenyl ethyl alcohol and pyridine, followed by identification testing of a standard battery of odorants *(45)*. A performance average on the two tests yields a composite score on a scale from 0 *(anosmia)* to 7 *(normosmia)*. Weiffenbach has provided a thorough review of the assessment of taste *(46)*, which should involve both subjective and objective tests since there can be discordance between the two. Generally, threshold, suprathreshold, and identification testing is performed for the four standard tastants: sucrose (sweet), sodium chloride (salty), citric acid (acidic), and quinine (bitter).

As with other variables that can have a nutritional impact, the nutritional consequences of diminished taste and smell are difficult to assess. An uncontrolled nutritional assessment of two cohorts (young: 25–43 yr, and elderly: >60 yr) of patients with smell dysfunction reported changes in eating habits and a decreased enjoyment of food, although there was little overall impact on nutritional intake compared to the RDA values *(47)*. These findings were confirmed in a mixed population of 310 patients referred for a chemosensory dysfunction (48 with no diagnosis, 64 subjects with hyposmia, 106 with anosmia, 30 with dysosmia, 31 with phantogeusia, and 31 with multiple diagnoses), where a reduction in food enjoyment was noted by 61–90% of the subjects, although overall there was no significant impact on the nutritional intakes by this population, as measured by 3-d dietary recalls and body weight changes, compared to a control group *(48)*. However, in both of these studies there was a wide variation of nutritional impact, and a dramatic impact was noted in some patients with chemosensory disorders; this variation likely depends on the type, duration, and cause of the disorder, and also by both the individual's diet and food-related activities before the onset of the disorder and his or her ability to compensate. Patients with aversive taste disorders may be more prone to lose weight because of the avoidance of certain foods, while, conversely, patients with diminished taste or smell may gain weight in an effort to find satisfying food combinations.

A common nutritional management strategy for patients with chemosensory disorders is to compensate for missing sensations by increasing the textural quality of foods and stimulating the sensory branches of the trigeminal nerves by adding hot foods such as pepper, horseradish, or mint. For patients with olfactory disorders who can detect primary taste qualities, compensation with salty, sweet, or acidic foods can greatly enhance food appreciation, although overuse of salty and sweet foods can have an impact on medical conditions such as hypertension or diabetes, respectively *(49)*.

2. CONCLUSIONS AND IMPLICATIONS FOR PRACTICE

Integration of nutrition and diet management with oral diseases and symptomatology will yield improved oral, nutritional, and systemic health. Diseases of the oral cavity as well as other systemic diseases with oral manifestations can impact nutritional well-being and ability to consume a regular diet. However, despite the significant impacts that compromised dentition and oral health can have on oral intake, dietary quality can be achieved when nutrition counseling is a routine component of dental practice *(8,20,43)*. In the dental office, tailored dietary guidelines on specific causes of eating difficulties (i.e., dentition, xerostomia, lesions) should be reviewed with and provided to patients (*see* Appendix E). In instances where nutrition status is also compromised or when the patient has other medically compromising conditions, a referral to a registered dietitian for medical nutrition therapy may be warranted. Similarly, in the dietetics practice setting, patients or clients exhibiting any of the oral manifestations covered should be provided with dietary guidance to maximize eating ability and reduce discomfort as well as with a referral to a dentist for oral intervention.

Nutrition risk may be minimized and/or avoided with early intervention, proper diet instruction, and referral to the appropriate health professional (*see* Chapter 17). The role of the dietetics and dental professional is similar: assess nutrition/oral implications and causes of complaints or findings, provide guidelines, and refer to the appropriate provider.

REFERENCES

1. Budtz-Jorgensen E, Chung JP, Mojon P. Successful aging: the case for prosthetic therapy. J Public Health Dent 2000; 60(4):308–312.
2. Wayler AH, Chauncey HH. Impact of complete dentures and impaired natural dentition on masticatory performance and food choice in healthy aging men. J Prosthet Dent 1983; 49(3):427–433.
3. Chauncey HH, Muench ME, Kapur KK, Wayler AH. The effect of the loss of teeth on diet and nutrition. Intl Dent J 1984; 34(2):98–104.
4. Joshipura KJ, Willett WC, Douglass CW. The impact of edentulousness on food and nutrient intake. J Am Dent Assoc 1996; 127(4):459–467.
5. Brodeur JM, Laurin D, Vallee R, Lachapelle D. Nutrient intake and gastrointestinal disorders related to masticatory performance in the edentulous elderly. J Prosthet Dent 1993; 70(5):468–473.
6. Greska LP, Parraga IM, Clark CA. The dietary adequacy of edentulous older adults. J Prosthetic Dent 1993; 70:468–473.
7. Kapur KK, Soman SD. Masticatory performance and efficiency in denture wearers. J Prosthet Dent 1994; 14:687–694.
8. Moynihan P, Bradbury J. Compromised dental function and nutrition. Nutrition 2001; 17:177–178.
9. Gunne HS. Masticatory efficiency and dental state: a comparison between two methods. Acta Odontolog Scand 1985; 43(3):139–146.
10. Joshipura KJ, Kent RL, DePaola PF. Gingival recession: intra-oral distribution and associated factors. J Periodontol 1994; 65(9):864–871.
11. American Dietetic Association. Position of the American Dietetic Association: Oral Health and Nutrition. J Am Diet Assoc 2003; 103:615–625.
12. Marcus SE, Drury TF, Brown LJ, Zion GR. Tooth retention and tooth loss in the permanent dentition of adults: United States, 1988–1991. J Dent Res 1996; 75(Spec No):684–695.
13. Thompson GW, Kreisel PS. The impact of the demographics of aging and the edentulous condition on dental care services. J Prosthet Dent 1998; 79(1):56–59.
14. Brodeur JM, Laurin D, Vallee R, Lachapelle D. Nutrient intake and gastrointestinal disorders related to masticatory performance in the edentulous elderly. J Prosthet Dent 1993; 70:468–473.

15. Manley RS, Shiere FR. The effect of dental deficiency on mastication and food preference. Oral Surg Oral Med Oral Pathol 1950; 3:674–685.
16. Touger-Decker R. Clinical and laboratory assessment of nutrition status. Dent Clin North Am 2003; 47(2):259–278.
17. Ettinger RL. Changing dietary patterns with changing dentition: how do people cope? Special Care Dent 1998; 18(1):33–39.
18. Allen F, McMillan A. Food selection and perceptions of chewing ability following provision of implant and conventional prostheses in complete denture wearers. Clin Oral Impl Res 2002; 13:320–326.
19. Shinkai RSA, Hatch JP, Sakai S, Mobley CC, Saunders MJ, Rugh JD. Oral function and diet quality in a community-based sample. J Dent Res 2001; 80(7):1625–1630.
20. Touger-Decker R, Schaeffer M, Flinton R, Steinberg L. Impact of diet counseling on diet and nutrition status post-denture. J Dent Res 1997; 76(AADR Abstract):172.
21. Nutrition Screening Initiative. DETERMINE Checklist. Washington DC: Nutrition Screening Initiative, 1992.
22. Shinkai RS, Hatch JP, Sakai S, Mobley CC, Saunders MJ, Rugh JD. Oral function and diet quality in a community-based sample. J Dent Res 2001; 80(7):1625–1630.
23. Burt BA, Eklund SA, Landis R, Larkin FA, Guire KE, Thompson FE. Diet and dental health, a study of relationships: United States, 1971–74. Vital & Health Statistics, Series 11: Data From the National Health Survey 1982; 11(225):1–85.
24. Baxter JC. The nutritional intake of geriatric patients with varied dentitions. J Prosthet Dent 1984; 51(2):164–168.
25. Joshipura KJ, Willett WC, Douglass CW. The impact of edentulousness on food and nutrient intake. J Am Dent Assoc 1996; 127(4):459–467.
26. Papas AS, Palmer CA, Rounds MC, Russell RM. The effects of denture status on nutrition. Special Care in Dentistry 1998; 18:17–25.
27. Sheiham A, Steele JG, Marcenes W, et al. The relationship among dental status, nutrient intake, and nutritional status in older people. J Dent Res 2001; 80(2):408–413.
28. Appollonio I, Carabellese C, Frattola A, Trabucchi M. Influence of dental status on dietary intake and survival in community-dwelling elderly subjects. Age Ageing 1997; 26(6):445–456.
29. Turner L, Jacobsen C, Humenczuk M, Singhal VK, Moore D, Bell H. The effects of lactation education and a prosthetic obturator appliance on feeding efficiency in infants with cleft lip and palate. Cleft Palate Craniofac J 2001; 38(5):519–524.
30. Pashayan HM, McNab M. Simplified method of feeding infants born with cleft palate with or without cleft lip. Am J Dis Children 1979; 133(2):145–147.
31. Brine EA, Rickard KA, Brady MS, et al. Effectiveness of two feeding methods in improving energy intake and growth of infants with cleft palate: a randomized study. J Am Diet Assoc 1994; 94(7): 732–738.
32. Cancer Facts and Figures 2002. Atlanta: American Cancer Society, 2002.
33. van Bokhorst-de van der S, van Leeuwen PA, Kuik DJ, et al. The impact of nutritional status on the prognoses of patients with advanced head and neck cancer. Cancer 1999; 86(3):519–527.
34. Svensson P, Arendt-Nielsen L, Houe L. Muscle pain modulates mastication: an experimental study in humans. J Orofac Pain 1998: 12:7–16.
35. Raphael K, Marbach J, Touger-Decker R. Dietary fiber intake in patients with MFP. J Orofac Pain 2002; 16:39–47.
36. Baum BJ, Bodner L. Aging and oral motor function: evidence for altered performance among older persons. J Dent Res 1983; 62(1):2–6.
37. Miller CS, Epstein JB, Hall EH, Sirois D. Changing oral care needs in the United States: the continuing need for oral medicine. Oral Surg Oral Med Oral Path Oral Rad Endodont 2001; 91(1):34–44.
38. Ship JA, Pillemer SR, Baum BJ. Xerostomia and the geriatric patient. J Am Geriatr Soc 2002; 50(3): 535–543.
39. Rhodus NL. Qualitative nutritional intake analysis of older adults with Sjogren's syndrome. Gerodontology 1988; 7(2):61–69.
40. Rhodus NL, Brown J. The association of xerostomia and inadequate intake in older adults. J Am Dietet Assoc 1990; 90(12):1688–1692.

41. Dormenval V, Budtz-Jorgensen E, Mojon P, Bruyere A, Rapin CH. Associations between malnutrition, poor general health and oral dryness in hospitalized elderly patients. Age Ageing 1998; 27:123–128.
42. Winkler S, Garg AK, Mekayarajjananonth T, Bakaeen LG, Khan E. Depressed taste and smell in geriatric patients. J Am Dent Assoc 1999; 130(12):1759–1765.
43. Ettinger RL. Changing dietary patterns with changing dentition: how do people cope? Special Care Dent 1998; 18(1):33–39.
44. Ship JA, Duffy V, Jones JA, Langmore S. Geriatric oral health and its impact on eating. J Am Geriatr Soc 1996; 44(4):456–464.
45. Cowart BJ. Relationships between taste and smell across the adult life span. Ann NY Acad Sci 1989; 561:39–55.
46. Weiffenbach JM. Assessment of chemosensory functioning in aging: subjective and objective procedures. Ann NY Acad Sci 1989; 561:56.
47. Ferris AM, Duffy VB. Effect of olfactory deficits on nutritional status: does age predict persons at risk? Ann NY Acad Sci 1989; 561:113–123.
48. Mattes RD, Cowart BJ. Dietary assessment of patients with chemosensory disorders. J Am Diet Assoc 1994; 94(1):50–56.
49. Duffy VB, Ferris AM. Nutritional management of patients with chemosensory disturbances. Ear Nose Throat J 1989; 68(5):395–397.

9 Complementary and Alternative Medical Practices and Their Impact on Oral and Nutritional Health

Ruth M. DeBusk and Diane Rigassio Radler

1. INTRODUCTION

Complementary and alternative medical (CAM) practices refer to those therapeutic choices that are outside of conventional, mainstream options within the United States and cover a broad range of approaches to healing. Although not widely accepted in the United States, many CAM practices are indigenous to other cultures worldwide and considered by those to be traditional health care practices. The increasing use of CAM practices within the United States has been documented since the early 1990s, but little is known about their efficacy or long-term safety. The ongoing challenge for the US health care system has been to assess the appropriateness of a variety of CAM modalities using the best research designs presently available. Several of these modalities have implications for dental practice and are the focus of this chapter.

1.1. What Is CAM?

The authoritative body for complementary and alternative medicine in the United States is the National Center for Complementary and Alternative Medicine (NCCAM) within the National Institutes of Health. NCCAM describes CAM as "those treatments and health care practices not taught widely in medical schools, not generally used in hospitals, and not usually reimbursed by medical insurance companies," and as "those health care and medical practices that are not currently an integral part of conventional medicine" *(1)*. NCCAM notes that the term "conventional medicine" refers to medicine as practiced by those with medical doctor (MD) or doctor of osteopathy (DO) degrees and may be called allopathy, Western, regular, or mainstream medicine *(1)*. "Complementary" refers to practices that are adjunctive to conventional practice. "Alternative" refers to practices that are used instead of conventional practices. "Integrative," an emerging term, refers to the practice of combining allopathic, complementary, and alternative approaches to deliver health care that is superior to any one modality alone *(1)*.

From: *Nutrition and Oral Medicine*
Edited by: R. Touger-Decker, D. A. Sirois, and C. C. Mobley © Humana Press Inc., Totowa, NJ

Table 1
Types of Complementary and Alternative Medicine Practice*

Type	Characteristics
Alternative medical systems	Include such approaches as homeopathy, natural medicine, and TOM.
Mind–body interventions	Focus on the mind's ability to influence the body's function and symptoms and include such approaches as hypnosis; meditation; dance, music, and art therapies; and prayer and mental healing.
Biologically based treatments	Include special diets, herbal and other dietary supplements, and orthomolecular therapy (use of vitamin regimens at levels significantly greater than the daily recommended intake).
Manipulative and body-based methods	Include methods involved in the manipulation or movement of the body, such as chiropractic, osteopathy, and massage.
Energy therapies	Refer to energy fields that may originate within the body (biofields) or those that originate outside the body, such as electromagnetic fields.

*Source: National Center for Complementary and Alternative medicine (Website: www.nccam.nih.gov).

NCCAM groups CAM practices into five domains: alternative medical systems, mind–body interventions, biologically based treatments, manipulative and body-based methods, and energy therapies (1). These are explained in more detail in Table 1.

1.2. Trends in CAM Usage in the United States

CAM has been increasing in popularity in the United States for the past two decades, with documented escalation in usage during the 1990s. A survey conducted in 1990 by Eisenberg and colleagues is widely considered to have served as a wake-up call for health care professionals concerning the growing popularity of CAM in the United States (2). In this landmark survey of 1539 respondents, the researchers disclosed that one in three Americans who participated in the survey had used at least one CAM therapy during the past year and that visits to CAM providers totaled 425 million, which exceeded the number of visits to all US primary care physicians that year. The majority of those who used CAM therapies for serious medical conditions also sought care from their conventional physicians, but approx 72% did not disclose their CAM activities to these physicians. Furthermore, most (estimated at 75%) of the expenditures associated with the use of CAM therapy were paid out of pocket.

When consumers were surveyed in 1997, an even greater number of participants had used a CAM modality (42 vs 34% in 1990), out-of-pocket expenditures were similar, and the same percentage of users did not share their CAM activities with their conventional physicians (3). In another survey in which lifetime use and age at onset were examined, 67.6% of 2055 respondents had used at least one CAM therapy in their lifetimes (4). For the population as a whole, lifetime use increased with age. This study concluded that the trend for CAM therapies was strong and that there would be a continuing demand for CAM therapies for the foreseeable future.

In a survey designed to examine CAM use in the United States, Astin found those most likely to be using CAM were white, well-educated, upper middle-class individuals with disposable income *(5)*. They were not necessarily dissatisfied with mainstream medicine; they were simply more comfortable with CAM options, which they found to be more congruent with their personal health philosophies. A similar conclusion was reached by Eisenberg and coworkers when they surveyed adults who saw a medical doctor and also used CAM therapies *(6)*. Of the 831 people surveyed, there was no widespread dissatisfaction with conventional medicine. Instead, 79% felt the combination was superior to either approach alone.

Patterns of CAM use in dentistry have not been surveyed but are assumed to be similar to the characteristics to those disclosed by prior research *(7)*. However, the lack of scientific support of alternative therapies in dentistry has given these remedies a poor reputation, and many consider the treatments to be quackery. Evidence should be sought, either in support of or against the use of a particular therapy and assessed by dental practitioners in patient care *(8)*.

1.3. Concerns About Efficacy and Safety of CAM Therapies

Among the key issues regarding CAM use that concern health care providers is the uncertainty over efficacy and safety of many CAM practices. Many of these modalities have been used in other cultures for centuries. In the United States, however, consumers are quick to adapt therapies that have not been validated through research, such as locally grown botanicals, that may differ from those of other countries in terms of species, soil, water, and growing conditions. The creation of NCCAM has been a major step forward in laying the groundwork for investigating efficacy and safety of various CAM modalities. The mission of NCCAM is to subject CAM practices to rigorous scientific scrutiny, train CAM researchers, and provide credible information to both consumers and health care professionals *(9–11)*. Primary attention is being given to studies that focus on the safety and efficacy of natural products, the pharmacological action of natural products and their interactions with commonly used medications, and the effectiveness of various CAM practices, such as acupuncture and chiropractic. For those CAM modalities that are found to be health promoting, the expectation is that they will be integrated into mainstream medicine. The rise in demand and availability, ease of obtaining products, and limited proof of efficacy and safety are cause for concern. Dental practitioners and consumers need to emphasize critical thinking and evaluation when considering CAM therapies *(7)*.

Among the clinical trials supported by NCCAM, several may be of interest to dental professionals *(12)*. One study is investigating the use of naturopathic medicine and traditional Oriental medicine (TOM) compared with usual care for women with temporomandibular disorders (TMDs). Another related study is assessing the ability of acupuncture, chiropractic therapy, and bodywork therapy compared with usual care in managing the pain associated with TMD in both men and women. A third study will assess the effectiveness of natural medicine for chronic periodontitis and explore the variables that influence successful outcomes when naturopathic approaches are combined with conventional care. A fourth study will examine the potential for herb–drug interactions and will focus on the ability of 10 of the most popular herbal products to affect (inhibit or induce) two key cytochrome P450 enzymes, the 3A4 and 2D6 isozymes, which are known to be major drug-metabolizing enzymes.

1.4. Dietary Supplement Health and Education Act of 1994

The growing interest in CAM by US consumers has been fueled in part by the explosion in the number of dietary supplements that have entered the market in the past decade since the passage of the Dietary Supplement Health and Education Act of 1994 (DSHEA, pronounced "de-SHAY"). Congress passed DSHEA as an amendment to the federal Food, Drug, and Cosmetic Act *(13)*. DSHEA included several provisions that set dietary supplements and dietary supplement ingredients apart from the usual regulations that apply to food and drugs. It defined "dietary supplement," established a new framework for ensuring safety, provided guidelines for the use of claims that could be made about dietary supplements and for literature that was displayed where supplements were sold, established labeling requirements for dietary supplements, and granted the Food and Drug Administration (FDA) the authority to establish good manufacturing practices (GMPs) for the production of dietary supplements.

DSHEA defined a dietary supplement as a product intended to supplement the diet that contains a vitamin, a mineral, an herb or other botanical, an amino acid, or a combination of these. Additionally, a dietary supplement is intended for ingestion in pill, capsule, tablet, or liquid form; is not represented for use as a conventional food or as the sole item of a meal or diet; and is labeled as a "dietary supplement" *(13)*. All dietary supplements must be labeled as such and must carry the following disclaimer: "This statement has not been evaluated by the Food and Drug Administration. This product is not intended to diagnose, treat, cure, or prevent any disease." This disclaimer is mandatory for all supplements, regardless of whether they are effective in improving health. It conveys no judgment on the part of the FDA as to whether the supplement is effective for its intended purpose.

To help consumers decipher how much is known about the intended purpose of a dietary supplement, DSHEA further established regulations for product claims. There are two types of claims that are of particular help to supplement users: health claims and structure–function claims. Health claims are the gold standard and make a direct linkage between a dietary ingredient and a health benefit and have substantial documentation, in the form of clinical study data, behind the claim. An example of a health claim is: "Diets high in calcium may reduce the risk of osteoporosis." Dietary supplements cannot claim to decrease risk of a disease unless the claim has been cleared by the FDA as a health claim.

The second type of claim, the structure–function claim, is more commonly seen and is more general, stating that a particular supplement may promote a healthier condition, but may not make a direct link between the supplement and a disease. Structure–function claims cannot state that a supplement will prevent, treat, or cure a disease. An example of an allowable structure–function claim would be: "Soy isoflavones promote bone health," because it makes no reference to a disease state.

The passage of DSHEA has had profound effects on the availability of dietary supplements to the public, and the number of supplements has greatly increased with consumer demand. Perhaps the primary concern among consumers and health care professionals is whether these supplements are safe. In contrast to drugs, dietary supplements are not subjected to premarket approval for safety and efficacy, nor are there, as yet, widespread stringent manufacturing standards for these products. The FDA, however, has the authority to implement GMP quality standards and to remove from the market any products that are found to be unsafe.

The main difference between how dietary supplements and drugs (both prescription and over the counter) are brought to market lies with the degree of scrutiny that products are given prior to being released to the market. Drugs undergo extensive safety and efficacy testing, which forms the basis for FDA approval of a drug's entry into the marketplace, whereas dietary supplements do not have to undergo this level of premarket testing and approval. As a result, there is considerably more room for an unscrupulous dietary supplement manufacturer to market an impure or ineffective product than for a drug manufacturer to do so and, indeed, several reports of such problems have been documented *(14)*. Information on dietary supplements with adverse effects can be found on the FDA website at www.fda.gov. In addition to safety concerns, there is often limited scientific documentation that a particular supplement is effective for its intended purpose. The present atmosphere in the natural products industry is one of "buyer beware." However, numerous high-quality manufacturers have voluntarily adopted GMPs similar to those of the pharmaceutical industry and are producing excellent products based on the scientific literature and tested in clinical studies. Further, the industry itself has moved to put in place protocols in which a company subjects its products, facilities, and manufacturing procedures to evaluation by independent third parties. Among the more rigorous certification programs are those offered by the US Pharmacopeia (www.usp.org) and NSF International (www.nsf.org).

2. DENTAL-RELATED CAM

Good oral health is an essential foundation for optimal overall health. The recognition that oral health is integral to general health is reinforced in a position of the American Dietetic Association and in Healthy People 2010 *(15,16)*. The Surgeon General's Report on Oral Health *(17)* underscores the fact that diseases and limitations of the oral cavity may impact general health and wellness. Dental practitioners are concerned with preventing disorders that affect the health of the oral cavity and alleviating or preventing symptomatic manifestations of systemic diseases.

2.1. Alternative Medical Systems

Among the more popular alternative medical systems are homeopathy, natural medicine, and TOM, which includes acupuncture.

2.1.1. HOMEOPATHY

The word "homeopathy" derives from the Greek *homeos*, meaning similar, and *pathos*, meaning suffering. Homeopathy *(18–21)* is a medical system developed in the late 18th century by the German physician Samuel Hahnemann and is based on the "law of similars," which refers to the concept of like curing like. When a homeopathic medication ("remedy") is administered to a healthy person, the individual will develop signs and symptoms. If an ill person with similar signs and symptoms is given the same remedy, the ill person often becomes well. The administration of a homeopathic remedy to a well person and the careful noting of all signs and symptoms is called a "proving." One of the fundamental principles of homeopathy is that only a single remedy is administered at a time.

A second principle of homeopathy is that the minimum dose is given, so that side effects are rare. The original solution is serially diluted until not even a single molecule of the original solute remains. At each dilution, the solution is shaken vigorously, a process called "dynamizing" or "succussion." Because, theoretically, no solute is present in the final dilution, which is the form used as the homeopathic medication, there is concern among Western scientists that any effect represents simply a placebo effect *(22)*. Some scientists have suggested that the process of preparing the remedy could alter the molecular structure of water, which may be an important factor in the efficacy of the remedy. In a systematic review of prospective clinical trials of homeopathy, Linde et al. *(23)* concluded that the majority of trials suggested positive results beyond that of a placebo effect but not conclusively so. However, the theory underlying homeopathy has not yet been explained by modern chemistry *(24)*.

2.1.1.1. Dental Implications

Homeopathic remedies are generally considered nontoxic and are not known to cause complications with dental procedures or surgery. Homeopathic preparations and indications for use are readily available on the Internet for sale by for-profit marketers. Dental practitioners should be concerned that patients may try to relieve symptoms themselves without consulting a homeopathic provider or in lieu of other proven treatments. Goldstein and Epstein argue that homeopathic philosophy lacks a rational basis and that, even though the preparations may pose no significant risk, irrational care may not be harmless *(25)*. If a patient wishes to use a homeopathic remedy, a referral to a qualified homeopath would be prudent.

2.1.2. NATURAL MEDICINE

Natural medicine *(26–29)* has been a Western medical system since the end of the 19th century. Unlike other health care systems, natural medicine is not associated with any one therapy or modality. Instead, it is an eclectic system of health care in which practitioners combine several elements of today's CAM with training in conventional medicine's basic and clinical sciences. Practitioners span the spectrum from using only "nature's cures" to extensive manipulation of the body's biochemistry and physiology using natural medicines. However, all have in common natural medicine's basic principles of "the healing power of nature" (*vis medicatrix naturae*), "first do no harm," "find the cause," "treat the whole person," preventive medicine, wellness, and the "doctor as teacher" *(28)*. Considerable focus is on teaching individuals how to prevent disease and to work within the body's natural ability to heal itself.

Natural medicine is licensed in many US states. Licensed practitioners can be expected to have completed a 4-yr graduate-level medical school whose curriculum is strikingly similar to that of allopathic medicine. In addition, the natural medicine physician is trained in clinical nutrition, acupuncture, homeopathy, botanical medicine, and psychology. Natural medicine physicians integrate many conventional and complementary approaches. Among the cornerstones of the natural medicine approach are food, dietary supplements, physical activity, and spirituality.

2.1.2.1. Dental Implications

Most natural medicines and therapies are noninvasive and designed to promote intrinsic healing and would not be expected to have negative side effects from a dental health perspective. However, the use of dietary supplements may have implications for dental care. Certain dietary supplements can promote bleeding or enhance the action of anesthetics (specifics follow in the Subheading 2.2.2.). It is important, therefore, that dental professionals discuss with the patient the dietary supplements being taken and identify potentially problematic ones prior to initiating dental care.

2.1.3. TRADITIONAL ORIENTAL MEDICINE

Traditional Oriental medicine *(30,31)* encompasses the ancient medical practices of China, Japan, and other Asian countries. TOM is a holistic practice in which the body is viewed as being in a state of harmony and balance, both within itself and with the environment in which it lives. Disharmony signals disease, and the therapeutic goal is to bring the individual back into balance. The body and mind are unified, and a universal life force of *chi* (pronounced "chee" in Chinese and "kee" in Japanese) is believed to flow throughout the individual along specific channels or "meridians." Maintaining the free flow of *chi* is essential for health. TOM practitioners use a combination of acupressure and acupuncture, herbal remedies, and meditative exercise to achieve balance.

TOM practitioners are keen observers and include parameters in their examinations not typically used in the West. Practitioners ask many questions and observe the voice, emotions, and general demeanor of the patient. They conduct a visual examination that includes body movement, facial colors, and the tongue. TOM practitioners believe they can tell much about the health of the inner organs by observing the health of the tongue: its color, moisture, coating, fit within the oral cavity, and presence of abnormalities. They are careful listeners and also rely on smell to detect disharmony within the body. Finally, they use a touching exam to determine the person's sensitivity to touch and to evaluate pulses, which provides insight into the state of the individual's *chi*.

In TOM, disharmony results when the flow of *chi* is out of balance. Acupressure and acupuncture are used to correct the balance of *chi*. Acupressure uses the pressure of the fingers, palm, or elbow to stimulate specific sites along the meridians, whereas acupuncture uses hair-thin needles to stimulate these sites. TOM practitioners also use dietary therapy and herbal medicines to rebalance the body.

2.1.3.1. Dental Implications

Individuals may seek acupressure or acupuncture for TMD, gagging, myofascial pain, or postoperative pain. Many find these treatments relaxing and helpful for pain relief, and they are not thought to present a health hazard as long as the acupuncture needles have been properly sterilized or the practitioner uses disposable single-use needles. The use of Chinese herbs, however, may potentially interfere with dental therapy. Because these mixtures are typically complex, it can be difficult to determine which active constituents are present and how these might interact with anesthetics and other medications. The dental practitioner may want to contact the TOM provider to determine what is in the mixture and for consultation in light of planned dental treatment.

2.1.4. ACUPUNCTURE

The flow of *chi* moves through 59 channels or "meridians" in the body. In an unhealthy individual, the flow of *chi* is impaired. As stated previously, the goal of acupuncture *(32–35)* is to rebalance the *chi* so that it flows freely along the meridians throughout the body.

Thin needles are inserted into specific points along the meridians. The select acupuncture points and the angle and depth of the needles are believed to be important. Needles are sometimes twirled or stimulated with electric current or heat to increase their effect. Acupuncture is particularly helpful in the treatment of chronic pain conditions. It is thought that the needles stimulate the release of natural endorphins that mitigate pain. In a 1997 consensus statement, a panel convened by NCCAM reviewed the existing research and concluded that, although the data were equivocal, acupuncture was a promising modality for a number of applications, including postoperative dental pain. They further recommended that acupuncture be incorporated into conventional medicine and that studies into its mechanism of action be conducted *(33)*.

2.1.4.1. Dental Implications

Acupuncture has become popular in the United States for the treatment of chronic pain, particularly low back pain but also for temporomandibular, myofascial, and postoperative dental pain. As an analgesic, acupuncture may be an alternative for patients with severe allergic reactions to conventional medications. In a review of scientific validity of acupuncture in dentistry, Rosted reported that the use of acupuncture in treating temporomandibular pain may be valuable but its use as a dental analgesic needs additional research to claim efficacy *(36)*.

Acupuncture has also been used to treat xerostomia *(37–39)*. Johnstone et al. reported preliminary results in 50 patients who had xerostomia following radiation therapy for head and neck malignancies *(38)*. Treatment (2–15 sessions, mean 5 sessions) provided substantive relief to 35 of the 50 patients studied. In a retrospective study of 70 patients with xerostomia of different etiologies, Blom and Lundeberg found that, after 24 acupuncture treatments, there was a significant difference in salivary flow rates *(39)*. Furthermore, continuing acupuncture therapy maintained the improvement in flow rate. Clinicians may find that acupuncture applied to a specific point on the wrist is effective in preventing the gagging reflex *(40)*. Even thumb pressure (acupressure) applied to this point has been shown to be somewhat effective.

2.1.5. MIND–BODY INTERVENTIONS

Mind–body medicine *(31,41–44)* recognizes that the mind plays a key role in health. It views the mind and the body as a unified whole and believes that they should not be treated as separate entities *(42,43)*. Animal and human research into the biochemistry of emotion is providing examples of how mind–body communication might take place *(44)*. A number of mind–body interventions are used to promote a state of relaxation in the body. Meditation, hypnosis, yoga, progressive muscle relaxation, biofeedback, and music therapy are perhaps the better-known applications to dental therapy. Meditation involves deep-breathing exercises and focused attention to effect muscle relaxation. Dr. Herbert Benson introduced the concept of the "relaxation response" in the early 1970s *(41)*. In this approach he brought together a number of different types of relaxation and meditation techniques, with a common outcome of a state of consciousness that reduced heart rate, blood pressure, breathing rate, brain-wave patterns, and, often, pain. Mindfulness meditation derives from the Buddhist tradition and is the concept of staying in the present moment. It underlies all of the mind–body interventions and promotes a state of enhanced relaxation and insightfulness. Hypnosis is a state between sleep and wakefulness that allows for relaxation and deep concentration. Yoga is often described as the "science of the spirit." Its postures, breathing exercises, and meditation have become popular forms of mind–body interventions in the United States. Progressive muscle relaxation makes one aware of the tension throughout the body by teaching methods to release that tension. Typically, one begins with deep breathing, followed by systematically tensing each part of the body from the toes to the head and then releasing the tension, generating a wave of relaxation over the entire body. Biofeedback is a process of monitoring the tension in the body in response to thoughts, feelings, and sensations. Electrodes are attached to the body area that is tense, and the monitoring equipment provides feedback to the patient through an audible or visual signal. The patient is told to use thoughts and feelings to affect the amount of tension in the area being monitored. As muscles contract, the signal is rapid; as muscles relax, the signal is slowed. With training, patients learn to slow the signal through thoughts, feelings, and actions. Music therapy is yet another effective method for reducing stress and pain levels *(45)*.

2.1.5.1. Dental Applications

Patients may use mind–body interventions to manage fear of dental therapy or to minimize pain. Published research and case reports have suggested that some individuals are helped by a combination of one or more of these approaches to control needle phobia, gag reflex, pain, or fear and may be used as an adjunct to conventional anesthesia *(46–48)*.

2.2. Biologically Based Treatments

2.2.1. DIETARY

In general, dietary strategies to reduce the risk of caries focus on limiting the number of times the teeth are exposed to fermentable carbohydrates without oral hygiene intervention. Individualized diet recommendations may be provided by a registered dietitian (RD) for those with inflammation, pain, or other limitations in mastication. There are no CAM-based diets developed specifically for dentistry. Individuals with cancer may be tempted to try various diet regimens that purport to reverse or cure the disease. Often these diets are too restrictive to meet nutrient needs, and the patient should be referred to an RD to ensure nutritional adequacy.

2.2.2. DIETARY SUPPLEMENTS

Dietary supplements can be conveniently divided into botanicals, which include herbs and other plant materials with potential health benefits, and nutritionals, which are essentially all other dietary supplements, such as vitamins, minerals, amino acids, fatty acids, and metabolites. Dietary supplements of primary interest to dental professionals fall mainly into the categories of anticoagulants, anti-inflammatory agents, antimicrobial agents, immune stimulants, and metabolic stimulants. Anti-inflammatory and antimicrobial agents have a direct application to oral health, whereas the anticoagulants and stimulants that increase immune response or metabolic rate may interfere with dental treatment. It is important to know which anticoagulant medication, botanical, or nutritional supplement, or combination of these, a patient may be taking because of a potential cumulative effect that may increase bleeding. The primary anticoagulant dietary supplements that patients may be taking are *Ginkgo biloba*, garlic, ginger, vitamin E in high doses, and omega-3 fatty acids such as α-linolenic acid, eicosapentaneoic acid, and docosahexaneoic acid. Similarly, the use of metabolic stimulants, such as ephedra, guarana, and maté, may enhance the effects of epinephrine. There are still many unknowns in the use of dietary supplements. It would be wise to adopt a policy of having patients discontinue all dietary supplements 2–3 wk prior to any procedures that require anesthesia (49).

2.2.2.1. Botanicals (Phytotherapy)

Patients presenting for dental care may be using botanicals (50,51) for the treatment of dental symptoms or for an unrelated chronic disease. If the supplement is used for an oral problem, the dental practitioner should be aware and ascertain if it is in lieu of a conventional treatment. Whether the botanical is being used for treatment of a systemic disease or for disease prevention, the practitioner should evaluate it for safety, efficacy, and potential interactions with planned procedures. Botanicals that may be of concern to the dental practitioner are listed in Table 2 (52–68).

2.2.2.2. Nutrition Supplements

Table 3 (53,68–74) includes various supplements with consumer uses and concerns relevant to the dental practitioner. Patients should be encouraged to consume a variety of foods for nutrient adequacy and be advised that it is the position of the American Dietetic Association that supplemental vitamins and minerals or both may be beneficial in the circumstance that a well-balanced diet cannot be maintained (69). No scientific evidence has been found in published literature that a select combination of vitamins and minerals in supplement form will enhance oral health or prevent oral disease.

2.3. Manipulative and Body-Based Methods

2.3.1. CHIROPRACTIC

Chiropractic (31, 75–78), like natural medicine, embraces the belief that the body has the inherent ability to heal itself and that the practitioner's role is to facilitate this natural propensity. Developed in the late 1800s by Daniel David Palmer, chiropractic is rooted in the belief that proper alignment of the spine impacts the health of the body. Wellness and prevention are the guiding principles in chiropractic. Treatment is noninvasive, and practitioners do not employ drugs or surgery. Instead, chiropractors focus on keeping the nervous system healthy and removing any musculoskeletal problems (called "subluxations") that may interfere with optimal functioning of the nervous system.

The term "chiropractic" derives from the Greek *chiropraktikos*, which means "effective treatment by hand." Chiropractors manually manipulate the body to promote optimal functioning of the nervous system by aligning the spine properly and relieving muscle tension. The chiropractic philosophy is based on two fundamental precepts: the importance of the influence that the structure and condition of the body have on its physiological functioning and the importance of the mind–body connection in promoting healing and maintaining health.

Chiropractic is a popular CAM modality, particularly for those seeking relief from chronic pain, such as low back pain or temporomandibular or fibromyalgia pain. Although popular with consumers, conventional medical practitioners remain skep-

Table 2
Botanical Supplements

Supplement	General use(s)	Oral use(s)	Concerns	Additional reference(s)*
Aloe vera	Anti-inflammatory	Mouth rinse	May cause diarrhea, malabsorption, electrolyte imbalance when ingested	
Bilberry	Relieve diabetic neuropathy, antioxidant, improve eyesight	As an astringent rinse to treat mildly inflamed mucous membranes of mouth and throat		(52)
Calendula	Anti-inflammatory, reduce swelling, improve wound healing	Applied topically to treat inflammation of oral mucosa	May cause allergic reactions in individuals sensitive to members of the Asteraceae (daisy) family	http://www.herbmed.org
Cayenne	Used topically for pain relief	Topical application for pain relief for toothache, trigeminal neuralgia. NIDCR to test effectiveness of capsaicin in pain control after third molar extraction	Capsaicin is active compound in chili/cayenne peppers; irritant to skin and eyes; topical use only	http://www.clinicaltrials.gov
Echinacea	Upper respiratory infections, wound healing	Locally applied as antimicrobial for oral health, inflammation of mouth	Research has not demonstrated efficacy in oral health; not to be used with immunosupressants or hepatotoxic drugs, or in patients with AIDS, tuberculosis, or autoimmune diseases; use to be discontinued prior to surgery	(49,53)
Ephedra	Stimulant, ergogenic aid		Tachycardia, hypertension, arrhythmias; possible additive effect with epinephrine; reduces effectiveness of prednisone	(49,54)

Continued on next page

Table 2 (Continued)
Botanical Supplements

Supplement	General use(s)	Oral use(s)	Concerns	Additional reference(s)*
Feverfew	Migraine headaches, menstrual symptoms, inflammation		If leaves are chewed, may cause mouth ulcers, sore tongue, swollen lips, and taste changes; may interfere with blood clotting; avoid with use of aspirin, NSAIDS; may cause allergic reactions in individuals sensitive to members of the Asteraceae (daisy) family	(53)
Garlic	Cardiovascular disease (decrease blood pressure and LDL cholesterol)	Inflammation of oral mucosa, or aqueous extract for the treatment and prevention of oral candidiasis	Additive effects with anticoagulant agents; halitosis unless using "odorless" preparations	(49,55,56)
Ginger	Nausea or vomiting	Antiemetic; stimulates saliva and gastric juices	Inhibits platelet aggregation	(57)
Ginkgo biloba	Increases peripheral and cerebral circulation		Inhibits platelet aggregation; discontinue at least 36 h prior to surgery	(49)
Ginseng, Panax	General tonic, stimulant, improve stress resistance		Interferes with platelet aggregation and possibly with other stimulants; may decrease blood glucose levels in type 2 diabetes; avoid use with estrogens or corticosteroids	(49,53)
Goldenseal	Anti-inflammatory		May increase saliva production; mouth and throat irritations in high doses	(58)
Green Tea	Cancer prevention	Oral and esophageal cancer prevention; reduce risk of dental caries	Additional research needed	(59,60)

154

Herb	Use	Notes/Interactions	Ref.
Guarana	Contains caffeine; used in weight loss aids, reduces fatigue	Avoid use with caffeine, ephedra, or other CNS stimulants; possible additive effect with epinephrine	(61)
Kava	Antianxiety	Additive effect with sedatives; implicated in liver failure	(49) http://nccam.nih.gov/
Maté	Stimulant to relieve mental and physical pain; headache	Additive effect with other CNS stimulants, may increase blood pressure, contains caffeine; possible additive effect with epinephrine	(62)
Mexican sanguinaria (*Polygonum aviculare L.*)	Astringent properties may be useful adjunct with usual oral hygiene to reduce gingivitis when applied topically or used as rinse		
Stevia	Sweetener	Use in place of sugar in food and beverages	(63)
St John's Wort (*Hypericum perforatum*)	Mild depression, viral infections	Topical application may relieve TMJ pain	
		Interaction with medications including digoxin, cyclosporin, indinavir, statins, oral contraceptives, and some preoperative drugs such as midazolam and diazepam; may also cause xerostomia	(49,66)
Tea Tree Oil (*Melaleuca alternifolia*)	Topical use for bacterial and fungal infections of the skin	Topically for bacterial and fungal infections of mucosa, including candidiasis	
		Oil should not be ingested; contact dermatitis has been reported	http://www.herbmed.org
Valerian	Antianxiety	Additive effect with barbiturates and other CNS depressants	(53)
Yohimbe	Impotence, exhaustion, diabetic neuropathy	To increase saliva flow in those with xerostomia	
		May elevate blood pressure; do not use in kidney or liver disease, anxiety or panic disorders, or with psychoactive drugs	

* General sources: refs. 67,68.
NIDCR, *National Institute of Dental and Craniofacial Research*; NSAIDs, nonsteroidal anti-inflammatory drugs; LDL, low-density lipoprotein; CNS, central nervous system; TMJ, temporomandibular joint.

Table 3
Nutritional Supplements

Supplement	General use(s)	Oral use(s)	Concerns	Additional reference(s)*
Calcium	Bone density	Integrity of maxilla and mandible	Inadequate calcium may be implicated in tooth loss and periodontal disease	(68)
Coenzyme Q10	Cardiovascular health, adjunctive therapy for symptoms of congestive heart failure	Periodontal disease treatment	Research has not demonstrated efficacy in treating periodontal disease	(69)
Lysine	An essential amino acid in human metabolism	Aphthous and herpes ulcers	Additional research is needed to determine effective dose	(70,71)
Omega-3 fatty acids	Decrease inflammation	TMD	Possible additive effect with anti-coagulants	http://www.OneMedicine.com
Vitamin C	Collagen formation, among others	Integrity of gingiva and improved healing	Research has not demonstrated benefit of vitamin C supplementation for periodontal disease or oral mucosa healing	(72)
Vitamin E	Lipid-soluble antioxidant	General antioxidant	Possible additive effect with anti-coagulants	
Zinc	Immune stimulant		Avoid use with immunosuppressives	(53)

*General sources: refs. 67,68.
TMD, temporomandibular disorders.

156

tical that spinal manipulation is connected with the body's ability to heal. NCCAM has established the Consortial Center for Chiropractic Research for the purposes of subjecting chiropractic to rigorous clinical trials and investigating whether chiropractic is an effective and safe therapeutic modality. All 50 states require chiropractors to be licensed, which involves completing a 4-yr program at a nationally accredited college of chiropractic and successfully passing a national certifying examination.

2.3.1.1. Dental Implications

Chiropractic is noninvasive and does not involve drugs. Practitioners may adjust the head and neck region to relieve chronic temporomandibular pain. They may also recommend dietary supplements that could have implications for dental care, particularly for those supplements that promote bleeding or enhance the action of anesthetics (refer to Subheading 2.2.2.). Dental professionals should discuss with the patient the dietary supplements being taken and identify potentially problematic ones prior to initiating dental care.

2.3.2. OSTEOPATHY

Osteopathy *(31,79)* is a holistic healing system first practiced by Andrew Taylor Still in the late 1800s. Similar to chiropractic, osteopathy includes a form of therapeutic manipulation that seeks to restore optimal flexibility and mobility to the body to relieve pain and promote well-being. Originally, osteopaths used long-lever manipulation, which involves the arms and legs as fulcrums for bending and twisting the body. Chiropractic, in contrast, used short-lever manipulation that focused on the protruding parts of the spinal vertebrae. Today, however, osteopathic medicine training is essentially the same as that of medical doctors except that osteopaths receive additional training in the musculoskeletal system. DOs are fully trained and licensed physicians who may prescribe drugs, perform surgery, and utilize all accepted modalities to maintain and restore health. Many osteopaths serve as primary care physicians because of their commitment to treating the whole person. Rather than being an alternative therapy per se, osteopathy is a conventional medical system that includes the alternative practice of therapeutic manipulation.

2.3.2.1. Dental Applications

A patient with myofascial pain or fibromyalgia may use osteopathic manipulation to minimize pain. Osteopathy would not be expected to interfere with dental therapy.

2.3.3. MASSAGE

Massage *(31)* is an ancient practice commonly used in Chinese, Greek, and Roman cultures. Using their fingers and palms, massage therapists knead or otherwise manipulate soft tissues to relax sore, tired muscles; dispel tension from the body; and improve lymphatic circulation. The benefits of massage are not well documented in the scientific literature, and it is not clear how much of the perceived benefit comes from the bodywork itself and how much to the attention and touch that are an integral part of massage therapy.

In the United States, three types of massage are commonly available: European massage, deep-tissue massage, and pressure-point techniques. Swedish massage, a type of European massage, is perhaps the best known in the United States. This type of massage involves long gliding strokes, kneading, and friction. Rolfing is a popular type of deep-tissue massage and involves working with the fascia to loosen the sheaths that cover the muscles, which is thought to allow the body to be held erect with less muscular effort. Acupressure is an example of pressure-point massage and involves pressing with the fingers on the acupressure points throughout the body (*see* Subheading 2.1.3. on Traditional Oriental Medicine). Shiatsu massage is a popular Japanese form of this pressure-point technique.

2.3.3.1. Dental Implications

Individuals may use massage therapy to ease chronic myofascial pain, fibromyalgia, or TMD. Research in the 1980s suggested that ice massage of the webbed area between the thumb and index finger was helpful in relieving dental pain, but the practice is not widely used *(80)*. Massage with aromatherapy has been suggested as an effective alternative in relieving symptoms of teething *(81)*. Massage is not known to cause harm and may actually provide relief to those with chronic pain and allow for relaxation prior to dental treatment.

3. PRACTICAL APPLICATIONS

3.1. Potential CAM–Medication Interactions

Many consumers believe it is safe to take herbs and supplements because they are "natural." However, it is important to keep in mind that dietary supplements are subject to the same mechanisms of interactions as pharmaceuticals. Pharmacokinetic or pharmacodynamic interactions may occur with food, medications, or other supplements. Pharmacokinetic interactions are related to absorption, displacement, and metabolism, while pharmacodynamic mechanisms refer to additive, opposing, or transport changes. For example, kava and valerian may have additive effects when combined with alcohol or prescribed sedatives; anticoagulants such as garlic can have additive effects with warfarin; and St John's wort has been implicated in pharmacokinetic interactions with several drugs using similar metabolic pathways *(49,82)*. Current information on drug interactions and advisories can be obtained from the NCCAM Website at http://nccam.nih.gov/health/.

3.2. Working With Patients Who Are Using CAM Modalities

The health practitioner has a professional responsibility to the patient to protect, permit, promote, and partner, described as follows. The practitioner must "first do no harm" and protect the patient from toxic or ineffective therapies that would be used in place of efficacious treatments. The practitioner should, however, also permit the patient to choose safe treatments and adjunctive treatments with no demonstrated side effects, as long as the therapy is accessible, not prohibitive in cost, and does not displace proven remedies *(83–85)*. Health practitioners can promote dialogue for safe and effective treatments and help consumers discern good information and reputable therapies and therapists. Finally, practitioners should partner with their patients to comanage illness, provide direction to resources and evidence, and provide professional input into the decision process. Partnership is advisable also for monitoring progress and response to treatment if a patient makes an informed decision to engage in CAM.

An open dialogue with all patients is essential and maintaining one should be discussed as part of routine care. Pertinent questions to ask are "what, why, when, where, and how," outlined as follows. The first question to ask is, "What are you taking?" Alternatively, the dental practitioner could ask, "Are you taking any supplements?" but that may put the patient on the defense. Assuming that patients are taking supplements may let the patients know that the practitioner is receptive to a discussion. This discussion should include use of any vitamins, minerals, botanicals, or other dietary supplements. It may be followed by a question about any other treatments or therapies used that may be considered complementary or alternative. A patient may not think to inform her dental provider about the acupuncture treatments she is having for headaches, but this may in fact lead you to discover other symptoms and therapies not previously disclosed. Also included in the "what" question is, "What dosage do you take?" This should include how much per tablet or capsule or how much of an herb is brewed in tea, and should also include the frequency with which the patient consumes the supplement or participates in treatment. Dental implications will differ in the patient who takes ginger tea occasionally for nausea versus another patient who takes concentrated ginger in capsules twice each day.

The second question is, "Why are you taking it?" Is it to remedy a symptom, to treat a disease, or is it for disease prevention? A practitioner may discover a patient who is taking garlic and would question whether he is taking it to treat oral candidiasis or for the prevention of cardiovascular disease, both of which would have very different implications to the practitioner.

The next question is, "When did you start taking it?" (or, in the case of a therapy, how long ago did the patient start using the treatment) to find out how long the patient has been on the regimen. Often in the case of dietary supplements, symptom relief or treatment may not appear noticeable for several months. If, however, the patient indicates that he has taken the supplement for 4 mo without any relief, it may be advisable to discontinue the regimen and try another approach. Another important consideration to ask is, "When in the day do you take it?" to discern whether there are potential pharmacokinetic interactions with food or medications or whether the patient takes a remedy at a particular time when symptoms seem most severe.

During the interview, the practitioner should ask, "Where did you obtain your information and where do you buy the product?" These are important questions to determine whether the patient regularly sees a CAM provider or whether the information was obtained from advertising or testimonials. The origin of purchase will disclose whether the patient is buying directly from the person making recommendations or selecting independently without guidance. Finally, the practitioner should ask, "How is it working?" Is the patient receiving the results that he thought he would? Have the symptoms been completely alleviated or just diminished? Are there any side effects attributable to the treatment?

These questions may at first seem daunting to a practitioner who is not fully knowledgeable about various supplements. It is intimidating to consider starting a dialogue about CAM therapies because of a limited knowledge base. The first step is to learn about common supplements most likely to be used in the population you serve. Familiarity with terminology may ease any tension in the discussion. Inquiry to the patient can also be educational to understand his or her rationale for using a treatment. Additionally, and perhaps most important, in order to increase the likelihood of honest responses, patients should understand why a dental practitioner inquires about CAM.

3.3. Choosing Quality CAM

3.3.1. CHOOSING QUALITY SUPPLEMENTS

In evaluating the potential for a supplement, consider the following five factors: method of action, available research, adverse effects, legality of use, and professional ethics *(86)*. If patients make an informed decision to take supplements, advise them to buy from well-known, reputable companies to reduce the risk of supplement contamination and adulteration *(87)*. Consumers should be educated to look for quality control standards. One example is the Dietary Supplement Verification Program (DSVP) set up in 2000 by the United States Pharmacopoeia (USP), an independent, nongovernmental organization, to respond to the need to assure consumers that dietary supplements contain the type and amount of ingredients listed on the label *(88)*. Manufacturers of dietary supplements voluntarily participate in this program. The rigorous program subjects products to scientific testing for purity, accuracy of ingredient labeling, and quality manufacturing practices. A product that passes the USP standards may bear the DSVP certification mark.

Another similar voluntary certification program for dietary supplements is offered by NSF International *(89)*. The certification process includes product testing, GMP inspections, and ongoing monitoring in exchange for the NSF mark.

The USP and NSF International certifications are rigorous and ensure quality at all levels of the manufacturing process. Another potentially useful source of information is ConsumerLabs.com. This company evaluates supplements for labeling accuracy and consistency of product units. ConsumerLabs.com is an independent testing laboratory that investigates whether the label accurately reflects what is in the product container, whether the product is free of contaminates, whether the product disintegrates in a reasonable amount of time so that it can be absorbed by the body, and whether there is consistency among each unit (such as a tablet or capsule) within the product. If a product successfully meets these criteria, ConsumerLabs.com awards its CL Seal of Approval to that product. Test results are available at Website: www.consumerlabs.com. Summaries of the findings are available for free; full reports are available by subscription for a modest fee *(90)*.

These types of certifications are useful to consumers and health care practitioners. They help to identify quality products and increase confidence in the product selected. Consumer and practitioner collaboration is critical to safe and rational use of supplements *(85)*.

3.3.2. EVALUATING A PRACTITIONER

The Website address, http://nccam.nih.gov/health/decisions/index.htm, within the NCCAM Website, has a number of tips for consumers who wish to explore CAM therapies. Topics include selecting complementary and alternative therapies, examining the practitioner's expertise, considering the cost, partnering with a health care provider, and finding credible sources of information about complementary and alternative therapies. Additionally, therapies requiring licenses for practice, such as natural medicine, have a credentialing organization that may include a referral system or a process to check the qualifications of a particular therapist. For example, licensed natural medicine practitioners can be located at Website: http://www.naturopathic.org. Dental practitioners should familiarize themselves with local CAM practitioners to get to know the resources likely used by patients and to establish a rapport for future consultation with these practitioners.

3.3.3. Legal Issues

All health practitioners must advise patients of potential harm or risk involved with any therapy, whether it is considered conventional or CAM. In order for health practitioners to continue to practice comprehensively and ethically, they must be familiar with CAM therapies related to dental practice and treatment *(91)*. Malpractice refers to treatment that deviates from the accepted standards of care, which, in dentistry, are based on scientific knowledge and proven practice. CAM may eventually prove to be scientifically valid and accepted into mainstream practice, but many of the therapies are not thoroughly studied at this time.

Informed consent is always obtained in medical or dental practice for conventional treatments and now needs to be considered for CAM therapy. The practitioner is faced with keeping up with contemporary findings in CAM research and use, communicating the risks and benefits of the therapy or of the lack of standard care if the patient should choose only the alternative therapy, and obtaining and documenting informed consent from a competent patient *(92)*. Working together for the optimal solution should provide the patient with the best options from which to choose and the best outcomes in patient care. For example, a patient undergoing dental surgery may use music therapy during the procedure to decrease anxiety and acupuncture following the procedure to reduce postoperative pain and minimize the need for pain medication.

4. SUMMARY

CAM health care practices are popular. There are five major categories of CAM: alternative medicine therapies (homeopathy, natural medicine, TOM); mind–body interventions (meditation, prayer, and spirituality); biologically based treatments (special diets, use of dietary supplements); body-based methods (chiropractic, massage, osteopathy); and energy therapies (energy healing, electromagnetism). Consumers typically use these approaches to augment rather than to substitute for conventional care. Among the CAM modalities likely to be encountered by dental professionals are the use of homeopathic remedies for pain, infection, or swelling; acupuncture for pain; mind–body therapies to reduce anxiety and pain; dietary supplements for general health promotion and to treat specific disorders; and manipulative techniques to decrease pain.

Homeopathic remedies are readily available to consumers and considered to be nontoxic. However, to maximize effectiveness, they should be used under the guidance of a qualified homeopathic provider rather than the patient using them to self-medicate. Acupuncture appears to be beneficial for postoperative dental pain and possibly for TMD and xerostomia. It, too, should be administered by a qualified provider. Osteopathic, chiropractic, and massage manipulation are also used to minimize pain. None of these modalities is invasive or known to interfere with dental therapy and may provide relief from myofascial pain or fibromyalgia for many patients. Numerous mind–body interventions are used by patients to minimize pain or decrease fear of dental therapy: biofeedback, hypnosis, meditation, programmed relaxation, music therapy, and yoga. The most popular biologically based therapies is the use of dietary supplements. The main classes of supplements that have implications to dental therapy are the anticoagulant, anti-inflammatory, and antimicrobial agents, and the immune and metabolic stimulants. It is important for the dental professional to ask patients what they are taking and to know how their supplements may potentially interact with anesthetics and other dental medications. Chinese herbs are often complex mixtures and may not be from reliable sources. Dental professionals should work with the patient's TOM provider to evaluate any potential problems, particularly with herbal mixtures.

Clearly, it is important for the dental professional to be aware of the CAM modalities being used by patients and to review whether they might interfere with dental therapy. An important finding in surveying CAM users is that they often do not volunteer information to their health care providers concerning their use of CAM therapies. A nonjudgmental approach to the patient's choices fosters a comfortable environment and provides an opportunity to educate patients about efficacy and safety of the various modalities and to provide credible resources for further self-education.

REFERENCES

1. National Center for Complementary and Alternative Medicine. What Is Complementary and Alternative Medicine (CAM)? Available at Website: (http://www.nccam.nih.gov/health/whatiscam/#1). Accessed July 15, 2002.
2. Eisenberg DM, Kessler RC, Foster C, et al. Unconventional medicine in the United States: prevalence, costs, and patterns of use. N Engl J Med 1993; 328:246–252.
3. Eisenberg DM, Davis RB, Ettner SL, et al. Trends in alternative medicine use in the United States, 1990–1997: results of a follow-up national survey. JAMA 1998; 280:1569–1575.
4. Kessler RC, Davis RB, Foster DF, et al. Long-term trends in the use of complementary and alternative medical therapies in the United States. Ann Intern Med 2001; 135:262–268.
5. Astin JA. Why patients use alternative medicine: results of a national study. JAMA 1998; 279:1548–1553.
6. Eisenberg DM, Kessler RC, Van Rompay MI, et al. Perceptions about complementary therapies relative to conventional therapies among adults who use both: results from a national survey. Ann Intern Med 2001; 135:344–351.
7. Goldstein BH. Unconventional dentistry. 2. Practitioners and patients. J Can Dent Assoc 2000; 66: 381–383.
8. Jacobsen PL, Epstein JB, Cohan RP. Understanding "alternative" dental products. Gen Dent 2001; 49:616–620.
9. Harlan WR Jr. New opportunities and proven approaches in complementary and alternative medicine research at the National Institutes of Health. J Altern Complement Med 2001; 7(Suppl. 1):S53–S59.
10. Harlan WR Jr. Research on complementary and alternative medicine using randomized controlled trials. J Altern Complement Med 2001; 7(Suppl. 1):S45–S52.
11. National Center for Complementary and Alternative Medicine. About the National Center for Complementary and Alternative Medicine. Available at Website: (http://nccam.nih.gov/about/aboutnccam/index.htm). Accessed July 15, 2002.
12. ClinicalTrials.gov. Linking patients to clinical research. Available at Website: (http://clinicaltrials.gov). Accessed June 28, 2002.
13. Food and Drug Administration, Center for Food Safety and Applied Nutrition. Dietary Supplement Health and Education Act of 1994. Public law 103-417.94. Available at Website: (http://vm.cfsan.fda.gov/~dms/dietsupp.html). Accessed June 28, 2002.
14. Food and Drug Administration. MedWatch: 2002 Safety Information. Available at Website: (http://www.fda.gov/medwatch/SAFETY/2002/safety02.htm). Accessed July 15, 2002.
15. Touger-Decker R, Mobley C. Oral health and nutrition: position of ADA. J Am Diet Assoc 2003; 103: 615–625.
16. US Department of Health and Human Services. Healthy People 2010: Understanding and Improving Health. 2nd Ed. Washington, DC: U.S. Government Printing Office, 2000.
17. US Department of Health and Human Services. Oral Health in America: A Report of the Surgeon General. Rockville, MD: US Department of Health and Human Services, National Institute of Dental and Craniofacial Research, National Institutes of Health, 2000.

18. Jacobs J, Moskowitz H. Homeopathy. In Micozzi MS, ed. Fundamentals of Complementary and Alternative Medicine. New York, NY: Churchill Livingstone, 1996, 67–78.
19. Lange A. Homeopathy. In Pizzorno JE, Murray MT, eds. Textbook of Natural Medicine. New York, NY: Churchill Livingstone, 1999, 335–343.
20. Reilly D. The puzzle of homeopathy. J Altern Complement Med 2001; 7(Suppl. 1):S103–S109.
21. Vickers A, Zollman C. ABC of Complementary Medicine: Homoeopathy. Br Med J 1999; 319:1115–1118.
22. Linde K, Clausius N, Ramirez G, et al. Are the clinical effects of homeopathy placebo effects? A meta-analysis of placebo-controlled trials. Lancet 1997; 350:834–843.
23. Linde K, Clausius N, Ramierez G, et al. Systematic Reviews of Complementary Therapies: An Annotated Bibliography. 3. Homeopathy. Available at Website: (http://www.biomedcentral.com/1472-6882/1/4). Accessed July 15, 2002.
24. Brunette DM. Alternative therapies: abuses of scientific method and challenges to dental research. J Prosthet Dent 1998; 80:605–614.
25. Goldstein BH, Epstein JB. Unconventional Dentistry. 4. unconventional dental practices and products. J Can Dent Assoc 2000; 66:564–568.
26. Bradley RS. Philosophy of naturopathic medicine. In Pizzorno JE, Murray MT, eds. Textbook of Natural Medicine. New York, NY: Churchill Livingstone, 1999, 41–49.
27. Pizzorno JE. Naturopathic Medicine. In Micozzi MS, ed. Fundamentals of Complementary and Alternative Medicine. New York, NY: Churchill Livingstone, 1996, 163–181.
28. Pizzorno JE, Murray MT, eds. Textbook of Natural Medicine. New York, NY: Churchill Livingstone, 1999.
29. Smith MJ, Logan AC. Naturopathy. Med Clin North Am 2002; 86:173–184.
30. Ergil KV. Chinese Medicine: China's Traditional Medicine. In Micozzi MS, ed. Fundamentals of Complementary and Alternative Medicine. New York, NY: Churchill Livingstone, 1996, 183–230.
31. Fugh-Berman A. Alternative Medicine: What Works. Tucson, AZ: Odonian Press, 1996.
32. National Center for Complementary and Alternative Medicine. Acupuncture Information and Resources. Available at Website: (http://nccam.nih.gov/health/acupuncture/). Accessed July 15, 2002.
33. Acupuncture. NIH Consensus Statement Online 1997; 15(5):1–34. Available at Website: (http://odp.od.nih.gov/consensus/cons/107/107_statement.htm). Accessed June 30, 2002.
34. Berman BM. Clinical applications of acupuncture: an overview of the evidence. J Altern Complement Med 2001; 7(Suppl. 1):S111–S118.
35. Linde K, Clausius N, Ramierez G, et al. Systematic Reviews of Complementary Therapies: An Annotated Bibliography. 1. Acupuncture. Available at Website: (http://www.biomedcentral.com/1472-6882/1/3). Accessed July 15, 2002.
36. Rosted P. The use of acupuncture in dentistry: a review of the scientific validity of published papers. Oral Dis 1998; 4:100–104.
37. Rydholm M, Strang P. Acupuncture for patients in hospital-based home care suffering from xerostomia. J Palliat Care 1999; 15(4):20–23.
38. Johnstone PA, Niemtzow RC, Riffenburgh RH. Acupuncture for xerostomia: clinical update. Cancer 2002; 94:1151–1156.
39. Blom M, Lundeberg T. Long-term follow-up of patients treated with acupuncture for xerostomia and the influence of additional treatment. Oral Dis 2000; 6:15–24.
40. Lu DP, Lu GP, Reed JF 3rd. Acupuncture/acupressure to treat gagging dental patients: a clinical study of anti-gagging effects. Gen Dent 2000; 48:446–452.
41. Benson H. The Relaxation Response. New York: Outlet Books, 1993.
42. Jacobs GD. Clinical applications of the relaxation response and mind–body interventions. J Altern Complement Med 2001; 7(Suppl. 1):S93–S101.
43. Jacobs GD. The physiology of mind–body interactions: the stress response and the relaxation response. J Altern Complement Med 2001; 7(Suppl. 1):S83–S92.
44. Pert CB, Dreher HE, Ruff MR. The psychosomatic network: foundations of mind–body medicine. Altern Ther Health Med 1998; 4:30–41.
45. Kerkvliet GJ. Music therapy may help control cancer pain. J Natl Cancer Inst 1990; 82:350–352.
46. Gardea MA, Gatchel RJ, Mishra KD. Long-term efficacy of biobehavioral treatment of temporomandibular disorders. J Behav Med 2001; 24:341–359.
47. Patel B, Potter C, Mellor AC. The use of hypnosis in dentistry: a review. Dent Update 2000; 27:198–202.

48. Shaw AJ, Welbury RR. The use of hypnosis in a sedation clinic for dental extractions in children: report of 20 cases. J Dent Child 1996; 63:418–420.

49. Ang-Lee MK, Moss J, Yuan CS. Herbal medicines and perioperative care. JAMA 2001; 286:208–216.

50. Linde K, Clausius N, Ramierez G, et al. Systematic Reviews of Complementary Therapies: An Annotated Bibliography. 2. Herbal Medicine. Available at Website: (http://www.biomedcentral.com/1472-6882/1/5). Accessed July 15, 2002.

51. Vickers A, Zollman C. ABC of complementary medicine: herbal medicine. Br Med J 1999; 319: 1050–1053.

52. Anonymous. Monograph. *Vaccinium myrtillus* (bilberry). Altern Med Rev 2001; 6:500–504.

53. Miller LG. Herbal medicinals: selected clinical considerations focusing on known or potential drug–herb interactions. Arch Intern Med 1998; 158:2200–2211.

54. Haller CA, Benowitz NL. Adverse cardiovascular and central nervous system events associated with dietary supplements containing ephedra alkaloids. N Engl J Med 2000; 343:1833–1838.

55. Ghannoum MA. Inhibition of Candida adhesion to buccal epithelial cells by an aqueous extract of *Allium sativum* (garlic). J Appl Bacteriol 1990; 68:163–169.

56. Ankri S, Mirelman D. Antimicrobial properties of allicin from garlic. Microbes Infect 1999; 1:125–129.

57. Ernst E, Pittler MH. Efficacy of ginger for nausea and vomiting: a systematic review of randomized clinical trials. Br J Anaesth 2000; 84:367–371.

58. Anonymous. Monograph. Berberine. Altern Med Rev 2000; 5:175–177.

59. Hamilton-Miller JM. Anti-cariogenic properties of tea (*Camellia sinensis*). J Med Microbiol 2001; 50:299–302.

60. Hsu S, Lewis JB, Borke JL, et al. Chemopreventive effects of green tea polyphenols correlate with reversible induction of p57 expression. Anticancer Res 2001; 21:3743–3748.

61. Haller CA, Jacob P 3rd, Benowitz NL. Pharmacology of ephedra alkaloids and caffeine after single-dose dietary supplement use. Clin Pharmacol Ther 2002; 71:421–432.

62. Gonzalez Begne M, Yslas N, Reyes E, et al. Clinical effect of a Mexican sanguinaria extract (*Polygonum aviculare* L.) on gingivitis. J Ethnopharmacol 2001; 74:45–51.

63. Kinghorn AD, Kaneda N, Baek NI, Kennelly EJ, Soejarto DD. Noncariogenic intense natural sweeteners. Med Res Rev 1998; 18:347–360.

64. Moore LB, Goodwin B, Jones SA, et al. St. John's wort induces hepatic drug metabolism through activation of the pregnane X receptor. Proc Natl Acad Sci U S A 2000;97:7500–7502.

65. Piscitelli SC, Burstein AH, Chaitt D, et al. Indinavir concentrations and St John's wort. Lancet 2000; 355:547–548.

66. Ruschitzka F, Meier PJ, Turina M, et al. Acute heart transplant rejection due to Saint John's wort. Lancet 2000; 355:548–549.

67. Jellin JM, Gregory P, Batz F, et al. Pharmacist's Letter/Prescriber's Letter Natural Medicines Comprehensive Database. 4th ed. Stockton, CA: Therapeutic Research Faculty; 2002; Website: (http://www.naturaldatabase.com). Accessed July 15, 2002.

68. Blumenthal M, Goldberg A, Brinckmann, J. Herbal Medicine. Expanded Commission E Monographs. Austin, TX: American Botanical Council; and Boston: Integrative Medicine Communications, 2000.

69. American Dietetic Association. Position on Food Fortification and Dietary Supplements. J Am Diet Assoc 2001; 101:115. Available at Website: (http://www.eatright.com/positions.html#4). Accessed July 15, 2002.

70. Nishida M, Grossi SG, Dunford RG, Ho AW, Trevisan M, Genco RJ. Calcium and the risk for periodontal disease. J Periodontol 2000; 71:1057–1066.

71. Al-Hasso S. Coenzyme Q10: a review. Hosp Pharm 2001; 36:51–55.

72. Poland JM. Current therapeutic management of recurrent herpes labialis. Gen Dent 1994; 42:46–50.

73. Wright EF. Clinical effectiveness of lysine in treating recurrent aphthous ulcers and herpes labialis. Gen Dent 1994; 42:40–42.

74. Nishida M, Grossi SG, Dunford RG, et al. Dietary vitamin C and the risk for periodontal disease. J Periodontol 2000; 71:1215–1223.

75. Cherkin DC, Mootz RD, eds. Chiropractic in the United States: training, practice and research. AHCPR Publication No. 98-N002. published 1997. Available at Website: (http://www.chiroweb.com/archives/ahcpr/uschiros.htm). Accessed June 30, 2002.

76. Redwood D. Chiropractic. In Micozzi MS, ed. Fundamentals of Complementary and Alternative Medicine. New York, NY: Churchill Livingstone, 1996:91–110.
77. Vickers A, Zollman C. ABC of complementary medicine: the manipulative therapies: osteopathy and chiropractic. Br Med J 1999; 319:1176–1179.
78. Berman BM, Swyers JP. Complementary medicine treatments for fibromyalgia syndrome. Baillieres Best Pract Res Clin Rheumatol 1999; 13:487–492.
79. Wagner GN. Osteopathy. In Micozzi MS, ed. Fundamentals of Complementary and Alternative Medicine. New York, NY: Churchill Livingstone, 1996:79–89.
80. Melzack R, Guite S, Gonshor A. Relief of dental pain by ice massage of the hand. Can Med Assoc J 1980; 122:189–191.
81. McIntyre GT, McIntyre GM. Teething troubles? Br Dent J 2002; 192:251–255.
82. Fugh-Berman A. Herb–drug interactions. Lancet 2000; 355:134–138.
83. Eisenberg DM. Advising patients who seek alternative medical therapies. Ann Intern Med 1997; 127: 61–69.
84. Delbanco TL. Bitter herbs: mainstream, magic, and menace. Ann Intern Med 1994; 121:803–804.
85. Bauer BA. Herbal therapy: what a clinician needs to know to counsel patients effectively. Mayo Clin Proc 2000; 75:835–841.
86. Stephens MB. Ergogenic aids: powders, pills and potions to enhance performance. Am Fam Physician 2001; 63:842–843.
87. Scott GN, Elmer GW. Update on natural product–drug interactions. Am J Health Syst Pharm 2002; 59:339–347.
88. US Pharmacopeia. Dietary Supplement Verification Program Overview. Available at Website: (http://www.usp-dsvp.org/background/overview.html). Accessed May 28, 2002.
89. NSF International. Dietary Supplement Certification Program. Available at Website: (http://www.nsf.org/Dietary/). Accessed May 28, 2002.
90. ConsumerLab.com. Independent tests of herbal, vitamin, and mineral supplements. Available at Website: (http://www.consumerlabs.com). Accessed July 15, 2002.
91. Goldstein BH. Unconventional dentistry. 5. Professional issues, concerns and uses. J Can Dent Assoc 2000;66: 608–610.
92. Ernst E, Cohen MH. Informed consent in complementary and alternative medicine. Arch Intern Med 2001; 161:2288–2292.

ADDITIONAL RESOURCES

Selected Print Resources

McGuffin M, Hobbs C, Upton R, Goldberg A eds. American Herbal Products Association's Botanical Safety Handbook: Guidelines for the Safe Use and Labeling for Herbs of Commerce. Boca Raton, FL: CRC Press, 1997.
Blumenthal M, Busse WR, Goldberg A, et al. eds. The Complete German Commission E Monographs: Therapeutic Guide to Herbal Medicines. Klein S, Rister RS, trans. Austin, TX: American Botanical Council; Boston: Integrative Medicine Communications, 1998. Also available from the American Botanical Council Website: (http://www.herbalgram.org).
Blumenthal M, Goldberg A, Brinckmann, J. Herbal Medicine. Expanded German Commission E Monographs. Austin, TX: American Botanical Council; Boston: Integrative Medicine Communications, 2000.
DeBusk RM, Treadwell PR. Herbs as Medicine: What You Should Know. Tallahassee, FL: DeBusk Communications, 2000.
DeSmet PAGM. The safety of herbal products. In Jonas WB, Levin JS, eds. Essentials of Complementary and Alternative Medicine. Philadelphia, PA: Lippincott Williams and Wilkins, 1999.
Foster S, Tyler VE. Tyler's Honest Herbal: A Sensible Guide to the Use of Herbs and Related Remedies. 4th Ed. New York, NY: Haworth Press, 1999.
PDR for Herbal Medicines. 2nd Ed. Montvale, NJ: Medical Economics Company, 2000.
PDR for Nutritional Supplements. Montvale, NJ: Medical Economics Company, 2001.

American Botanical Council; quarterly publication, subscription information available at Website: (www.herbalgram.com).
Herr SM. Herb–Drug Interaction Handbook. 2nd Ed. Nassau, NY: Church Street Books, 2002.
Integrative Medicine Access. Professional Reference to Conditions, Herbs, and Supplements. Boston: Integrative Medicine Communications, 2000.
Jellin JM, Gregory P, Batz F, et al. Pharmacists Letter/Prescribers Letter Natural Medicines Comprehensive Database. 4th Ed. Stockton, CA: Therapeutic Research Faculty, 2002; updated daily online available by subscription at Website: (http://www.naturaldatabase.com). Micozzi MS, ed. Fundamentals of Complementary and Alternative Medicine. New York, NY: Churchill Livngstone,1996.

Selected Websites

Agricultural Research Services' Dr. Duke's Phytochemical and Ethnobotanical Database
http://www.ars-grin.gov/duke/index.html
American Botanical Council
http://www.herbalgram.org
Alternative Medicine Homepage (University of Pittsburgh)
http://www.pitt.edu/~cbw/altm.html
Bratman, S. ed. The Natural Pharmacist Encyclopedia
http://www.tnp.com
CAM Clearinghouse
http://nccam.nih.gov
NCCAM Clearinghouse, PO Box 7923, Gaithersburg, MD 20898-7923;
Toll Free: 1-888-644-6226; International: 301-519-3153 TTY;
(for deaf or hard-of-hearing callers): 1-866-464-3615; (Toll-free) Fax: 1-866-464-3616;
(Toll-free) Fax-on-Demand Service: 1-888-644-6226;
Email: info@nccam. nih.gov
CAM on PubMed (a subset of the National Library of Medicine's Pub Med free literature search service limited to CAM literature)
http://www.nlm.nih.gov/nccam/camonpubmed.html
IBIDS database; includes consumer or peer review searches
http://lobo.nal.usda.gov/WebZ/Authorize?sessionid=0
FDA-authorized health claims for food and dietary supplements
http://www.cfsan.fda.gov/~dms/flg-6c.html
NCCAM Fact Sheets
http://nccam.nih.gov/fcp/factsheets
NCCAM Fact Sheets: Questions and Answers About Coenzyme Q10
http://cis.nci.nih.gov/fact/9_16.htm
National Center for Complementary and Alternative Medicine–sponsored studies
http://nccam.nih.gov/ne/clinical-trial
Natural Medicines Comprehensive Database
http://www.naturaldatabase.com
WHO Traditional Medicine Strategy 2002–2005
http://www.who.int/medicines/organization/trm/orgtrmmain.shtml

10 Emerging Research and Practices Regarding Nutrition, Diet, and Oral Medicine

Shelby Kashket and Dominick P. DePaola

1. INTRODUCTION

The field of nutrition had its early heyday in the first half of the 20th century, only to be superseded by the rapidly growing fields of biochemistry, molecular biology, immunology, and genomics in the latter part of the century. At the present time, questions are once again being asked about nutrients, but this time they are being directed toward genomics, proteomics, cell signaling, developmental biology, cancer biology, tissue engineering, and much more. Like much of science, the questions relating nutrition to specific states of health and disease that have not yet been defined are the most intriguing. The aim of this chapter, therefore, is to guide the reader to areas of uncertainty and to leave the development of new approaches to defining the nutrition–disease relationship to the imagination and genius of the student, scientist, clinical practitioner, or entrepreneur.

2. ORAL HARD TISSUES

2.1. Dental Caries

Caries have been investigated for many years and the role of fluoride in preventing caries is well described. However, the focus has shifted to include the deleterious effects of the agent on tooth development. Fomon et al. *(1)* examined the effects of dosage in infants and young children and concluded that the prevalence of fluorosis is likely to continue to increase. Fluorosis has increased in communities with water fluoridation as well as in communities without fluoridation. Recommendations to limit the occurrence of fluorosis included the use of low-fluoride water in the preparation of infant formulas, adult supervision of brushing, and the application of stringent criteria to the administration of fluoride supplements to children. Measures of the toxic effects of fluoride appear to be an area that will continue to require further research. It is critical to point out, however, that the introduction of fluoride to the communal water supply is still the most effective way to prevent dental caries and has been hailed as one of the world's ten greatest public health advances.

From: *Nutrition and Oral Medicine*
Edited by: R. Touger-Decker, D. A. Sirois, and C. C. Mobley © Humana Press Inc., Totowa, NJ

Alvarez and Navia and their coworkers *(2)* described the delayed eruption of the dentition in malnourished children and the increased incidence of caries in these teeth. Even one mild to moderate malnutrition episode during the first year was sufficient to increase caries in both the deciduous and permanent dentition. Malnutrition is widespread throughout the world and affects millions of children and adults and, as a result, further study of the phenomenon would be very worthwhile.

In more affluent countries, the effects of nutrition take on quite another aspect, namely, the increased frequency of consumption of sugars and other fermentable carbohydrates in the diet. Added to the frequent suboptimal level of oral care in certain communities, this leads to an increased prevalence of caries despite the widespread availability of fluoride.

Konig *(3)* referred to studies showing that most adolescents can remain caries-free if oral hygiene is practiced, despite a reported persisting, high per capita level of sugar consumption. Lingstrom et al. *(4)* stressed the role of starches in caries etiology. The different forms of starch and their differential susceptibilities to amylolytic degradation probably determine their bioavailability and potential cariogenicity. Studies on the relation between the glycemic indices (i.e., the effect of the ingestion of a given food on blood glucose levels) of starchy foods and cariogenicity could help to better understand the relative contributions of starches in caries etiology. Investigations continue on the effects of simple (extrinsic) sugars *(4–6)* and on the development of new non- or low-cariogenic sugar replacers (i.e., sugar alcohols or polyols) and sweeteners *(7)*.

Konig *(3)* concluded that the risks from high-carbohydrate foods, under conditions of proper oral hygiene, do not require any dietary recommendations other than those that are already prescribed for good general health. Indeed, Soderling *(8)*, in summarizing a symposium on nutrition, diet, and oral health in the 21st century, pointed out that in most central and eastern European countries, current and expected future improved oral hygiene and the use of fluoride-containing toothpaste have made recommendations on cariogenic foods less necessary at population levels. Furthermore, targeted intervention involving dietary recommendations was seen as best directed at individuals and population groups with existing dental health problems.

2.2. Remineralization

Highly promising research in recent years involves the study of enamel remineralization and the reversibility of the demineralization process *(9)*. The application of microradiographic and other new procedures, in combination with intraoral assay devices, has made such studies possible *(10)*. Calcium-containing foods have been found to enhance remineralization and, indeed, milk and cheeses have been shown to be effective both in reducing demineralization and enhancing remineralization *(11)*. In addition, gum chewing has been shown to rapidly reverse the drop in plaque pH that is induced after the consumption of a wide variety of foods *(12)* and to enhance remineralization *(13)*. Szoke et al. *(14)* demonstrated that after-meal gum chewing reduced the rate of caries development, whereas Machiulskiene et al. *(15)* reported that the effect was caused by the chewing process itself and was not influenced by the nature of the sugar-free sweetener (i.e., sorbitol or xylitol) in the gum.

Root caries has drawn increasing attention especially as the older population grows in number, as teeth are retained into the older years, and as the use of diuretics and other medications continues to increase. Concern is being expressed about the role of cariogenic foods, as well as erosive foods and beverages, on the relatively soft dentinal mineral. The techniques used to study enamel caries are being applied to the study of root caries.

2.3. Vaccines

Caries vaccines have been under development for many years and are close to clinical testing and development for commercial application *(16)*. There is a serious need for such vaccines both in developing and more affluent countries. Pockets of dental disease exist in underserved and low-income populations in Europe and the United States despite the widespread availability of fluoride. Interestingly, the influence of nutrients on the response to these vaccines has not been studied, although it is possible that the impact of malnutrition on the effectiveness of such vaccines may be serious inasmuch as nutrients can affect the immune response (*see* Subheading 3.1.5.).

2.4. Tissue Engineering

Tissue-engineering techniques are being used to create viable tooth substitutes *(17)*. In this procedure, cells that were enzymatically dissociated from a tooth germ were seeded into a polyglycollic acid scaffold and implanted into a rat omentum or into a third molar tooth socket. Analyses showed that, after 20–30 wk, a variety of enamel and dentin structures had formed. The procedure, when developed further, could be highly suitable for the study of nutritional factors in tooth formation.

3. ORAL SOFT TISSUES

3.1. Periodontal Tissues

Periodontal disease is an infectious process and the search for nutritional factors and intervention have generally proven to be of limited significance. Most information relates to severe nutritional deficiencies in humans and animals, while minor nutritional deficiencies in animal studies have not been found to convincingly affect periodontal health. However, Enwonwu *(18)* has pointed out that good nutrition may be a useful adjunct in delaying and/or mitigating severe inflammatory lesions while at the same time promoting healing, but is of very limited value if the chronic inflammatory stimuli from dental plaque are not removed. Munoz et al. *(19)* assessed the effects of a multivitamin supplement simply as an adjunct to home care in patients with periodontal disease and found significant reductions in clinical parameters after 60 d. Gingival indices and pocket depths were reduced but no changes were found in bleeding indices or attachment loss. Enwonwu *(20)* has further reviewed the potential role of malnutrition in the pathogenesis of inflammatory periodontal disease and has concluded that malnutrition influences the oral microbial ecology, the reparative process, the host inflammatory response, and/or the invasion and/or destruction of the periodontium. Furthermore, since inflammatory periodontal diseases are episodic in nature, syntheses and/or availability of factors and nutrients that are compromised by malnutrition can have a powerful effect on the progress of periodontal diseases *(21,22)*. These factors and nutrients include essential amino acids, essential fatty acids, dietary energy, and several micronutrients, such as zinc, calcium, retinol, and ascorbate *(20)* (*see* Fig. 1).

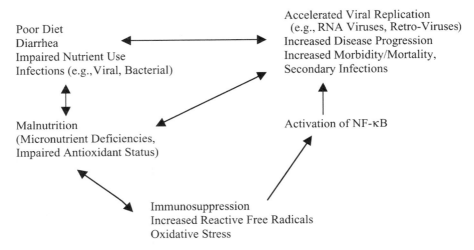

Fig. 1. Model of complex interactions of infections, nutritional status, and immune function*(20)*. Reprint permission from the Compendium of Continuing Education in Dentistry.

In addition, cellular depletion of antioxidant nutrients, such as zinc, α-tocopherol, β-carotene, ascorbic acid, and glutathione, promotes immunosuppression, accelerated replication rate of RNA viruses and increased disease progression *(20)*. Therefore, malnutrition can intensify oral infection severity, which leads to life-threatening conditions *(20)*. New correlates with systemic diseases and new modeling of biological mechanisms have opened the way for a new look at the role of nutrition in periodontal and other soft-tissue diseases that promise exciting future research advancements.

3.2. Relation to Systemic Diseases

A highly promising and active area of research that has developed in recent years deals with the study of the apparent interrelation between periodontal disease and a variety of systemic diseases, including cardiovascular disease, diabetes mellitus, stroke, and chronic degenerative diseases such as ulcerative colitis, as well as pregnancy outcomes. In one such recent report, Wu et al. *(23)* examined the association between periodontal disease and cerebrovascular accidents (CVA). Data taken from the first National Health and Nutrition Examination Survey (NHANES) and its follow-up study found periodontitis to be a significant risk factor for CVA, in particular nonhemorrhagic stroke. Hazard ratios for relative risks of association were lower for gingivitis and endentulousness. Ratios for total and fatal CVA were lower but similar to those for nonhemorrhagic stroke. Increased relative risks were found for white men and women and African Americans.

Genco et al. *(24)* reviewed the epidemiologic studies reporting an association between periodontal and cardiovascular diseases and concluded that there appears to be a moderate association. However, a causal relationship between the two has not been studied. Genco points out that animal and laboratory studies have provided evidence to support the view that subgingival pathogenic microorganisms are associated with myocardial infarction. Other studies from the same laboratory *(25)* reported evidence that a number of inflammatory mediators were elevated in the sera of subjects with periodontal disease, cardiovascular disease, or both, supporting the premise that local infection can lead to changes in the inflammatory mediators and that these, in turn, can impact inflammation-associated atherosclerosis. However, the relationship has been questioned, and Genco et al. *(24)* wondered whether the treatment of periodontal disease could reduce the risk for heart disease. A multisite clinical study, funded by the National Institute of Dental and Craniofacial Research to assess whether intervention can reduce risk for cardiovascular disease is currently ongoing.

Joshipura et al. *(26)* have drawn attention to the possibility of confounding factors (i.e., shared risk factors for oral and systemic diseases) that could result in oversimplified associations between periodontal and cardiovascular diseases. Thus, missing teeth, themselves markers of previous dental disease, may lead to dietary alterations and thus to increased systemic disease. Common elements such as bacteremia and inflammatory mediators (e.g., cytokines) *(24)* offer possible mechanisms whereby one factor contributes to both. Indeed, Saito et al. *(27)* argued that cardiovascular disease and periodontitis are both associated with increased levels of visceral fat and the latter may be a confounding factor. Nevertheless, the current evidence suggests causal associations between chronic periodontal disease and tooth loss with cardiovascular disease, bacterial endocarditis, pregnancy outcomes, and all-cause overall mortality. Joshipura *(28)* reviewed epidemiologic studies relating oral conditions with stroke and peripheral vascular disease and found some significant associations in seven out of nine studies that evaluated tooth loss and periodontal disease as risk factors for the vascular diseases. It was not clear whether any causal relationship existed. There appears to be general agreement that further studies are needed to clearly demonstrate that such associations are real and independent of common risk factors. It is too early to draw clinical recommendations from the current data.

Tsai et al. *(29)* attempted to eliminate a number of potentially confounding variables in a study of the association between diabetes mellitus and periodontal disease. Such an association has been proposed for many years but the evidence has not been consistent *(30)*. Reviews *(31,32)* point out the similar incidences of both diseases in the population, and the apparently higher incidence and severity of periodontitis in diabetic patients. Conversely, the prevalence of diabetes is higher in patients with periodontitis than in periodontally healthy individuals. However, studies are not always consistent and the relation becomes less clear when attempts are made to correlate glycemic control and the severity of periodontal disease. Soskolne and Klinger *(31)* outlined two possible mechanisms to explain associations: (a) a direct relationship such that the metabolic abnormalities of diabetes directly exacerbate the bacteria-induced, localized inflammation, and (b) a genetic predisposition in which a given individual will develop one or both diseases. Grossi and Genco *(30)* proposed an up-regulation of cytokine production by lipopolysaccharides and other products of periodontal microorganisms that may amplify advanced glycation end product (AGE)-mediated responses (*see* below) that would, in turn, exacerbate tissue destruction as seen in diabetes. They considered this to be a two-way relationship between diabetes and periodontal disease. The role of diet in maintaining good control in diabetes is well known, and studies such as this point to the need for a continuing examination of the role of diet in periodontitis under conditions of systemic disease.

Krall *(33)* reviewed the implications for the connection between periodontal disease and osteoporosis (*see* Chapter 15). Hormone replacement therapy and nutritional supplements such as vitamin D and calcium are used to treat osteoporosis and appear also to reduce the rate of alveolar bone loss in postmenopausal women, as well as in men. Tooth retention is improved and the risks for edentulism are correspondingly reduced. Nishida et al. *(34)* assessed the role of calcium intake as a potential modulator of periodontal disease by examining the data from the third National Health and Nutrition Examination Survey (NHANES III). They found a statistically significant association of lower dietary calcium intake with periodontal disease in young males and females and in older males (40–59 yr). Conversely, a calcium intake of 800 mg or more per day appeared to reduce the risk of periodontal disease in females. These results are consistent with the commonality of pathology in oral and the systemic diseases, and the parallel response to dietary factors. They stress the importance of assessing oral effects especially for new medications that are being developed for the treatment of osteoporosis.

3.3. Plaque Microbiota

The significance of microbial biofilms and microbial diversity has only recently become a focus for the general biologist, yet oral biologists have been investigating these systems (i.e., dental plaque) for a long time and have contributed greatly to our understanding of the impact of nutrition on biofilms. Earlier studies involved mainly the microbiota of supragingival plaque and the nutritional effects on these and their relation to the development of caries. However, considerable attention has been placed in recent years on determining the composition of the microorganisms of subgingival plaque and attempting to understand the role of the numerous species and strains, and their interactions, in the initiation and progression of periodontal disease. The use of molecular probes has greatly enhanced the rapid identification of these microorganisms in subgingival plaque and a number of putative pathogens have been identified *(35)*. However, little attention has been given to the possible nutritional effects on the subgingival microbiota. These microorganisms derive nutrients from the host tissues but are also subjected to the food elements that are delivered to the gingival tissue via the blood. It is not known what influence these blood-borne nutrients may have on the subgingival microorganisms. Interestingly, Maiden et al. *(36)* demonstrated the partial inhibitory effect of glucose on the growth of *Bacteroides forsythus* in vitro, with the concomitant release of high levels of the toxic metabolite methylglyoxal. The latter was also found to be elevated in the gingival crevicular fluid from periodontitis pockets *(37)*, leading one to speculate about the possibility that the protein-reactive agent may contribute to inflammatory episodes in patients with periodontitis. Since blood sugar levels vary with time, the effects on periodontal tissues may be episodic and not readily detectable, yet these may be cumulative and of major significance. Indeed, diabetic patients who are known to experience fluctuating blood sugar levels have been found to exhibit signs of tissue damage with increased levels of AGEs. Glucose (or some of its oxidation products), as well as methylglyoxal, can interact with proteins nonenzymatically to form AGEs. Lalla et al. *(38)* proposed that cellular receptors for advanced glycation end products play a central role in oral infection, exaggerated inflammatory host responses, and destruction of alveolar bone in diabetes. Similarly, cytokines and other inflammatory mediators, while known to accumulate with increasing bacterial load *(39,40)*, may be significantly affected by transient blood sugar and nutrient levels. These and other findings point strongly to the need to reevaluate the role of nutrients in periodontal diseases. The relation may be quite complex and not obvious to the casual observer.

3.4. Obesity

Saito et al. (41) reported a significant association between obesity and periodontitis and suggested that the latter may be exacerbated by some conditions associated with obesity. Subsequent studies by this group showed that waste–hip ratio (i.e., upper body obesity), body mass index (BMI), and body fat were significant risk indicators for periodontitis and, more specifically, that risk increased primarily in subjects with high waist–hip ratios and elevated BMI (27). Obesity is a known risk factor for Type 2 diabetes, cardiovascular disease, and other chronic diseases (42) and, not surprisingly, Grossi and Genco (30) reported the interrelationship between obesity, diabetes, and periodontal disease. Preliminary studies at the Forsyth Institute (43) have shown that obese individuals, as determined by elevated BMI, were more likely to exhibit periodontitis and had higher proportions of B. forsythus in their subgingival plaque than nonobese individuals. Thus, the evidence for an association between obesity and periodontal disease appears to be growing, although the nature of the association is not known at present. A number of mechanisms are possible. Other systemic diseases may exacerbate the conditions that favor the development of periodontal disease as suggested by Saito and coworkers. On the other hand, periodontal disease may be yet another manifestation of a common set of mechanisms involving increased caloric intake with a concomitant increased exposure to specific sugars or other nutrients, the uptake of specific fats, or the shared exposure to inflammatory mediators resulting from increased metabolic stresses. Obesity may result in decreased blood flow to the periodontal tissues and may generally affect the host immune responses (44). Gemmell et al. (45) reported that adipose tissue can secrete tumor necrosis factor (TNF)-α, which mediates endotoxin-induced tissue injury in periodontal tissue, whereas Grossi and Genco (30) found that periodontal treatment resulted in improved diabetic control. These disparate observations, and others, tend to support the view that the interrelationship between periodontal disease and a variety of systemic conditions or diseases does indeed exist and is complex, and requires more careful study.

3.5. Immune Responses

It has long been accepted that nutrients can have a profound effect on immune function (46). However, this relationship is most easily seen in instances of malnutrition (20). Thus, protein energy malnutrition is probably the most common cause of immunodeficiency, while scurvy leads to readily observable effects on the gingiva. In vitro studies have supplemented clinical observations and have provided mechanisms whereby the specific roles of given nutrients have been explained. The focus has generally been on antioxidants such as vitamin E and selenium as well as on vitamins A and D, zinc, and fatty acids. These have been shown to regulate immune function, and studies have shown the benefits of increasing the intake of such nutrients. The review by Field et al. (46) covers specifics of some these findings, and reference to such observations (especially the interesting results with polyunsaturated fatty acids) have been made in this text. Two points stand out from many studies: (a) clinical studies on the efficacy of nutrient additives on the immune system are complex, inconsistent, and difficult to interpret even when mechanisms have been worked out at the cellular laboratory animal level; and (b) even less is known about effects on the oral system.

Studies with polyunsaturated fatty acids (PUFA), specifically *n*-3 PUFA, illustrate the current state of the field *(4)*. Feeding PUFA to animals has resulted in reductions in tumor growth and survival; however, high levels of *n*-3 PUFA (>10% of total fat) fed to animals or humans can suppress lymphocyte proliferation or activation, natural killer cell activity, macrophage activation, and TNF-α production. More moderate amounts may enhance immune functions so that there appears to be a transition between positive and negative effects that depends on concentration, and probably also on the disease load. Dietary *n*-3 PUFA can lead to changes in cell membrane composition, alterations in eicosanoid production and signal transduction, and modulations in gene expression (*see* below). Despite increasing knowledge about the function of *n*-3 PUFA, it is clear that more work has to be done to delineate the optimal conditions under which *n*-3 PUFA can stimulate the immune response in healthy subjects as well as in patients suffering from various diseases. The same conclusions apply to other macro- and micronutrients. Grimble *(22)* carried out a meta-analysis of a number of large randomized placebo-controlled trials using immunonutrition (i.e., supplementation with nutrients known to modulate inflammatory response to injury and infection) in humans and found improvements in patient recovery. However, the author was concerned about the difficulty in demonstrating effectiveness of immunonutrition and pointed to uncertainties in antioxidant status of subjects as well as genotypic variations. The data suggested that not all genotypes respond the same way to the nutritional therapy. Clearly, new factors are being discovered and all of these must be taken into consideration before meaningful clinical applications can be developed and tested.

3.6. Gene Expression

The findings that nutrients can regulate gene expression has brought about a renewed interest in nutrition and stimulated the interest of researchers in genomics, medicine, and various other disciplines but has not yet brought about much interest in oral biology. These approaches and concepts have been applied to studies of diabetes, obesity, cardiovascular disease, and numerous other health issues. Amino acids, fatty acids, steroids, and trace minerals, among numerous plant and animal products, have been shown to regulate key target genes generally involved in their metabolism *(47–50)*. Clark *(51)* and Jump and Clark *(52)* showed that PUFAs down-regulate genes that control fatty acid synthesis and storage, and up-regulate genes that enhance fatty acid oxidation. This shift in partitioning of fatty acids between storage and catabolism can serve to explain many dietary observations on the beneficial effects of linoleic acid *(50)*. Furthermore, such mechanisms may play critical roles in obesity and diabetes, two conditions that have been associated with periodontal disease. Gene regulation may be one of the common factors that play a vital role in all of these conditions. Furthermore, gene polymorphism has been shown to modulate the response to nutrients *(53)* and may help to explain the differences observed in the responses of different individuals toward nutrient and other therapies. Studies such as these clearly fall into the new field of "nutrigenomics" *(54)* (Table 1).

Within this field, nutrients are seen as "dietary signals that ... influence gene and protein expression and, subsequently, metabolite production." High-throughput genomics, as well as proteomics and metabolomics tools, are used to study the effects of

Table 1
Transcription-Factor Pathways Mediating Nutrient–Gene Interactions

Nutrient	Compound	Transcription factor
Macronutrients		
Fats	Fatty acids	PPARs, SREBPS, LXR, HNF4, ChREBP
	Cholesterol	SREBPs, LXRs, FXR
Carbohydrates	Glucose	USFs, SREBPs, ChREBP
Proteins	Amino acids	C/EBPs
Micronutrients		
Vitamins	Vitamin A	RAR, RXR
	Vitamin D	VDR
	Vitamin E	PXR
Minerals	Calcium	Calcineurin/NF-ATs
	Iron	IRP1 IRP2
	Zinc	MTF-1
Other food components		
	Flavonoids	ER, NF–κB, AP1
	Xenobiotics	CAR, PXR

AP1, activating protein 1; CAR constitutively active receptor; C/EBP, CAAT/enhancer binding protein; ChREBP, carbohydrate responsive element binding protein; ER, estrogen receptor; FXR, farnesoid X receptor; HNF, hepatocyte nuclear factor; IRP, iron regulatory protein; LXR, liver X receptor; MTF1, metal-responsive transcription factors; NF–κB, nuclear factor–κB; NF-AT, nuclear factor of activated T cells; PPAR, peroxisome proliferator-activated receptor; PXR, pregnane X receptor; RAR, retinoic acid receptor; RXR, retinoid X receptor; SREBP, sterol-responsive-element binding protein; USF, upstream stimulatory factor; VDR, vitamin D receptor. (From ref. *54*.)
Reprint permission from *Nutrition Reviews*.

dietary constituents. Micro- and macronutrients and the effects of genotypic diversity on the responses to these can be studied in these systems. In other words, nutrigenomics bridges the gap between current gene research and traditional nutrition research. Muller and Kersten *(54)* reviewed the work done so far on gene expression profiling, including studies on aging, diabetes, and cancer but did not list studies on oral biological systems, although they urge a systems-wide approach. The application of these new tools to oral systems is needed and will undoubtedly lead to new understandings of the mechanisms by which nutrients regulate homeostasis and modulate oral disease processes.

3.7. Polyphenols/Antioxidants

Polyphenols exist widely in the plant kingdom and are major constituents of many of the foods that humans eat *(55,56)*. Despite earlier concerns about the adverse effect of certain polyphenols on protein digestibility, interest in polyphenols has been revived in recent years because of the antioxidant and free-radical scavenging activities of many of these plant metabolites. Thus, phenolic antioxidants can interfere with the oxidation of lipids by reacting with free radicals to form relatively stable phenoxy radical intermediates. In addition, polyphenols are effective metal chelators and so can interfere with the formation of free oxygen radicals. As a result, their use in the prevention of cardiovascular diseases, cancer, and other diseases has been actively pursued. However, relatively little attention has been given to plant antioxidants, their use in the treatment of oral disease, and the effects of nutrition on the levels of these factors in the oral cavity.

Waddington et al. *(57)* and Sculley and Langley-Evans *(58)* reviewed the evidence for the participation of reactive oxygen species (ROS) in the destruction of periodontal tissue in disease. ROS oxidation products such as connective tissue metabolites have been detected in gingival crevicular fluid, consistent with the role of ROS in tissue destruction. In vitro studies showing the deleterious effects of ROS on the extracellular matrix support these findings. Microorganisms such as *Porphyromonas gingivalis* can trigger the release of cytokines (e.g., interleukin [IL]-8 and TNF-α), leading to increases in tissue polymorphonucleocyte numbers and activity, which, in turn, produce ROS. Although blood plasma contains levels of antioxidants such as ascorbate, albumin, and urate that reflect dietary intake, the primary antioxidant in saliva is urate and its relation to diet is unclear. It is significant that levels of salivary antioxidant activity have been found to be reduced in periodontal patients *(59)*. There is a need to understand more about the effects of antioxidants in periodontal disease and the efficacy of diet in delivering these compounds especially to the sites of active periodontal damage.

Plant polyphenols are known also to bind to proteins and to inhibit enzymes, as well as to be antibacterial. Considerable work has been done on the effects of tea, cocoa, and other plant polyphenols on cariogenic microorganisms *(60–64)*. Several of the studies showed that the polyphenols inhibited the glucosyltransferase of *Streptococcus mutans* *(61,62)* and salivary amylase *(60)*. Ho *(65)* recently reported the inhibitory effects of certain tannins from *Vaccinium vitis-idaea* L on *P. gingivalis* and *Prevotella intermedia*. Mao et al. *(66)* showed that polyphenols (more specifically, flavonols) from cocoa modulated IL-1β, IL-2, IL-4, and IL-5 production by peripheral blood mononuclear cells, whereas Song et al. *(67)* reported that polyphenols (procyanidin oligomers) inhibited several metalloproteinases in gingival crevicular fluid and the trypsinlike enzymes from *Treponema denticola* and *P. gingivalis*. It remains unclear whether dietary polyphenols play a role in vivo in modulating subgingival enzymes such as those examined in the latter study, and whether alterations in diet could improve the outcome. Interestingly, in a pilot study Hirasawa et al. *(68)* applied cellulose strips containing a green tea polyphenol (catechin) in pockets of periodontal patients once a week for 8 wk and found that pocket depth and the proportion of black pigmented rods were significantly reduced. Peptidase activity in the gingival crevicular fluid was also reduced.

3.8. Vitamin C

Reports on the modulating effect of vitamin C on periodontal disease have been in the literature for a long time; however, the data are not entirely convincing. In a study by Nishida et al. *(69)* on vitamin C as a risk factor, the authors found a weak but statistically significant effect for the overall study population, especially in current and former smokers. Odds ratios fell from 1.30 for those taking 0–29 mg vitamin C/d, to 1.16 for those taking 100–179 mg/d, compared to those taking 180 mg vitamin C/d.

Neiva et al. *(70)* reviewed the data in the literature on the effects of the nutritional elements vitamin B complex, vitamin C, and dietary calcium on wound healing, periodontal disease status, and response to periodontal therapy. They found that a number of studies reported associations between nutritional supplements and periodontal status, while others reported positive effects on therapeutic outcomes. However, their conclusion was that the efficacy of such supplementation has yet to be determined.

4. ORAL FUNCTION AND NUTRITION

The link between oral health status and diet, especially when dental function is compromised, has long been accepted. However, recent studies suggest that the relation is not clear. Shinkai et al. *(71)* reported that masticatory variables, including masticatory performance, bite force, number of posterior functional tooth units, temporomandibular joint disorder, and dentition status, were not related to diet quality in a general community-based sample. Walls et al. *(72)*, however, found in a review of the literature a progressive alteration in food choice with decreasing numbers of teeth that were associated with altered blood levels of key nutrients. Sheiham et al. *(73)* studied an older population (65 yr and older) and found that, while the intakes of most nutrients, including nonstarch polysaccharides, protein, calcium, nonheme iron, niacin, and vitamin C, were lower in edentate subjects than dentate subjects, the differences did not appear to affect hematological constituents. Moynihan and Bradbury *(74)* reviewed recent research and noted that improvement of chewing ability with the introduction of new dentures and implant-supported prostheses did not significantly improve diet. An interesting insight was given by the authors: they concluded that individuals, once compromised by edentulism, may no longer be aware of dietary insufficiencies and may require dietary counseling if good eating habits are to be regained.

Ritchie et al. *(75)* evaluated 56 publications from 1966 through July 2001 that related oral conditions with nutrition, the limits being that the articles were in English, sampled more than 30 subjects, and used objective oral health measures. The data suggested that tooth loss affected nutrient intake such that the risk for several systemic diseases could be affected. Xerostomia and altered taste appeared to result in poorer nutrition, but there was little information relating periodontal disease and nutrition. The authors concluded that, altogether, there is a paucity of well-designed studies addressing oral health and nutrition and that more studies are needed with larger sample sizes and better control of confounders before the relation between oral health and nutrition can be understood. The need for a better understanding is made more compelling by the recent findings of relationships between oral health and systemic diseases.

5. INTERDISCIPLINARY RESEARCH

A recurring theme in the discussion so far has been the relationship between oral and systemic health. At the very least, such relationships have already been shown to exist in a number of specific cases. These relatively recent findings bring home the point that studies in oral health/dentistry have to become more closely tied to studies in systemic disease—that is, oral and systemic research must become interdisciplinary. Not only do studies in oral health have to encompass nutrition, molecular biology, immunology, genomics, proteomics, and the other sciences, but they must reach out and become involved in studies in medicine and its related sciences. Indeed, this was one of the major conclusions of a workshop on nutrition and oral infectious disease that was held in 2000 at the Forsyth Institute. In summary, the goal was put forward that mechanistic studies aimed at understanding the connection between oral infections, immunity/inflammation, and systemic diseases should involve multidisciplinary projects with interdisciplinary collaborations using modern technologies.

Such an approach should open many new avenues of research. Questions arise about the commonality of the determinants of systemic and oral disease. Not only can systemic disease be caused by infectious agents of oral origin, but both types may have a common source in the genetic profile of an individual. The expression of molecular markers may not be limited to systemic diseases but may have counterparts in the mouth. By considering oral diseases from this point of view, it becomes clear that the oral biologist/dentist must begin to utilize the new technologies that are becoming available at an ever-increasing rate. New markers of inflammation, infection, genetic polymorphisms, tissue destruction, and the like can lead to new insights into oral and related systemic diseases.

From this perspective, the study of the effects of nutritional status may be seen as affecting both the oral and the systemic status of an individual. It follows that clinical studies of nutrition would be most productive if both aspects are examined. Additionally, the technologies that are already being used in many studies of the systemic components could be made available for the study of the oral biology with the result that entirely new patterns might be detected. A similar approach for the study of nutritional supplements or dietary additives—that is, the simultaneous examination of systemic and oral sequellae with the use of up-to-date biomarkers—could be most productive and save time in the long run. New dietary products, including, for example, genetically modified foods, antioxidants, and phytochemicals, will make this multidisciplinary approach not only desirable, but necessary. In addition, the newer findings in the neurosciences and behavioral sciences are opening new approaches to the understanding of dietary habits and the therapeutic modification of diet. The connection between oral biology and nutrition and these newly developing areas cannot be ignored and may lead to entirely new and exciting ways of studying and treating nutritional deficiencies, especially those associated with systemic disease.

6. INTERNATIONAL PERSPECTIVE

The third goal that came out of the workshop on nutrition and oral infectious disease was the collaboration between scientists and investigative clinicians on an international scale. The problems that face researchers in developed countries are encountered and often exacerbated in less-developed countries. The same approaches that could lead to better understanding of nutritional diseases can be applied in the latter. Indeed, conditions in the less-developed nations offer new opportunities for studying the interrelational effects of nutrition on oral and systemic diseases. In addition, ethnic and religious practices can often be examined in local quasi-isolated conditions and open the possibilities for gaining new insights into the effects of these practices on health and disease. Also, the effects of genetic variation in response to diet and the effects of newly introduced foods (including genetically modified foods) can be evaluated on the whole individual. The opportunities for new, innovative, and socially important studies are considerable and would be best achieved if carried out with a multidisciplinary, high-technology approach.

7. THE SCIENTIST AND THE COMMUNITY

It is important that, as scientists, we speak out on scientific issues. The scientific and health communities have an obligation to educate the public about scientific studies, results, and work in progress in the simplest, most direct, and easy-to-understand fashion. It will continue to be our responsibility not only to carry out the best, most imaginative research, but also to keep the public informed. In addition, it will be increasingly important to inform government agencies, as well as companies that produce foods and related products, of the benefits that nutrition research has for humanity and the need for them to continue to support this research. Nutrition researchers and practitioners will be needed with special talents in these areas, who will be able to speak responsibly to and for the community.

REFERENCES

1. Fomon SJ, Ekstrand J, Ziegler EE. Fluoride intake and prevalence of dental fluorosis: trends in fluoride intake with special attention to infants. J Public Health Dent 2000; 60:131–139.
2. Alvarez JO. Nutrition, tooth development, and dental caries. Am J Clin Nutr 1995; 61(Suppl.):410S–416S.
3. Konig KG. Diet and oral health. Int Dent J 2000; 50:162–174.
4. Lingstrom P, van Houte J, Kashket S. Food starches and dental caries. Crit Rev Oral Biol Med 2000; 11: 366–80.
5. Moynihan P. The British Nutrition Foundation Oral Task Force Report: issues relevant to dental health professionals. Br Dent J 2000; 188:308–312.
6. Sheiham A. Dietary effects on dental disease. Public Health Nutr 2001; 4:569–591.
7. McNutt K. Sugar replacers and the FDA noncariogenicity claim. J Dent Hygiene 2000; 74:36–40
8. Soderling E. Summary Report: Nutrition, diet and oral health in the 21st century. Int Dent J 2001; 51: 389–391.
9. Kashket S. Historical review of remineralization research. J Clin Dent 1999; 10:56–63.
10. Proceedings, Workshop on Technological Advances in Intra-oral Model Systems Used to Assess Cariogenicity. J Dent Res 1992; 71(Spec Issue):801–956.
11. Kashket S, DePaola DP. Cheese consumption and the development and progression of dental caries. Nutr Rev 2002; 60:97–103.
12. Jensen ME, Wefel JS. Human plaque pH responses to meals and the effects of chewing gum. Br Dent J 1989; 167:204–208.
13. Hall AF, Creanor SL, Strang R, et al. The effect of sucrose-containing chewing-gum use on *in situ* enamel lesion remineralization. Caries Res 1995; 29:477–482.
14. Szoke J, Banoczy J, Proskin HM. Effect of after-meal sucrose-free gum-chewing on clinical caries. J Dent Res 2001; 80:1725–1729.
15. Machiulskiene V, Nyvad B, Baelum V. Caries preventive effect of sugar-substituted chewing gum. Community Dent Oral Epidemiol 2001; 29:278–288.
16. Smith DJ. Dental caries vaccines: prospects and concerns. Crit Rev Oral Biol Med 2002; 13:335–349.
17. Young CS, Vacanti JP, Terada S, Bartlett JD, Yelick PC. Immunohistochemical analyses of bioengineered tooth tissues. J Dent Res 2002; 81(Spec Issue A):A-146.
18. Enwonwu CO. Interface of malnutrition and periodontal diseases. Am J Clin Nutr 1995; 61(Suppl.): 430S–436S.
19. Munoz CS, Kiger RD, Stephens JA, Kim J, Wilson AC. Effects of a nutritional supplement on periodontal status. Compend Contin Educ Dent 2001; 22:425–428.
20. Enwonwu CO, Phillips RS, Falkler WA. Nutrition and oral infectious diseases: state of the science. Compend Contin Educ Dent 2002; 23:431–448.
21. Enwonwu CO. Cellular and molecular effects of malnutrition and their relevance to periodontal disease. J Clin Periodontol 1994; 21(10):643–657.
22. Grimble, RF. Nutritional modulation of immune function. Proc Nutr Soc 2001; 60:389–397.
23. Wu T, Trevisan M, Genco RJ, Dorn JP, Falkner KL, Sempos CT. Periodontal disease and risk of cerebrovascular disease: the first national health and nutrition examination survey and its follow-up study. Arch Intern Med 2000; 160:2749–2755.
24. Genco R, Offenbacher S, Beck J. Periodontal disease and cardiovascular disease: epidemiology and possible mechanisms. J Am Dent Assoc 2002; 133(Suppl.):14S–22S.
25. Glurich I, Grossi S, Albini B, et al. Systemic inflammation in cardiovascular and periodontal disease: comparative study. Clin Diag Lab Immunol 2002; 9:425–432.

26. Joshipura K, Ritchie C, Douglass C. Strength of evidence linking oral conditions and systemic disease. Compend Contin Educ Dent 2000; 21(Suppl.):12–23.

27. Saito Tssimazaki Y, Koga T, Tsuzuki M, Oshima A. Relationship between upper body obesity and periodontitis. J Dent Res 2001; 80:1631–1636.

28. Joshipura K. The relationship between oral conditions and ischemic stroke and peripheral vascular disease. J Am Dent Assoc 2002; 133(Suppl.):23S–30S.

29. Tsai C, Hayes C, Taylor GW. Glycemic control of type 2 diabetes and severe periodontal disease in the US adult population. Community Dent Oral Epidemiol 2002; 30:182–192.

30. Grossi SG, Genco RJ. Periodontal disease and diabetes mellitus: a two-way relationship. Ann Periodontol 1998; 3:51–61.

31. Soskolne WA, Klinger A. The relationship between periodontal diseases and diabetes: an overview. Ann Periodontol 2001; 6:91–98.

32. Salvi GE, Lawrence HP, Offenbacher S, Beck JD. Influence of risk factors on the pathogenesis of periodontitis. Periodontol 2000 1997; 14:173–201.

33. Krall EA. The periodontal–systemic connection: implications for treatment of patients with osteoporosis and periodontal disease. Ann Periodontol 2002; 6:209–213.

34. Nishida M, Grossi SG, Dunford RG, Ho AW, Trevisan M, Genco RJ. Calcium and the risk for periodontal disease. J Periodontol 20001; 71:1057–1066.

35. Socransky SS, Haffajee AD, Cugini MA, Smith C, Kent RL Jr. Microbial complexes in subgingival plaque. J Clin Periodontol 1998; 25:134–144.

36. Maiden MFJ, Pham C, Kashket S. Glucose toxicity effect and accumulation of methylglyoxal by the periodontal anaerobe *Bacteroides forsythus*. Anaerobe 2004; 10:27–32.

37. Kashket S, Maiden M, Haffajee A, Kashket ER. Accumulation of methylglyoxal in the gingival crevicular fluid of chronic periodontitis patients. J Clin Periodontol 2003; 30:364–367.

38. Lalla E, Lamster IB, Stern DM, Schmidt AM. Receptor for advanced glycation end products, inflammation, and accelerated periodontal disease in diabetes: mechanisms and insights into therapeutic modalities. Ann Periodontol 2001; 6:113–118.

39. Heasman PA, Collins JG, Offenbacher S. Changes in crevicular fluid levels of interleukin-1 beta, leukotriene B4, prostaglandin E2, thomboxane B2 and tumour necrosis factor alpha in experimental gingivitis in humans. J Periodontol Res 1993; 28:241–247.

40. Zhang J, Kashket S, Lingstrom P. Evidence for the early onset of gingival inflammation following short-term plaque accumulation. J Clin Periodontol 2003; 29:1082–1085; 30:278.

41. Saito T, Shimazaki Y, Yamashita Y, Koga T, Tsuzuki M, Sakamoto M. Association between periodontitis and exercise capacity. Periodontal Insights 1999; 62:9–12.

42. Kopelman PG. Obesity as a medical problem. Nature 2000; 404:635–643.

43. Haffajee AD, Socransky SS, Carpino EA, Teles RP. Relation of BMI to periodontal, microbial and host parameters. J Dent Res 2004; 83(Spec Iss A)abstract 173.

44. Das UN. Is obesity an inflammatory condition? Nutrition 2001; 17:953–966.

45. Gemmell E, Marshall RJ, Seymour GJ. Cytokines and prostaglandins in immune homeostasis and tissue destruction in periodontal disease. Periodontol 2000 1997; 14:112–143.

46. Gemmell E, Marshall RJ, Seymour GJ. Cytokines and prostaglandins in immune homeostasis and tissue destruction in periodontal disease. Periodontol 2000 1997; 14:112–143.

47. Averous J, Bruhat A, Mordier S, Fafournoux P. Recent advances in the understanding of amino acid regulation of gene expression. J Nutr 2003; 133(Suppl. 1):2040S–2045S.

49. Moore JB, Blanchard RK, Cousins RJ. Dietary zinc modulates gene expression in murine thymus: results from a comprehensive differential display screening. Proc Natl Acad Sci USA 2003; 100: 3883–3888.

49. Hesketh JE, Villette S. Intracellular trafficking of micronutrients from gene regulation to nutrient requirements. Proc Nutr Soc 2002; 61:405–414.

50. Olson RE. Nutrition and genetics: an expanding frontier. Am J Clin Nutr 2003; 78:201–208.

51. Clark SD. Polyunsaturated fatty acid regulation of gene transcription: a mechanism to improve energy balance and insulin resistance. Br J Nutr 2000; 83(Suppl.):S59–S66.

52. Jump DB, Clark SD. Regulation of gene expression by dietary fat. Annu Rev Nutr 1999; 19:63–90.

53. Loktionov A. Common gene polymorphisms and nutrition: emerging links with pathogenesis of multifactorial chronic diseases (review). J Nutr Biochem 2003; 14:426–451.
54. Muller M, Kersten S. Nutrigenomics: goals and strategies. Nature Rev (Genetics) 2003; 4:315–322.
55. Battino M, Bullon P, Wilson M, Newman H. Oxidative injury and inflammatory periodontal diseases: the challenge of anti-oxidants to free radicals and reactive oxygen species. Crit Rev Oral Biol Med 1999; 10:458–476.
56. Bravo L. Polyphenols: chemistry, dietary sources, metabolism, and nutritional significance. Nutr Rev 1998; 56:317–333.
57. Waddington RJ, Moseley R, Embery G. Reactive oxygen species: a potential role in the pathogenesis of periodontal diseases. Oral Dis 2000; 6:136–137.
58. Sculley DV, Langley-Evans SC. Salivary antioxidants and periodontal disease status. Proc Nutr Soc 2002; 61:137–143.
59. Diab-Ladki R, Pellat B, Chahine R. Decrease in the total antioxidant activity of saliva in patients with periodontal diseases. Clin Oral Investig 2003; 7:103–107.
60. Zhang J, Kashket S. Inhibition of salivary amylase by black and green teas and their effects on the intraoral hydrolysis of starch. Caries Res 1998; 32:233–238.
61. Paolino VJ, Kashket S. Inhibition by cocoa extracts of biosynthesis of extracellular polysaccharides by human oral bacteria. Arch Oral Biol 1985; 30:359–363.
62. Hattori M, Kusumoto IT, Namba T, Ishigami T, Hara Y. Effect of tea polyphenols on glucan synthesis by glucosyltransferase from Streptococcus mutans. Chem Pharm Bull (Tokyo) 1990; 38:717–720.
63. Hara Y. Antioxidative action of tea polyphenols. 1. Am Biotechnol Lab 1994; 12:48.
63a. Wu CD, Wei GX. Tea as a functional food for oral health. Nutrition 2002; 18:443–444.
64. Hwang BY, Roberts SK, Chadwick LR, Wu CD, Kinghorn A. Antimicrobial constituents from goldenseal (the rhizomes of *Hydrastis canadensis*) against select oral pathogens. Planta Med 2003; 69: 623–627.
65. Ho KY, Tsai CC, Huang JS, Chen CP, Lin TC, Lin CC. Antimicrobial activity of tannin components from Vaccinium vitis-idaea L. J Pharm Pharmacol 2001; 53:187–191.
66. Mao TK, Van der Water J, Keen CL, Schmitz HH, Geshwind ME. Effect of flavonols and their related oligomers on the secretin of interleukin-5 in peripheral blood mononuclear cells. J Med Food 2002; 5:17–22.
67. Song SE, Choi BK, Kim SN, et al. Inhibitory effect of procyanidin oligomer from elm cortex on the matrix metalloproteinases and proteases of periodontopathogens. J Periodontal Res 2003; 38:282–289.
68. Hirasawa M, Takada K, Makimura M, Otake S. Improvement of periodontal status by green tea catechin using a local delivery system: a clinical pilot study. J Periodontal Res 2002; 37:433–438.
69. Nishida M, Grossi SG, Dunford RG, Ho AW, Trevisan M, Genco RJ. Dietary vitamin C and the risk for periodontal disease. J Periodontol 2000b; 71:1215–1223.
70. Neiva RF, Steigenga J, Al-Shammari KF, Wang HL. Effects of specific nutrients on periodontal disease onset, progression and treatment. J Clin Periodontol 2003; 30:579–589.
71. Shinkai RS, Hatch JP, Sakai S, Mobley CC, Saunders MJ, Rugh JD. Oral functions and diet quality in a community-based sample. J Dent Res 2001; 80:1625–1630.
72. Walls AW, Steele JG, Sheiham A, Marcenes W, Moynihan PJ. Oral health and nutrition in older people. J Public Health Dent 2000; 60:304–307.
73. Sheiham A, Steele JG, Marcenes W, et al. The relationship among dental status, nutrient intake, and nutritional status in older people. J Dent Res 2001; 80:408–413.
74. Moynihan P, Bradbury J. Compromised dental function and nutrition. Nutrition 2001; 17:177–178.
75. Ritchie CS, Joshipura K, Hung HC, Douglass CW. Nutrition as a mediator in the relation between oral and systemic disease: associations between specific measures of adult oral health and nutrition outcomes. Crit Rev Oral Biol Med 2002; 13:291–300.

IV SELECT DISEASES AND CONDITIONS WITH KNOWN NUTRITION AND ORAL HEALTH RELATIONSHIPS

11 Diabetes Mellitus

Nutrition and Oral Health Relationships

Riva Touger-Decker, David A. Sirois, and Anthony T. Vernillo

1. INTRODUCTION

Diabetes mellitus (DM) is the most common endocrine metabolic disorder and its diagnosis is increasing at an alarming rate *(1)*. No definitive cure exists for this disorder, which is the third leading cause of mortality and morbidity in the United States. In 1980, slightly less than 6 million Americans were diagnosed with diabetes. In 2000, this number doubled to about 12 million reported cases. Adults age 65 and older account for approx 40% of the population with diabetes. In 2002, this number rose to about 13 million individuals diagnosed with diabetes, with roughly 5 million individuals with undiagnosed diabetes *(2)*. This increased incidence is multifactorial in nature: increased screening efforts, rising rates of obesity, and longer life spans have all contributed to the rising incidence of diabetes in the United States.

DM is a pernicious disease. The relative risk for individuals with diabetes acquiring end-stage renal disease is 25 times that of individuals without diabetes. The relative risk for patients with diabetes having a limb amputated because of diabetic complications is more than 40 times that of normal. More than 20,000 amputations per year are performed on patients with DM, representing nearly 50% of all nontraumatic amputations. The relative risk of an individual with diabetes becoming blind is 20 times greater than for other individuals *(3)*. Myocardial infarction is 10 times more likely in the patient with DM.

The dental professional is in a prime position to improve the detection of undiagnosed diabetes (approx 25% of patients with diabetes are undiagnosed) and the surveillance of glycemic control: 70% of all adults visit the dentist at least once a year. Because diet management is the cornerstone of diabetes management, medical nutrition therapy provided by a registered dietitian (RD) is an essential component of effective diabetes management. Effective health care partnerships between dentists, dietitians, and physicians is the ideal scenario for optimal disease management. The role for each health care provider is included in the most recent recommendations for diabetes surveillance (Table 1). Earlier detection, treatment, and management of diabetes will improve quality of life and reduce disease-associated morbidity and mortality.

From: *Nutrition and Oral Medicine*
Edited by: R. Touger-Decker, D. A. Sirois, and C. C. Mobley © Humana Press Inc., Totowa, NJ

Table 1
Recommended Diabetes Surveillance Program

At each regular diabetes visit:
- Measure weight and blood pressure
- Inspect feet
- Review self-monitoring glucose record
- Review/adjust medications
- Recommend regular use of aspirin for cardiovascular disease prevention
- Review self-management skills, dietary needs, and physical activity
- Determine Medicare benefits eligibility for MNT and diabetes self-management education
- Counsel on smoking cessation and alcohol use

Twice a year:
- Obtain HbA1C in patients meeting treatment goals with stable glycemia (quarterly if not)
- Refer for oral/dental exam

Annually:
- Obtain fasting lipid profile
- Obtain serum creatinine and urinalysis for protein and microalbumin
- Refer for dilated eye exam
- Perform comprehensive foot exam
- Administer influenza vaccine

Usually only once:
- Administer pneumococcal vaccination

From the National Diabetes Education Program, NIH Publication NDEP-12, Website: (www.ndep.nih. gov), revised February 2003. MNT, medical nutrition therapy.

In addition to the systemic complications of diabetes (hypertension, neuropathy, nephropathy, impaired immunity, coronary artery disease), several important oral complications may develop or be worsened as a result of poorly controlled diabetes: candidiasis, caries, gingivitis, periodontitis, xerostomia, mucosal disease, and oral burning and other dysesthesias. Conversely, there is evidence indicating that poor oral health can affect glycemic control. This chapter reviews the relationships between oral, systemic, and nutritional risk factors for diabetes and diabetes-related oral disorders, which have also been extensively reviewed in a supplement of the *Journal of the American Dental Association (4)*.

2. CLINICAL CLASSIFICATIONS OF DIABETES MELLITUS, ETIOLOGY, AND PATHOGENESIS

2.1. Type 1 Diabetes Mellitus

The presentation of hyperglycemia is the hallmark of DM, as are its chronic metabolic complications; these are generally more severe in the person with Type 1 diabetes mellitus (T1DM). Such complications include increased susceptibility to infection and delayed healing; microvascular disease and associated neuropathy, retinopathy, and nephropathy; and accelerated atherosclerosis with associated myocardial infarction, stroke, atherosclerotic aneurysms, and amputation (macrovascular disease). The development of these secondary lesions in the diabetic patient relates largely to the severity and chronic duration of hyperglycemia. In general, the major classic findings of hyperglycemia with polyuria, polydipsia, polyphagia, weight loss, and fatigue occur in the setting of new-onset diabetes in young patients whose disease is caused by profound insulin deficiency (Type 1) *(5)*. T1DM, or insulin-dependent diabetes mellitus (IDDM), constitutes approx 3–5% of all cases of diabetes mellitus and is related to autoimmune-mediated destruction of the insulin-producing β-pancreatic islet cells. Thus, these patients are prone to diabetic ketoacidosis, an acute and potentially life-threatening metabolic complication, and are completely dependent on exogenous insulin to sustain life. Ketoacidosis may develop rapidly and lower the pH of the blood, leading to coma and death. The onset of signs and symptoms of diabetes in these patients is relatively abrupt and usually occurs at a young age (mean of 15 yr), although T1DM may arise at any age. The destruction of the β-cells in T1DM has been linked to the presence of certain major histocompatibility locus antigens (HLA), some of which are also associated with other autoimmune diseases *(5)*. These autoimmune diseases include Hashimoto's thyroiditis (hypothyroidism) and Addison's disease (primary chronic adrenal insufficiency). The only genes definitely associated with T1DM are those of the major HLA. In T1DM, 95% of persons affected express either HLA-DR3 or HLA-DR4, or both, compared with 40% of the general population *(6)*. Thus, the overall clinical management of the individual with Type 1 diabetes must take into careful consideration the potential for the development of other autoimmune-mediated endocrine diseases characterized by hypofunction.

2.2. Type 2 Diabetes Mellitus

Type 2 diabetes mellitus (T2DM) accounts for approx 95% of all cases of diabetes. The insulin levels of affected patients may be normal, increased, or decreased, but there is no profound insulin deficiency. However, over many years, the majority of individuals with T2DM show a continual decrease in their insulin levels. The etiology and pathogenesis of T2DM may be more heterogeneous with multiple biochemical or molecular lesions *(5)*. These lesions may include impaired insulin secretion; a defect at the insulin receptor; a defect distal to the insulin receptor; or a defect in the hepatic uptake of glucose, contributing to insulin intolerance. These patients are not prone to ketoacidosis under basal conditions and are not completely dependent on exogenous insulin to sustain life. However, insulin treatment for patients with T2DM (25–30% of cases) can improve control of hyperglycemia.

The hyperglycemia in T2DM is not caused by autoimmune destruction of β-cells; it is rather a failure of those cells to meet an increased demand for insulin (impaired insulin secretion). Obesity is an overwhelming risk factor and is frequently associated with T2DM *(6)*. Obesity and its associated high serum cholesterol can also further exacerbate accelerated atherosclerosis that is frequently a preexisting component of clinical diabetes. The diagnosis of T2DM usually occurs after age 40. Eighty percent of adult diabetics are obese or have a history of obesity. Among adults who are at least 25% over their ideal body weight, one out of five has elevated fasting blood sugar levels, and three out of five have abnormal oral glucose tolerance tests *(5)*. Obesity increases insulin levels and decreases the concentration of insulin receptors or their sensitivity in tissue, including skeletal muscle and fat (clinical insulin resistance). Exercise increases the number of insulin receptors and improves insulin sensitivity, whereas a sedentary lifestyle is associated with glucose intolerance. Regular exercise with weight loss is associated with a decreased incidence of T2DM after adjusting for body mass index *(5)*.

Multifactorial inheritance is also a clinical factor in the development of T2DM *(6)*. However, a family history is not an absolute prerequisite for the development of diabetes. In fact, patients develop diabetes without any known family history. There is usually a stronger family history in T2DM than in T1DM. Sixty percent of patients with T2DM have either a parent or a sibling with the disease. In some populations, notably the Pima Indians of Arizona and the natives of Nauru in the Gilbert Islands of the Pacific, one-third to one-half of all persons are afflicted with T2DM. When one member of a monozygotic twinship has the disease, the second identical twin is almost invariably affected (90% concordance). However, there is no association with genes of the major histocompatibility complex similar to that occurring in T2DM. Despite the high familial prevalence of T2DM, the precise mode of inheritance remains undefined. As stated above, constitutional factors such as obesity and the amount of exercise influence the expression of this disease.

3. ORAL COMPLICATIONS OF DIABETES MELLITUS

The oral complications of uncontrolled DM may include, but are not necessarily limited to, infection, poor healing, increased incidence and severity of caries, candidiasis with its protean presentations, gingivitis and periodontal disease, periapical abscesses, xerostomia, altered taste, and burning mouth *(3)*. The oral complications in patients with uncontrolled DM are most likely related to the excessive loss of fluids through excessive urination (polyuria), the altered response to infection, the microvascular changes, and possibly the increased glucose concentrations in saliva (salivary hyperglycemia). Careful evaluation of glycemic control is critical in determining the risk assessment for progression to the oral complications from diabetes.

3.1. Xerostomia

A high percentage of persons with diabetes experience xerostomia and its related complications *(7–10)*. When the normal environment of the oral cavity is altered because of a decrease in salivary flow or alterations in salivary composition, a healthy mouth can become more susceptible to painful dental caries. Dry and atrophic oral mucosa can also result from xerostomia, potentially accompanied by mucositis, ulceration, and desquamation as well as opportunistic bacterial, viral, or fungal infections and an inflamed, depapillated tongue. Coupled with impairment in cell-mediated immunity, xerostomia is thus a devastating oral complication. Difficulty in lubricating, masticating, tasting, and swallowing are among the most serious complications of xerostomia and may contribute to impaired nutritional intake. Nutrition management for xerostomia focuses on adequate fluid with all meals and snacks and use of moist foods (see the appendix for nutrition guidelines). Aside from topical treatments for xerostomia, improved metabolic control of diabetes may mitigate against its complications. Therefore, it is critical that the dentist and nutritionist work together to develop an effective dietary management plan for the diabetic patient with xerostomia.

3.2. Caries

The relationship between DM and caries has been investigated with conflicting conclusions. Risk factors for caries that may be influenced by diabetes include the quality and quantity of saliva, and salivary immune surveillance. Additionally, salivary hyperglycemia may contribute to increased caries risk *(11,12)*. Several studies have shown caries incidence that is higher *(13–20)* or lower *(21–25)* in individuals with diabetes compared to those without diabetes. This contradiction is most likely the result of study design, cohort characteristics, and degree of diabetes control.

Regular oral and dental examination, as an integral component of diabetes care, is imperative to detect caries and render corrective and preventive therapy at the earliest opportunity. Any patient with three or more carious lesions during a 12-mo period should be considered at the highest risk for future caries, and preventive steps should be taken: sealants, fluoride, and diet evaluation or modification as needed.

3.3. Oral Candidiasis

Oral candidiasis is an opportunistic fungal infection commonly associated with hyperglycemia and is a frequent complication of diabetes *(26)*. Oral lesions associated with candidal infection include median rhomboid glossitis (central papillary atrophy), atrophic glossitis, denture stomatitis, pseudomembranous candidiasis (thrush), and angular cheilitis *(26)*. *Candida albicans* is a constituent of the normal oral microflora. It rarely colonizes and infects the oral mucosa unless there are predisposing factors. These include immunologically compromised conditions, as seen prototypically in malignancy, chemotherapy, human immunodeficiency virus infection and acquired immunodeficiency syndrome, or, particularly, poorly or marginally controlled diabetes mellitus; individuals who wear dentures and practice poor oral hygiene; and the chronic use of broad-spectrum antibiotics. The contribution of xerostomia with the loss of saliva and its protective mechanisms, compromised immune function, and salivary hyperglycemia that provides a potential substrate for fungal growth are the major contributing factors for oral candidiasis in diabetes.

Guggenheimer *(28)* showed that more subjects with T1DM than control subjects without T1DM (15.1 vs 3.0%) were found with clinical manifestations of candidiasis, including median rhomboid glossitis (MRG), denture stomatitis, and angular cheilitis. Subjects with T1DM were also more likely to have *Candida pseudohyphae* in their cytologic smears as well as increased pseudohyphae in their counts. Diabetic subjects with MRG had a longer duration of T1DM as well as the microvascular complications of nephropathy and retinopathy. Denture stomatitis was associated with smoking, retinopathy, higher counts of candidal pseudohyphae, poor glycemic control, and a longer duration of T1DM. Three factors in this particular study were significantly associated with the presence of candidal pseudohyphae: cigarette smoking, the use of dentures, and elevated HbA1c levels, indicative of marginal to poor metabolic control *(28)*. Clearly, cigarette smoking and glycemic control are modifiable risk factors. The dentist must provide the patient with information on smoking cessation and monitor that patient's progress carefully and must also work closely with the patient's physician and nutritionist to ensure improved glycemic control and minimize the risk for these opportunistic fungal infections. Management strategies for oral candidiasis are summarized in Table 2.

3.4. Noncandidal-Associated Oral Lesions

A number of soft tissue abnormalities other than candidal infections have also been reported with DM *(30)*. These include aphthous stomatitis *(31,32)*, benign migratory glossitis (geographic tongue) *(33)*, fissured tongue *(34)*, hyperplastic gingivitis *(35)*,

Table 2
Regimens for Treatment of Oral Candidiasis

Agent	Duration	Label
Treatment for Oral Candidiasis		
Topical		
• Clotrimazole troches [a]	2 wk	Dissolve 1 10 mg troche in mouth 5 times a day
• Nystatin vaginal suppositories [b]	2 wk	Dissolve 1 tablet (100,000 U) in mouth 6 to 8 times a day
Systemic		
• Fluconazole	2 wk	100 mg/d
• Ketoconazole [c]	2 wk	200 mg/d
• Itraconazole [d]	2 wk	200 mg/d
Treatment for Angular Cheilitis		
Antifungal cream	2 wk	Apply to affected area 4 times a day
• Clotrimazole 1%		
• Miconazole 2%		
• Ketoconazole 2%		
Combination creams [e]	2 wk	Apply to affected area 3 times a day
• Hydrocortisone-iodoquinol cream		
• Betamethasone-dipropionate-clotrimazole cream		
• Triamcinolone-nystatin cream		

[a] Use with caution because of sugar content

[b] Although this preparation is not designed for oral use, clinicians have found it useful for the treatment of oral candidiasis when the sugar content of other topical anticandidal medications is of concern. A sugarless flavored lozenge maybe dissolved simultaneously in the mouth to mask the taste of Nystatin.

[c] Must use with caution; monitor for hepatotoxicity with liver function tests.

[d] Should be used for resistant strains of *C. albicans*.

[e] Some clinicians have found combination creams more effective than antifungal medications alone in the treatment of angular cheilitis. These include combination preparations of topical hydrocortisone, antifungal agents, and hydrocortisone-iodoquinol cream, which combines an antifungal–antibacterial agent with an anti-inflammatory antipruritic.

lichen planus *(36,37)*, and parotid gland enlargement *(38)*. Although many studies have evaluated oral lesions in patients with DM, there have been conflicting findings concerning the prevalence of some noncandidal associated conditions *(39–41)*. It is not clear whether the type of diabetes, the duration, or the degree of glycemic control account for some of these contradictory findings. Another recent study examined the prevalence and characteristics of noncandidal oral lesions in T1DM *(30)*. Nearly twice as many subjects with diabetes as those without the disease were found with one or more oral soft tissue lesions (44.7 vs 25.0%), and all had elevated HbA1c levels. Subjects with diabetes also had significantly higher prevalence rates for noncandidal lesions such as fissured tongue, irritation fibroma, and traumatic ulcers. Elevated glycosylated hemoglobin levels were noted in all patients, indicating marginal to poor glycemic control. Working with the registered dietitian (RD), the dentist can provide the patient with effective diet guidelines to minimize the recurrence of oral complications and promote healing from trauma or infection. It is equally imperative to treat traumatic ulcers with antibiotics to prevent secondary infections, particularly in the poorly controlled individual with diabetes. Patients with persistent noncandidal oral lesions should be referred to a dental oral medicine specialist for evaluation and treatment.

3.5. Periodontal Disease

The relationship between DM and periodontal disease and infection is bidirectional, with evidence for worsening of one disease being correlated with poor control of the other. Periodontal infection may complicate the severity of DM and the degree of metabolic glucose control *(24,25,27,42–47)*. Individuals with diabetes are more likely to develop periodontal disease: the longer the duration of the diabetes, the greater the severity of the periodontal disease *(19,29,31,48–52)*. Indeed, periodontal disease has been referred to as the "sixth complication of DM" *(53)*. The susceptibility to periodontal disease in diabetes, although related primarily to the presence of dental bacterial plaque, may also be related to several diabetes-associated pathological events. These include impairment in cell-mediated immunity such as neutrophil (polymorphonucleocyte) chemotaxis and macrophage function *(54,55)* and vascular disease. In most cases, the dental clinician can manage the well-controlled person with T1DM or T2DM in a manner consistent with a healthy individual without diabetes. The well-controlled person with diabetes generally does not require antibiotics following surgical procedures. However, the administration of antibiotics during the postsurgical phase is appropriate, particularly if there is significant infection, pain, and stress. Several papers have reported an additional therapeutic benefit from tetracyclines, principally as inhibitors of human matrix metalloproteinase activity (e.g., collagenase) and bone resorption; this inhibitory effect is independent of the antimicrobial action of tetracyclines, providing an added dimension to the therapeutic management of periodontitis *(56–62)*. Preventive periodontal therapy must be included in the comprehensive care of the patient with diabetes. Therapy includes an initial assessment of the risk of oral disease progression, explicit oral hygiene instruction, dietary assessment and instruction, and frequent periodic examinations and prophylactic dental cleaning.

The dentist can perform periodontal surgical procedures, although it is important for the patient to maintain a normal diet during the postsurgical phase to avoid hypoglycemia and ensure effective healing and repair. The practitioner should review any previous history of diabetic complications, determine the most recent test results (e.g., glycosylated hemoglobin and postprandial blood glucose levels), and maintain an ongoing dialogue with the patient's physician and nutritionist. Supportive periodontal therapy should be provided at relatively close intervals (2–3 mo) because some studies indicate a slight, but persistent, tendency to progressive periodontal destruction, despite effective metabolic control *(19,29,31,48,50,52)*. The dentist, nutritionist, and physician can work as a team to closely monitor oral hygiene maintenance, diet, and glycemic control in the diabetic patient.

3.6. Oral Burning/Dysesthesia

Patients with diabetes may complain of a continuous burning sensation, usually involving the tip and dorsum of the tongue or the palate. Associated underlying mucosal disorders (lichen planus, candidiasis) should be identified and treated, resulting in relief of the burning sensation. Burning may also be a sign of vitamin deficiency (B_{12}, zinc), and these levels should be examined and corrected if abnormal. Burning in the absence of physical or biochemical changes may represent a diabetes-related oral sensory neuropathy, and several reports have explored this possibility, although none in a rigorous and valid manner *(63–66)*. When a physical or biochemical abnormality cannot be found, the symptoms of burning mouth can be improved using adjuvant neuropathic analgesic

Table 3
Treatment Goals for the ABCs of Diabetes

A_1C <7%			
Preprandial plasma glucose	90–130 mg/dL		
Peak postprandial plasma glucose	<180 mg/dL		
Blood Pressure (mmHg)			
	Systolic		Diastolic
Hypertension definition	>140	and/or	>90
Treatment goal	<130	and	<80
Cholesterol: Lipid Profile (mg/dL)			
LDL	<100		
HDL	Men >40		Women >50
Triglycerides	<150		

From the American Diabetes Association Clinical Practice Recommendations, Diabetes Care 2003; 26 (Suppl. 1):S3–S50.

medications such as a tricyclic antidepressant or clonazepam. However, an unfortunate side effect of these medications is xerostomia, which may compound any existing alterations in saliva and increase risk of candidiasis and dental caries.

3.7. Altered Taste

Dysgeusia can occur in patients with diabetes and may adversely affect food choices and intake of nutrients. Altered taste in individuals with diabetes is often caused by altered salivary chemistry (secondary to diabetes out of control), xerostomia, burning mouth or tongue, and/or candidiasis; all possibilities should be explored to determine any possible underlying disorder. Possible approaches for relief from dysgeusia include increased use of flavoring agents during food preparation, substituting alternative protein sources if unable to tolerate meat, and use of artificial saliva as needed.

4. MANAGEMENT GOALS FOR THE PATIENT WITH DIABETES

The dietitian, dentist, and physician each have specific roles in optimal care for the patient with diabetes. Responsibilities include screening for nutritional, oral, and systemic disease as well as surveillance of glycemic control. Tables 1 and 3 summarize the goals of diabetes management and a recommended surveillance program, respectively, for patients with diabetes.

4.1. Oral/Medical Screening

Both disciplines should incorporate medical history questions consistent with the *Standards of Medical Care for Patients with Diabetes Mellitus (67)*. Specific questions regarding prior activity, metabolic control, and diet prescriptions are important. Questions regarding metabolic control will yield important information regarding past and potential future episodes of hyper- or hypoglycemia. Such information should include the following laboratory data: HbA1C; total, low- (LDL) and high-density lipoprotein (HDL) cholesterol; triglycerides; and fasting glucose as well as weight and any history of weight change. Previous diet and medication controls, frequency, severity and cause of episodes of hyper- and hypoglycemia, and other medications and over-the-counter products should be routinely asked of patients on initial and periodic follow-up exams. Prior diet prescriptions should be compared to current dietary habits based on the diet history taken; this will provide some level of assessment of patient compliance and health attitude. In addition to the oral exam, an overall physical exam including height and weight, blood pressure, skin, and cranial nerves should be conducted. Subsequent referrals to appropriate health professionals should be provided on the basis of the exam findings and patient needs. Tables 1 and 3 (from the National Diabetes Education Program) summarize current recommended diabetes surveillance and management strategies; important roles are clearly stated for dentist and RD.

4.2. Team Approach to Diabetes Management

All health professionals must be cognizant of the medical, dental, and nutrition goals for management of diabetes, be aware of the resources available and refer the patient to the appropriate health care provider. No discipline functions within a vacuum; in particular, in regard to dentistry and nutrition, there is sufficient evidence to support the need for awareness of diabetes management goals, screening, and referral mechanisms.

It is incumbent on dietetic and dental professionals to screen individuals with diabetes for nutrition and oral health risk, provide appropriate education, and refer to other health professionals as needed. The relationship between oral manifestations of diabetes and diet/nutrition is a complex two-way street. Oral manifestations of diabetes challenge and compromise eating ability and consequently diet quality and nutrient intake, ultimately impacting nutrition status. Clearly, the role of each discipline is different in this process; both roles are outlined below. A detailed review of oral nutrition risk assessment may be found in Chapter 17.

5. CO-MORBIDITIES AND DIABETES

The term "diabesity" has been coined to refer to the strong relationship between diabetes and obesity. Diabetes and obesity incidence are increasing at escalating proportions across the life span; T2DM in children, once considered rare, is becoming increasingly common with the increased incidence of obesity in children. Obesity remains a dominant modifiable risk factor for diabetes for adults and children.

Metabolic syndrome refers to the combination of the following risk factors: abdominal obesity, T2DM, insulin resistance, dyslipidemia, and hypertension (68). Obesity and central abdominal adiposity (waist circumference of 40 in for men, 35 in for women) are two independent predictors of metabolic syndrome that have an additive effect on risk factors for metabolic syndrome (68).

5.1. Screening

5.1.1. THE ROLE OF THE RD

Medical nutrition therapy (MNT) for individuals with all types of DM is a recognized essential component of care. The American Diabetes Association Clinical Practice Recommendations focus on treatment and prevention of diabetes and the related complications (69) and are described in the subsequent section of this chapter. Qualified dietetics professionals need to incorporate questions and guidelines on dental sequelae of diabetes into MNT as well as refer patients for dental care *(70)*. As a component of the health history and review of systems, the RD can ask about difficulties with biting, chewing, and swallowing, and the presence and severity of oral diseases and conduct a brief oral exam *(70,71)*. The oral exam by the RD should include a screen of the head and neck area, cranial nerves, and intraoral area to note integrity of the soft tissue, dentition, and occlusion *(71,72)*. Although it is not the role of the RD to diagnose or treat oral symptomatology or disease, it is incumbent on the RD to note any "nonnormal" finding, determine its impact on eating ability, and refer patients appropriately to the dentist *(72)*.

The RD will also complete a medical history and screen as described in the previous section and an in-depth diet history. The diet history taken by the RD differs from that suggested for the dentist. As clearly elucidated in the American Diabetes Association's nutrition guidelines *(73,74)*, it is the role of the RD to provide MNT but "it is essential that all team members be knowledgeable about nutrition therapy and supportive of the person with diabetes." The outcome of the RD screen will be one or more of the following: provide MNT for the patient, refer the patient to a dentist for evaluation and treatment, refer the patient to his or her primary care provider, or refer the patient to another health professional. MNT is described in a subsequent section.

5.1.2. The Role of the Dentist

The role of the dentist in screening individuals for nutrition risk includes questions about metabolic control of their disease, history of hypo- and hyperglycemia incidents, and questions regarding diet. Sample diet history questions are outlined in Chapter 17, Table 4 and Appendix A.

Patient responses to questions regarding difficulties with biting, chewing, and swallowing provide insight into the functional abilities of the oral cavity. Although the dental professional will address these issues as part of a dental treatment plan, it is likewise his or her responsibility to provide some guidelines on how to eat when dentition or oral function is compromised and refer patients as appropriate to an RD. Common scenarios where masticatory function can be compromised in a patient with diabetes and appropriate consultation or referral to an RD is justified include partial or complete edentulism, removable prostheses, postoperative periods when pain may significantly affect oral intake of nutrients, and chronic disorders affecting mastication such as xerostomia and chronic orofacial pain of myofascial, musculoskeletal, neuropathic, or mucosal origins.

6. GOALS OF MEDICATION MANAGEMENT OF DIABETES MELLITUS

6.1. Tight Control: Revisiting and Redefining an Established Concept

Current diabetes treatment goals are summarized in Table 3. Both acute and chronic, prolonged exposure to hyperglycemia is the primary factor responsible for the development of diabetic complications *(75)*. The common biochemical basis for complications is hyperglycemia-mediated formation of nonenzymatic advanced glycation end products (AGEs). AGEs are chemically irreversible, glucose-derived compounds that form slowly and continuously in plasma and tissues as a function of blood glucose concentration and have been linked to the development of diabetic complications such as renal failure *(76)*.

The glycated or glycosylated hemoglobin test (HbA1c) is widely used to assess glycemic control *(77)*. It also has prognostic value as shown in the the Diabetes Control and

Table 4
Correlation Between Glycosylated
Hemoglobin and Mean Plasma Glucose Level

Glycosylated hemoglobin (%)	Mean plasma glucose (mg/dL)
6	135
7	170
8	205
9	240
10	275
11	310
12	345

Complications Trial (DCCT) in 1993 *(78)*; the randomized prospective 6-yr study in Japan (Kumamoto study, 1995) *(79)*; and in the UK Prospective Diabetes Study Group in 1998 *(80)*. The HbA1c measures glucose that binds to blood hemoglobin within the circulating erythrocytes and remains attached for the life cycle of the red blood cell. Thus, hemoglobin is a marker to measure the glucose pool. Hence, it is the preferred test for the medical evaluation of diabetic control because it measures the blood glucose levels over a period of 8 to 12 wk. Continuous or prolonged hyperglycemia as measured by the glycated hemoglobin test is associated with chronic toxicity and tissue damage. The glycated hemoglobin can be elevated significantly with prolonged, severe hyperglycemia. Target therapeutic ranges for the HbA1C are below 7% (American Diabetes Association) or 6% (American College of Endocrinolgy); Table 4 summarizes the correlation between glycated hemoglobin and mean plasma glucose *(77)*. However, the glycated hemoglobin is not the most complete expression of the degree of hyperglycemia; the HbA1c measurement alone is not sufficient to assess diabetes control.

In 1995, the DCCT showed that other features of diabetic glucose control not reflected in the HbA1c might add to or modify the risk of complications *(81)*. For example, clinical data show that the risk and severity of complications may be even more highly dependent on the extent of 1 to 2 h postprandial (after meal) excursions of blood glucose (acute glycemia and toxicity) *(76)*. Hyperglycemia after a meal is associated with increased free radical production that can lead to tissue damage. Hyperglycemia 2 h postload is associated with an increased risk of death, independent of fasting blood glucose *(82)*. Data also show that the risk of microvascular (nerve, eye, and kidney) disease increases with progression in postprandial glucose levels from 180 to 260 mg/dL *(79)*. Hence, tight control in current therapy now includes a shift to a new focus: constant, daily, glucose monitoring (a battery-operated glucometer) often before and after meals to target postprandial levels (Table 3) and minimize the occurrence of acute hyperglycemia and acute toxicity. The battery-operated glucometer is a home monitoring device that enables the patient to obtain and record blood glucose data. The patient should perform this test, on average, at least four to six times per day. Walking this metabolic tightrope also carries risk: the patient may fall into profound hypoglycemia (insulin shock) with multiple insulin injections, or severe hyperglycemia with ketoacidosis (diabetic coma) on the insulin pump.

Oral hypoglycemic agents and insulin preparations currently available for treating diabetes mellitus are summarized in Tables 5 and 6 *(87)*.

Table 5
Oral Hypoglycemic Agents

Class	Drug	Dosage	Doses/day
Insulin Secretogogues			
Sulfonylureas	Chlorpropramide	100–500 mg	1
	Glibizide	5–40 mg	1–2
	Glyburide	1.5–2 mg	1–2
	Glimedpride	1–8 mg	1
Nonsulfonylureas	Nateglinide	180–360 mg	2–4
	Repaglinide	0.5–16 mg	2–4
Insulin Sensitizers			
Biguanides	Metformin	500–2250 mg	2–3
Thiazolidinediones	Pioglitazone	15–45 mg	1
	Rosiglitazone	4–8 mg	1–2
Delay Carb Absorption			
α-glucosidase inh	Acarbose	25–300 mg	3
	Miglitol	25–300 mg	3
Combination Agents	Rosiglitazone + Metformin		2
	Metformin + Glyburide		1–2
	Metformin + Glipizide		1–2

Table 6
Insulin Preparations

Type	Action	Onset time (h)	Peak time (h)	Duration (h)
Human				
Regular	Short–intermed	0.5	2–4	6–12
NPH	Intermed	1.5	4–6	14–16
Lente	Intermed	3.0	7–9	14–20
Ultralente	Intermed–long	4.0	8–14	24
Analogs				
Lispro	Rapid	0.25	1.25	2.5
Insulin Aspart	Rapid	0.25	1.25	2.5
Glargine	Long acting	2.00	none	>24
Insulin Mixtures				
Humulin 70/30	NPH 70% + Regular 30%	0.50	4.0	14–16
Novolin 70/30	NPH 70% + Regular 30%	6.50	4.0	14–16
Humulin 50/50	NPH 50% + Regular 50%	0.50	4.0	14–16
Humalog 75/25	NPH 75% + Humalog 25%	0.25	2.5	14–16
Novolog 70/30	NPH 70% + Novolog 30%	0.25	2.5	14–20

6.2. Medical Nutrition Therapy (MNT)

Diet management is the cornerstone of diabetes management. Clearly, there are several approaches to diet management of diabetes. Independent of the strategy selected is the need for MNT with a qualified provider, namely the RD. Goals of MNT are outlined in Table 7 *(73)*. MNT in diabetes care includes a comprehensive nutrition assessment

Table 7
Goals of Medical Nutrition Therapy

Goals for all persons with diabetes

- Attain and maintain desirable metabolic outcomes
  - Normal blood glucose values
  - Lipid profile consistent with risk reduction for macrovascular complications
  - Blood pressure levels associated with reduced risk for vascular disease
- Prevent and treat associated chronic complications of diabetes
  - Modify nutrient intake and lifestyle to prevent obesity, dyslipidemia, cardiovascular disease, hypertension, nephropathy
- Improve health through healthy food choices and physical activity
- Address individual nutritional needs considering personal and cultural preferences and lifestyle

Goals for specific situations

- In youth with T1DM, provide adequate energy for normal growth and development, integrate insulin regimens into usual eating and physical activity habits
- In youth with T2DM, facilitate changes in eating and physical activity habits that reduce insulin resistance and improve metabolic status
- In women who are pregnant and lactating, provide adequate energy and nutrients needed for optimal outcomes
- In older adults, provide for the nutritional and psychological needs of an aging individual
- In individuals treated with insulin or insulin secretagogues, provide self-management education for treatment (and prevention) of hypoglycemia, acute illnesses, and exercise-related blood glucose problems
- In people at risk for diabetes, decrease risk via encouraging physical activity and promotion of food choices that facilitate moderate weight loss or at least prevent weight gain

Adapted from ref. *74.*

that addresses current diet intake, eating patterns, lifestyle, metabolic status and control, readiness to change, goal-setting, diet instruction, and monitoring of response to therapy. Individuals at increased risk should be referred to an RD for MNT. The high-risk patient population includes persons at risk for oral problems because of poor glycemic control and those with diabetes who face dental (oral) procedures that will affect their functional ability to eat. Examples include individuals undergoing oral surgical procedures in which eating ability will be compromised for several days or longer (dental implants, extensive periodontal surgery, multiple extractions), those getting full dentures, or those getting reconstructive surgery.

Medicare reimbursement for MNT for individuals with diabetes supports referrals to an RD by dental professionals for individuals with diabetes. In most states, MNT by an RD with several follow-up visits is a benefit covered by all third-party payers and Medicaid. In addition to referring patients as appropriate to an RD, the oral health professional should reinforce the need to adhere to the diabetic diet, integrate oral hygiene into daily routines, and modify diet consistencies as needed to manage oral conditions and surgeries.

6.3. Nutrition Goals of Diabetes Management

The nutrition goals for diabetes management of the American Diabetes Association *(73,74)* are stated in Table 7. The evidence supporting these goals is provided for each of the macro- and micronutrients, alcohol, and energy needs is clearly stated as "A level" (strongest) to "B" and "C" level (weakest).

General recommendations regarding energy intake and obesity focus on provision of calories to promote weight loss and improve insulin resistance and glycemic control in individuals with insulin resistance (A-level evidence). Lifestyle modification programs including education, reduced fat (<30% of total calories) and energy intake, regular physical activity, and ongoing contact between participant and provider can promote long-term weight loss. Additionally, behavior modification and exercise are useful adjunctive therapies to support weight-loss initiatives. Energy intake should be determined based on weight management goals.

Expert consensus indicates that carbohydrate should comprise 60 to 70% of energy intake. However, the metabolic profile and need for weight loss should be considered when determining the macronutrient composition. A-level evidence for carbohydrate indicates that foods containing whole grains, fruits, vegetables, and low-fat milk should be included. The total amount of carbohydrate at meals and snacks should be considered as more important than the source or type of the carbohydrate. Glycemic response is influenced by many factors including the amount of carbohydrate, type of sugar (fructose, glucose, lactose, sucrose), nature of the starch, food processing, and cooking and form as well as the presence of other food components. The literature at this time *(73,74)* does not support use of glycemic index as a strategy to control diabetic diets, rather total carbohydrate. Sucrose-containing foods may be included but they should be substituted for other types of carbohydrates or covered with insulin. Nonnutritive sweeteners may be used. Dietary fiber recommendations are similar to those for the general population.

Expert consensus regarding protein intake indicates that it should comprise 15 to 20% of the total energy intake when renal function is normal. There is no A-level evidence regarding protein in the diabetic diet; B-level evidence indicates that although the protein requirement for individuals with diabetes may be more than the recommedned dietary allowance, it should not be greater than "usual" intake. The primary goal regarding dietary fat in the diet for diabetes is limitation of dietary saturated fat and cholesterol. A-level evidence supporting fat intake indicates that less than 10% of total energy intake should come from saturated fats and that those with an elevated LDL-C (>100mg/dL) may benefit by less than 7% from saturated fat. Dietary cholesterol should be less than 300 mg/d (those with a LDL-C >100mg/dL should have less than 200 mg/d). B-level evidence supports that total energy intake from saturated fat should be reduced when weight loss is a goal and intake of transunsaturated fatty acids should be minimized. B-level evidence also supports the fact that reduced-fat diets over time can contribute to a "modest" loss of weight and improvement in lipid levels. C-level evidence regarding fat supports a polyunsaturated fat intake of less than 10% of total energy needs.

Although there is no A-level evidence supporting added levels of micronutrient or antioxidant intake for individuals with diabetes, B-level evidence indicates no evidence of benefit from vitamin, mineral, or trace-element supplementation for individuals with diabetes in the absence of a deficiency. The exceptions to this include folate for the prevention of neural tubular birth defects and calcium for prevention of bone disease, both recommendations for all individuals independent of diabetes. In addition, the B-level evidence also indicates that routine supplementation of antioxidants is not advised as there are no data regarding the long-term efficacy or safety of supplemental doses. B-level evidence regarding alcohol indicates that intake should be limited to one drink per day for women and two for men.

The reader is encouraged to consult the references for more detailed discussion on management of T1DM and T2DM and special situations. Other recommended clinical resources include the American Diabetes Association (Website: www.diabetescare.org) and the American Dietetic Association (Website: www.eatright.org).

6.4. The Diabetic Diet

Individuals with diabetes should be seen by an RD for MNT on diagnosis in order to determine the appropriate diabetic diet and establish individualized goals and meal plans. In addition to the traditional diabetes exchange system diet, there is also carbohydrate counting, the diabetes food guide pyramid, and the glycemic index.

The diabetes food guide pyramid *(83)* is similar to the US Food Guide Pyramid but is composed of six food groups. The largest group, grains and starchy vegetables, forms the base of the pyramid, and fats, sweets, and alcohol are the smallest group is at the tip, indicating that one should consume the least amount of servings from each group. The remaining groups—vegetables, fruits, dairy, and protein foods—form the middle of the pyramid. An individualized diabetes diet care plan will include a specific number of servings from each group depending on the individual's goals and energy and nutrient needs. It is important to distribute food groups at each meal and snack.

The diabetes exchange lists are published by the American Dietetic Association and American Diabetes Association *(84)* and are another guide often used for individualized meal planning. Exchange systems are also available for several nationalities to facilitate keeping to one's ethnic food preferences. The exchange system is based on distribution of foods on the basis of their nutrient composition and includes a carbohydrate group that contains starch, fruit, milk, and other carbohydrates; and vegetable lists; a meat and meat substitutes group that includes categories based on the fat content; a fat group; and lists for vegetarian alternatives, fast foods, and other carbohydrates, including cakes, pies, puddings, and cookies.

Carbohydrate counting is another tool for individuals with diabetes to use in making food choices and planning meals *(85)*. It is based on the principle that total carbohydrate intake influences blood glucose the most. Using this method, individuals with diabetes calculate the grams of carbohydrate they eat at meals and snacks. Individuals must learn to use carbohydrate counting along with the principles of balanced nutrition and the food guide pyramid in planning their meals.

The glycemic index (GI) of a carbohydrate is the rise in plasma glucose (above baseline) relative to that induced by a standard, usually 50 g, glucose or "white bread challenge" *(86)*. GI values are based on digestion and absorption postprandially. Clearly, dietary fiber content and other factors influence the GI of individual foods. There is no consensus as to its usefulness and practicality as means of dietary management of DM.

7. SUMMARY

Given the systemic nature of DM and its sequellae, it is clear that nutrition and oral health are central to health maintanence and prevention of complications in individuals with diabetes. Dietetics and dental professionals in collaboration with physicians can provide a coordinated approach to care. Recognition and appreciation of the role of each discipline in disease management is critical to successful patient care.

Guidelines for Practice

	Nutrition–Diet	*Oral Health*
Assessment	• Nutrition risk evaluation • Determine level of risk and need for intervention (registered dietician [RD], dentist, medical, other) • Medical nutrition therapy (MNT) to include diet, clinical, anthropometric, and biochemical assessment	• Intra/extra oral exam of hard and soft tissue, cranial nerves • Determine level of risk and need for intervention (RD, dentist, medical, other)
Prevention	• Periodic comprehensive assessment and MNT to determine compliance • Reinforce guidelines for care	• Periodic oral examinations and prophylaxis • Reinforce guidelines for care
Intervention	• MNT	• Dental care as needed

REFERENCES

1. Diabetes Public Health Resource. Centers for Disease Control. Website: (http://www.cdc.gov/diabetes/statistics/prev/national/fig1.htm). Accessed December 23, 2003.
2. Centers for Disease Control and Prevention. National diabetes fact sheet: general information and national estimates on diabetes in the United States, 2002. Atlanta, GA: U.S. Department of Health and Human Services, Centers for Disease Control and Prevention, 2003. Website: (http://www.diabetes.org/info/facts/facts_natl.jsp). Accessed December 23, 2003.
3. Diabetes. In Little JW, Falace DA, Miller CS, Rhodus NL, eds. Dental Management of the Medically Compromised Patient. St. Louis, MO: Mosby, 1997, 387–409.
4. Special Supplement. J Am Dent Assoc 2003; 134.
5. Mullen AG Jr. Endocrinologic problems. In Goroll AH, May LA, Mulley AG Jr, eds. Primary Care Medicine: Office Evaluation and Management of the Adult Patient. Philadelphia, PA: J.B. Lippincott, 1995, 524–527.
6. Whitehead C. Diabetes. In Rubin E, Farber JL, eds. Pathology. Philadelphia, PA: J.B. Lippincott, 1994, 1148–1160.
7. Field EA, Longman LP, Bucknall R, et al. The establishment of a xerostomia clinic: a prospective study. Br J Oral Maxillofac Surg 1997; 35(2):96–103.
8. Chavez EM, Bornell LN, Taylor GW, Ship JA. A longitudinal analysis of salivary flow in control subjects and older adults with type 2 diabetes. Oral Surg Oral Med Oral Pathol Oral Radiol Endod 2001; 91:166–173.
9. Gilbert GH, Heft MW, Duncan RP. Mouth dryness as reported by older Floridians. Community Dent Oral Epidemiol 1993; 21:390–397.
10. Moore PA, Guggenheimer J, Etzel KR, Weyant RJ, Orchard T. Type I diabetes mellitus, xerostomia, and salivary flow rates. Oral Surg Oral Med Oral Pathol Oral Radiol Endod 2001; 92:281–292.
11. Feller RP, Shannon IL. The secretion of glucose by the parotid gland. J Am Assoc Dent Res 1975; 54:570.
12. Tenovuo J, Alanen P, Larjava H, Vilikari J, Lehtonen OP. Oral health of patients with insulin-dependent diabetes mellitus. Scand J Dent Res 1986; 94:338–346.

13. Moore PA, Weyant RJ, Etzel KR, et al. Type 1 diabetes mellitus and oral health: assessment of coronal and root caries. Community Dent Oral Epidemiol 2001; 29:183–194.
14. Lin BP, Taylor GW, Allen DJ, Ship JA. Dental caries in older adults with diabetes mellitus. Spec Care Dent 1999; 19:8–14.
15. Twetman S, Johansson I, Birkland D, Nederfors T. Caries incidence in young type 1 diabetes mellitus patients in relation to metabolic control and caries-associated risk factors. Caries Res 2002; 36: 31–35.
16. Tewtman S, Nedefors T, Stahl B, Aronson S. Two year longitudinal observations of salivary status and dental caries in children with diabetes mellitus. Pediatr Dent 1992; 14:184–188.
17. Tavares M, Depaola P, Soparkar P, Joshipura K. The prevalence of root caries in a diabetic population. J Dent Res 1991; 70:979–983.
18. Karajalainen KM, Knuuttila ML, Kaar ML. Relationship between caries and level of metabolic balance in children and adolescents with insulin dependant diabetes mellitus. Caries Res 1997; 31:13–18.
19. Emrich L, Schlossman M, Genco R. Periodontal disease in non-insulin dependant diabetes mellitus. J Periodontol 1991; 62:123–131.
20. Canepari P, Zerman N, Cavalleri G. Lack of correlations between salivary *Streptococcus mutans* and lactobacillicounts and caries in IDDM children. Minerva Stomatol 1989; 43:501–505.
21. Kirk JM, Kinirons MJ. Dental health of young insulin dependant diabetic subjects in Northern Ireland. Community Dent Health 1991; 8:335–341.
22. Matsson L, Koch G. Caries frequency in children with controlled diabetes. Scand J Dent Res 1975; 83:327–332.
23. Meurman JH, Collin HL, Niskaken L, et al. Saliva in non-insulin dependant diabetic patients and control subjects: the role of the autonomic nervous system. Oral Surg Oral Med Oral Pathol Oral Radiol Endod 1998; 86:69–76.
24. Taylor GW. Bidirectional interrelationships between diabetes and periodontal diseases: an epidemiological perspective. Ann Periodontol 2001; 6:99–112.
25. Grossi SG, Skrepcinski FB, DeCaro T, Zambon JJ, Cummins D, Genco RJ. Response to periodontal therapy in diabetics and smokers. J Periodontol 1996; 67(Suppl. 10):1094–1102.
26. Samarananayake LP. Host factors and oral candidosis. In Samarananayake LP, MacFarlane TW, eds. Oral Candidosis. London, UK: Wright, 1990, 66–103.
27. Grossi SG, Skrepcinski FB, DeCaro T, Zambon JJ, Cummins D, Genco RJ. Treatment of periodontal disease in diabetics reduces glycated hemoglobin. J Periodontol 1997; 68:713–719.
28. Guggenheimer J, Moore PA, Rossie K, et al. Insulin-dependent diabetes mellitus and oral soft tissue pathologies. II. Prevalence and characteristics of Candida and candidal lesions. Oral Surg Oral Med Oral Pathol Oral Radiol Endod 2000; 89:570–576.
29. Tervonen T, Oliver RC. Long term control of diabetes mellitus and periodontitis. J Clin Periodontol 1993; 20:431–435.
30. Guggenheimer J, Moore PA, Rossie K, et al. Insulin-dependent diabetes mellitus and oral soft tissue pathologies. 1. Prevalence and characteristics of non-candidal lesions. Oral Surg Oral Med Oral Pathol Oral Radiol Endod 2000; 89:563–569.
31. Ryan ME, Oana C, Kamer A. The influence of diabetes on the periodontal tissues. J Am Dent Assoc 2003; 134(Suppl.):34S–39S.
32. Lorini R, Scaramuzza A, Vitali L, et al. Clinical aspects of celiac disease in children with insulin dependant diabetes mellitus. J Pediatr Endocrinol Metab 1996;9(Suppl. 1):101–111.
33. Wysocki GP, Daley TD. Benign migratory glossitis in patients with juvenile diabetes. Oral Surg Oral Med Oral Pathol 1987; 63:68–70.
34. Farman AG. Atrophic lesions of the tongue: a prevalence study among 176 diabetic patients. J Oral Pathol 1976; 5:255–264.
35. Van Dis ML, Allen CM, Neville BW. Erythematous gingival enlargement in diabetic patients: a report of four cases. J Oral Maxillofac Surg 1988; 46:794–798.
36. Bagan-Sebastian JV, Milian-Masanet MA, Penarrocha-Diago M, Jiminez Y. A clinical study of 205 patients with oral lichen planus. J Oral Maxillofac Surg 1992; 50:116–118.
37. Petrou-Amerikanou C, Markopoulos AK, Belazi M, Karamitsos D, Papanayotou P. Prevalence of oral lichen planus in diabetes mellitus according to the type of diabetes. Oral Dis 1998; 4:37–40.

38. Russotto SM. Asymptomatic parotid gland enlargement in diabetes mellitus. Oral Surg Oral Med Oral Pathol 1981; 52:594–598.

39. Ben-Aryeh H, Serouya R, Kanter Y, Szargel R, Laufer D. Oral health and salivary composition in diabetic patients. J Diabetes Comp 1993; 7:57–62.

40. Borghelli RF, Pettinari IL, Chuchurru JA, Stirparo MA. Oral lichen planus in patients with diabetes. Oral Surg Oral Med Oral Pathol 1993; 75:498–500.

41. Van Dis ML, Parks ET. Prevalence of oral lichen planus in patients with diabetes mellitus. Oral Surg Oral Med Oral Pathol 1995; 79:696–700 .

42. Taylor GW. The effects of periodontal treatment on diabetes. J Am Dent Assoc 2003; 134(Suppl.): 41S–48S.

43. Grossi SG, Genco RJ. Periodontal disease and diabetes mellitus: a two-way relationship. Ann Periodontol 1998; 3(1):51–61.

44. Taylor GW. Periodontal treatment and its affect on glycemic control: a review of the evidence. Oral Surg Oral Med Oral Pathol Oral Radiol Endod 1999; 87:311–316.

45. Stewart JE, Wager KA, Friedlander AH, Zadeh HH. The effect of periodontal treatment on glycemic control in patients with type 2 diabetes mellitus. J Clin Periodontol 2001; 28:306–310.

46. Taylor GW, Burt BA, Becker MP. Severe periodontitis and risk for poor glycemic control in patients with non-insulin dependant diabetes mellitus. J Periodontol 1996; 67(Suppl. 10):1085–1093.

47. Iacopino AM. Periodontitis and diabetes interrelationships: role of inflammation. Ann Periodontol 2001; 6:125–137.

48. Taylor GW, Burt BA, Becker MP, Genco RJ, Schlossman M. Glycemic control and alveolar bone loss progression in type 2 diabetes. Ann Periodontol 1998; 3:30–39.

49. Grossi S. Treatment of periodontal disease and control of diabetes: an assessment of the evidence and need for future research. Ann Periodontol 2001; 6:138–145.

50. Tsai C, Hayes C, Taylor GW. Glycemic control of type 2 diabetes and severe periodontal disease in the US adult population. Community Dent Oral Epidemiol 2002; 30:182–192.

51. Oliver RC, Tervonen T. Diabetes: a risk factor for paeriodontitis in adults? J Periodontol 1994; 65 (Suppl. 5):530–538.

52. Moore PA, Weyant RJ, Mongelluzzo MB, et al. Type 1 diabetes mellitus and oral health: assessment of periodontal disease. J Periodontol 1999; 70:409–417.

53. Loe H. Periodontal disease: the sixth complication of diabetes mellitus. Diabetes Care 1993; 16:329–334.

54. Genco R, VanDyke TE, Levine MJ, Nelson RD, Wilson ME. Molecular factors influencing neutrophil defects in periodontal disease. J Dent Res 1986; 65:1379–1391.

55. Drell DW, Notkins AL. Multiple immunological abnormalities in patients with type-I (insulin-dependent) diabetes mellitus. Diabetologica 1987; 30:132–143.

56. Vernillo AT, Ramamurthy NS, Golub LM, Greenwald RA, Rifkin BR. Tetracyclines as inhibitors of bone loss in vivo. In Cohen MM Jr, Baum BJ, eds. Studies in Stomatology and Craniofacial Biology. Amsterdam, The Netherlands: IOS Press, 1997, 499–522.

57. Rifkin BR, Vernillo AT, Golub LM, Ramamurthy NS. Modulation of bone resorption by tetracyclines. Annals NY Acad Sci 1994; 732:165–180.

58. Vernillo AT, Ramamurthy NS, Golub LM, Rifkin BR. The nonantimicrobial properties of tetracycline for the treatment of periodontal disease. Curr Opin Periodontol 1994; 2:111–118.

59. Rifkin BR, Vernillo AT, Golub LM. Blocking periodontal disease progression by inhibiting tissue-destructive enzymes: a potential therapeutic role for tetracyclines and their chemically-modified analogs. J Periodontol 1993; 64:819–827.

60. Ramamurthy NS, Vernillo AT, Greenwald RA, et al. Reactive oxygen species activate and tetracyclines inhibit rat osteoblast collagenase. J Bone Min Res 1993; 8:1247–1253.

61. Golub LM, Ramamurthy NS, McNamara TF, Greenwald RA, Rifkin BR. Tetracyclines inhibit connective tissue breakdown: new therapeutic implications for an old family of drugs. Crit Rev Oral Biol Med 1991; 2:297–321.

62. Golub LM, Suomalainen K, Sorsa T. Host modulation with tetracyclines and their chemically modified analogues. Curr Opin Dent 1992; 2:80–90.

63. Ship JA, Grushka M, Lipton J, Mott A, Sessle B, Dionne R. Burning mouth syndrome: an update. J Am Dent Assoc 1995; 126:842–853.

64. Grushka M, Epstein JB, Gorsky M. Burning mouth syndrome Am Fam Physician 2002; 65:615–620.
65. Kalina RE. Seeing into the future: vision and aging. West J Med 1997; 167:253–257.
66. Ship JA, Duffy V, Jones JA, Langmore S. Geriatric oral health and its impact on eating. J Am Geriatr Soc 1996; 44:456–464.
67. American Diabetes Association. Standards of medical care for patients with diabetes mellitus. Diabetes Care 2002; 25(Suppl. 1):S33–S49.
68. Hauer H. Insulin resistance and the metabolic syndrome: a challenge of the new millennium. Eur J Clin Nutr 2002; 56(Suppl. 1):S25–S29.
69. American Diabetes Association. Evidence-based nutrition principles and recommendations for the treatment and prevention of diabetes and related complications. Diabetes Care 2003; 26(Suppl. 1): S51–S61.
70. Touger-Decker R, Sirois D. Dental care of the person with diabetes. In Powers MA, ed. Handbook of Diabetes Nutrition Management. 2nd Ed. Rockville, Md: Aspen Publishers, 1996.
71. American Dietetic Association. American Dietetic Association Position Paper: Nutrition and Oral Health. Journal of the American Dietetic Association 2003; 103(5):615–625.
72. Rigassio D, Touger-Decker R. Physical assessment skills for the R.D. Today's Dietitian 2000; 2(9): 24–26.
73. American Diabetes Association. Evidence-based nutrition principles and recommendations for the treatment and prevention of diabetes and related complications. Diabetes Care 2003; 26(Suppl. 1): S51–S61.
74. American Diabetes Association. Evidence-based nutrition principles and recommendations for the treatment and prevention of diabetes and related complications. Diabetes Care 2002; 25(Suppl. 1): S50–S60.
75. Diabetes Control and Complications Trial Research Group. Epidemiology of severe hyperglycemia in the diabetes control and complications trial. Am J Med 1991; 90:450–459.
76. Ceriello A. The emerging role of postprandial hyperglycemic spikes in the pathogenesis of diabetic complications. Diabet Med 1998; 15(3):188–193.
77. American Association of Clinical Endocrinologist and the American College of Endocrinology. Medical guidelines for the management of diabetes mellitus: the AACE system of intensive diabetes self-management—2002 update. Endocr Pract 2002; 8(Suppl. 1)41–82.
78. Diabetes Control and Complications Trial Research Group. The effect of intensive treatment of diabetes on the development and progression of long-term complications in insulin-dependent dependent mellitus. N Engl J Med 1993; 329:977–986.
79. Ohkubo Y, Kishikawa H, Araki E, et al. Intensive insulin therapy prevents the progression of diabetic microvascular complications in Japanese patients with noninsulin dependent diabetes mellitus: a randomized prospective 6-year study. Diabetes Res Clin Pract 1995; 28:103–117.
80. UK Prospective Diabetes Study Group (UKPDS). Lancet 1998; 352:837–853.
81. Diabetes Control and Complications Trial Research Group. Effect of intensive diabetes management on macrovascular and microvascular events and risk factors in the diabetes control and complications trial. Diabetes 1995; 44:968–983.
82. Hanefeld M, Temelkova-Kurktschiew T. The postprandial state and the risk of atherosclerosis. Diabet Med 1997; 14:S6–S11.
83. Diabetes Food Guide Pyramid. American Diabetes Association. Website: (http://www.diabetes.org/health/nutrition/foodpyramid/foodpyramid.jsp). Accessed December 23, 2003.
84. Meal Planning Exchange Lists. American Diabetes Association. http://www.diabetes.org/health/nutrition/exchanges/exchangelist.jsp. Accessed December 23, 2003.
85. Diabetes Care and Education Dietetic Practice Group. Website: (http://www.dce.org/). Accessed December 23, 2003.
86. Jenkins D, Kendall C, Augustin L, et al. Glycemic index: overview of implications in health and disease. Am J Clin Nutr 2002; 76(Suppl.):266S–73S.
87. Robertson C, Drexler A, Vermillo A. Update on diabetes diagnosis and management. J Am Dent Assn 2003; 134(5):165–235.

Selected Websites

American Diabetes Association
   www.diabetes.org
Centers for Disease Control: Division of Diabetes Translation
   www.cdc.gov/diabetes/index.htm
Centers for Disease Control: Diabetes Project Children and Diabetes
   www.cdc.gov/diabetes/projects/diab_child.html
The Spanish Federation of Associations of Educators in Diabetes (F.E.A.E.D)
   http://www.feaed.org/
MEDLINEplus Diabetes
   www.nlm.nih.gov/medlineplus/diabetes.html
National Diabetes Education Program
   http://ndep.nih.gov
National Institute of Diabetes and Digestive and Kidney Diseases—Nutrition
   www.niddk.nih.gov/health/nutrition.htm

12 Oral and Pharyngeal Cancer

Douglas E. Morse

1. INTRODUCTION

Worldwide, in the year 2000, there were approx 450,000 new cases of and 240,000 deaths attributable to cancer of the lip, oral cavity, pharynx, and salivary glands (ICD-9 140–149) *(1)*. A diagnosis of cancer at these sites is important because it can result in facial disfigurement, speech impairment, chewing and/or swallowing difficulties, mental anguish, a decreased quality of life, and reduced survival.

In the United States, approx 75% of all newly diagnosed oral and pharyngeal cancers (OPCs) are attributable to tobacco and alcohol consumption *(2)*; however, other modifiable exposures, including diet and nutrition, mouthwash use, socioeconomic status, occupation, and oral hygiene, have also been evaluated as potential risk or preventive factors. This chapter reviews findings from studies that have investigated diet and nutrition in relation to OPC risk.

2. NUTRITIONAL EPIDEMIOLOGY

Before presenting the relevant findings, a brief description of the methodological approach utilized in epidemiological studies of diet and nutrition is provided. Most such investigations employ a case–control study design. Using this approach, investigators identify persons with the disease of interest (cases) and persons without the disease (controls). In a case–control study of OPC, the case group is made up of persons with OPC, whereas the control group is composed of persons without such a history.

Information on past exposures of interest (e.g., tobacco use, alcoholic beverage consumption, and diet/nutrition) is then obtained from the cases and controls, with food-frequency questionnaires often used to procure information on previous dietary habits. Typically, food-frequency questionnaires include questions on numerous food items and ask the study participants to estimate how many times a day, week, or month they ate, on average, certain foods (e.g., apples) during their adult life or during a specified time period. The specific food items included in such questionnaires can and do vary across studies.

In some instances, the investigators focus on a particular food item (e.g., tomatoes), whereas in other situations, the researchers define a food group for investigation (e.g.,

From: *Nutrition and Oral Medicine*
Edited by: R. Touger-Decker, D. A. Sirois, and C. C. Mobley © Humana Press Inc., Totowa, NJ

fruits and vegetables). In still other instances, researchers calculate the level of macro-
and micronutrients in the diet by multiplying the average nutrient content within a typical
serving of each food item included on the questionnaire and summing across the various
foods eaten.

On the basis of the dietary information provided by study subjects, researchers then
compare intake patterns in the case and control groups. If ingestion of a given food
increases the risk of disease, cases would be more likely than controls to report having
consumed that food in the past or to have consumed the food on a more frequent basis.
The reverse would be true if the food had a protective effect.

Findings from case–control studies of OPC are often reported in terms of odds ratios
(ORs). The OR is a measure of association and in the case of rare diseases such as OPC,
serves as a good estimate of another epidemiologic measure, the relative risk (RR). The
RR is a useful measure because it relates the risk of disease (in this instance, OPC risk)
among those subjects who have a history of a given exposure relative to the risk of disease
among those persons who did not have the exposure. Both ORs and RRs can range in
magnitude from 0 to infinity. An OR or RR equal to 1.0 suggests no relationship
between exposure and the disease. An OR or RR greater than 1.0 indicates a positive
association between exposure and disease—that is, people with the exposure of interest
are more likely to have developed the disease than persons without the exposure. On the
other hand, an OR or RR less than 1.0 indicates a negative, or inverse, relationship
between the exposure and disease being studied—that is, individuals with the exposure
are less likely to have developed the cancer than are those persons who were unexposed.

The *magnitude* of the OR and RR in studies of OPC also imparts additional information regarding the relationship between a given disease and exposure. As stated previously, in studies of OPC, the OR is a good estimate of the RR. In that instance, an OR of
2.0 indicates a twofold (100%) increase in the risk of cancer among persons with a
particular exposure relative to the risk among those persons who were unexposed. Similarly, an OR of 3.0 indicates a threefold (200%) increase in the risk of cancer among the
exposed relative to the unexposed. As already indicated, ORs falling below 1.0 are
interpreted as suggesting a protective effect between a given exposure and disease. In
case–control studies of OPC, an OR of 0.5 represents a 50% reduction in the risk of such
cancers among those persons with the exposure compared to those who are unexposed.
Similarly, an OR of 0.3 is interpreted as a 70% reduction in risk.

ORs and RRs are also often reported as having been *adjusted* for factors such as
smoking and alcoholic beverage consumption. Although the manner in which such
adjustment takes place is beyond the scope of this chapter, the purpose of adjusting ORs
and RRs is to remove the potentially confounding effect of these factors from the relationship being studied *(3)*. For example, one might hypothesize that coffee drinking is
related to the risk of oral cancer. However, smoking is known to increase the risk of oral
cancer, and smokers are more likely to drink coffee than are nonsmokers (i.e., the
association between coffee drinking and oral cancer could be confounded by smoking).
If a research project identified a positive association between coffee drinking and oral
cancer risk (i.e., OR >1.0), it would be important to remove the potentially confounding
effect of tobacco smoking from the estimated OR for coffee drinking and oral cancer;
otherwise, the unadjusted (crude) OR could merely reflect confounding by smoking. In
studies of diet and nutrition in relation to cancer of the oral cavity and pharynx, it is

imperative that the investigators take into consideration such potential confounders as tobacco and alcohol use. For that reason, each of the studies cited here has adjusted its reported ORs for tobacco and alcohol consumption, often in addition to other potential confounders.

One might question the usefulness of conducting a dietary study in which the data is self-reported. After all, most of us cannot remember what we ate 2 d or 1 wk ago. How then can we expect others to recall what they ate over the past year or over their adult lifetime? In fact, from a study perspective it would be ideal if we could remember and report everything we ever ate; however, that is clearly not feasible. Instead, nutritional epidemiologists often seek to obtain "best" estimates of dietary consumption and, on the basis of those estimates, form groups with various levels of reported ingestion. The groups are often defined on the basis of the frequency distribution of intake as reported within the control group. For example, if one-third of the controls reported eating fewer than four servings of fruit per week, study subjects (cases and controls) reporting that level of fruit consumption would be placed in the "low" fruit-intake group. Similarly, if one-third of the controls reported eating 10 or more fruit servings per week, the "high" fruit-intake group would be defined accordingly. In this example, the "intermediate" intake group would be composed of those cases and controls who reported consuming 4 or more, but fewer than 10, fruit servings per week. Although each subject's estimated fruit consumption is no doubt a little high or low, one could argue that persons in the low-intake group most likely eat less fruit than persons in the intermediate or high consumption groups. By examining trends in the risk (or odds) of developing a given disease over increasing consumption levels of a given food group or item (e.g., low, intermediate, high), epidemiologists can evaluate whether that food is associated with an increased, decreased, or no risk of disease. If, for example, the ORs for consuming increasing levels of fruit are 1.0 (the OR for low consumption relative to itself), 0.7 (the OR for intermediate relative to low consumption), and 0.5 (high relative to low consumption), evidence for a protective pattern of risk exists. If a statistical test reveals that the trend is unlikely to have occurred by chance (i.e., if the p value is <0.05), the trend is said to be statistically significant.

Still, one might argue that food intake data are simply based on guesses and do not reflect, or even approach, reality. If that is true, one would expect that trends in risk over various levels of food intake would appear randomly or not at all. On the other hand, if a trend is observed with consistency across studies even given the fuzziness of the data, support for a relationship is strengthened.

3. FINDINGS FROM STUDIES OF OPC IN RELATION TO DIET AND NUTRITION

A number of epidemiological studies have suggested that certain dietary factors, or the lack thereof, may be linked to the risk of OPC. Early studies linked Plummer-Vinson (or Patterson-Kelly) syndrome, a disease complex related to deficiencies in iron, riboflavin, and other vitamins, to the development of primarily hypopharyngeal cancer in women *(4,5)*, but other investigations prior to the 1980s provided little evidence relating diet to OPC risk *(6,7)*. Since the early 1980s, however, a number of epidemiologic studies in various regions of the world have reported associations between the intake of some foods or nutrients and the risk of OPC.

3.1. Food Groups and Items

3.1.1. FRUITS AND VEGETABLES

Among studies investigating a possible link between OPC and the intake of various food groups and items, the most consistent finding has been an inverse association between cancers at these anatomical sites and the consumption of fruits and/or vegetables *(8–25)*. That is, the risk of OPC tends to decrease with increased fruit and vegetable intake. Table 1 presents findings from selected studies that investigated the relationship between OPC and the consumption of fruits and vegetables.

3.1.1.1. Fruits

With few exceptions, high, relative to low, fruit consumption has been linked to a reduced risk of OPC. In a large case–control study conducted in the United States *(9,11)*, risk reductions on the order of 40 to 80% were observed for high, relative to low, total fruit consumption among both blacks and whites and among males and females. Moreover, when fruit subgroups were analyzed separately, high intakes of citrus, dark yellow, and other fruits—including watermelon, strawberries, apples, pears, and bananas— were always associated with a reduced OPC risk across the racial and gender groups *(9,11)*. In a more recent report from a prospective cohort study involving more than 34,000 Iowan women followed for 14 yr, total fruit intake was again associated with a protective effect in terms of upper aerodigestive tract (oral/pharyngeal, esophageal, gastric, and laryngeal) cancers, but the finding was not statistically significant (not shown in Table 1) *(21)*. A large case–control study conducted in northeastern and central Italy also linked most types of fruit to a reduced risk of OPC, although the reduction associated with high consumption was greater for citrus (50%) than noncitrus (30%) fruits and statistically significant for citrus fruits only *(23)*. Notably, the beneficial effects associated with citrus-fruit intake in that study were derived from the consumption of both the whole fruit and fruit juices.

3.1.1.2. Vegetables

Findings regarding vegetable intake have also suggested a protective effect, but not necessarily across all studies or across all vegetable and population subgroups. In the large US case–control study, patterns of OPC risk reduction were seen for total vegetable consumption among black males, to a lesser extent among females, but not among white males, whose ORs remained at or near 1.0 for each level of consumption *(9,11)*. In that study, however, vegetables most likely to be eaten raw, including lettuce, cucumbers, fresh tomatoes, carrots, and coleslaw, were associated with 60 to 80% reductions in OPC risk among high, relative to low, consumers in both races and genders. In the cohort study of Iowan women, an inverse relationship was observed for total vegetable intake in relation to the risk of upper aerodigestive tract cancer, although, as with fruits, the finding was not statistically significant *(21)*. That study did, however, report a statistically significant reduction in cancer risk with regard to the intake of yellow and orange vegetables. In the Italian case–control study *(23)*, a high intake of both raw and cooked vegetables was associated with approx 50% reductions in OPC risk.

Although individual vegetable items have not been consistently included across studies, carrots *(9,12,16,20,23,25,26)* and tomatoes *(9,12,16,17,20,23,24)* have emerged as

Table 1
Selected Studies Investigating an Association Between OPC and the Consumption of Fruits and Vegetables

Author	Geographic region	Gender studied / Food group/item	Adjusted odds ratios by consumption level				Trend p-value
			1 (low)	2	3 (high)		
Winn et al.	Southern,	Females					
1984	USA	Fruits & vegetables	1.0	0.7	0.5 [a]		0.002
			1 (low)	2	3	4 (high)	
McLaughlin et al.	USA	White males					
1988		Fruits	1.0	0.6	0.4	0.4 [b]	<0.001
		Vegetables	1.0	1.1	1.0	1.0	0.69
		White females					
		Fruits	1.0	0.9	0.8	0.5	0.01
		Vegetables	1.0	1.1	0.7	0.8	0.20
Gridley et al.	USA	Black males					
1990		Fruits	1.0	0.8	0.9	0.2 [c]	0.006
		Vegetables	1.0	0.9	0.4	0.3	0.004
		Black females					
		Fruits	1.0	0.6	0.5	0.6	0.66
		Vegetables	1.0	0.4	1.1	0.8	0.92
			1 (low)	2	3 (high)		
Zheng et al	China,	Males					
1992	Shanghai	Fruits					
		Oranges/tangerines	1.0	0.40	0.40 [d]		≤0.05
		Other fruits	1.0	0.44	0.66		NS
		Vegetables					
		Dark yellow	1.0	0.52	0.32		≤0.05
		Dark green (except bok choy)	1.0	0.41	0.42		≤0.05
		Females					
		Fruits					
		Oranges/tangerines	1.0	0.33	0.42		≤0.05
		Other fruits	1.0	0.31	0.83		NS
		Vegetables					
		Dark yellow	1.0	0.79	0.78		NS
		Dark green (except bok choy)	1.0	0.87	0.69		NS
De Stefani et al.	Uruguay	Males					
1994		Fresh Fruits	1.0	0.7	0.6 [e]		NR
		Vegetables	1.0	0.4	0.4		NR

Continued on next page

Table 1 *(Continued)*
Selected Studies Investigating an Association Between
OPC and the Consumption of Fruits and Vegetables

Author	Geographic region	Gender studied / Food group/item	Adjusted odds ratios by consumption level					Trend p-value
			1 (low)	*2*	*3 (high)*			
Levi et al.	Switzerland,	Males & females						
1998	Vaud	Fruits						
		Citrus fruits	1.0	0.34	0.38 [f]			<0.01
		Other fruits	1.0	0.42	0.22			<0.01
		Vegetables						
		Raw vegetables	1.0	0.63	0.30			<0.01
		Cooked vegetables	1.00	0.42	0.14			<0.01
			1 (low)	*2*	*3*	*4*	*5 (high)*	
Franceschi et al.	Italy,	Males & females						
1999	Northeast	Fruits						
	& Central	Citrus Fruits	1.0	0.8	0.7	0.6	0.5 [g]	<0.01
		Other Fruits	1.0	0.7	0.7	0.8	0.7	NS
		Vegetables						
		Raw vegetables	1.0	0.4	0.5	0.5	0.4	<0.01
		Cooked vegetables	1.0	0.8	1.0	0.7	0.5	<0.01
Garrote et al.	Cuba	Males & females						
2001		Fruits	1.0	0.71	0.43 [h]			<0.05
		Vegetables	1.0	0.67	0.78			0.49

[a] Crude ORs, but the logistic model which adjusted simultaneously for race, education, tobacco use, alcohol consumption, interview respondent type, relative weight, dentures, missing teeth, gum-tooth quality, mouthwash use, 3+ meals per day, residence, urban/rural residence, and other food groups simultaneously, "yielded adjusted RRs not different from the crude RRs."
[b] Adjusted for smoking and drinking.
[c] Adjusted for smoking and drinking, and calories.
[d] Adjusted for smoking and education. "After adjustment for smoking and education, adjustment for other factors such as age, alcohol consumption, and income did not substantially change the ORs of oral cancer with dietary factors."
[e] Adjusted for smoking (pack-yrs), total alcohol consumption, education, age, and residence.
[f] Adjusted for smoking, alcohol, education, age, sex, and non-alcohol total energy.
[g] Adjusted for smoking, alcohol, education, age, sex, center, and total energy.
[h] Adjusted for smoking, alcohol, education, age, sex, residence, and other major food groups.
NR: Not reported; NS: Not statistically significant

potentially protective in a majority of studies, although the findings have not always been statistically significant. There is also evidence to suggest that diversity in terms of the fruits and vegetables consumed is inversely related to the risk of OPC *(18)*.

Not all investigations have evaluated the association between fruit and/or vegetable consumption and the risk of OPC in smokers and drinkers; however, among those studies that have, findings suggest that the effect of both smoking and drinking may be attenuated among persons with a diet high in these foods *(8,9,11,13,24–26)*. For example, in one case–control study of OPC in southern US women, smokers with a low consumption of fruits and vegetables had over a 300% increase in cancer risk relative to nontobacco users with a low intake of fruits and vegetables (the referent group). However, smokers with a high consumption of fruits and vegetables had only a 60% increase in risk (again relative to the referent group) *(8)*. In other words, smoking increased the risk of OPC among these women, but a high consumption of fruits and vegetables was associated with a notable reduction in that excess risk.

3.1.2. BREADS, GRAINS, AND CEREALS

Some studies suggest that bread, grain, and cereal consumption may also be related to the risk of OPC. In the case–control study of OPC among women living in the southern United States, Winn et al. reported a statistically significant protective effect associated with a high, relative to low, consumption of breads and cereals *(8)*. In the subsequent large US case–control study, however, no clear pattern of increased or decreased risk was observed in relation to overall grain consumption among whites, while among blacks, an increased intake was associated with nonsignificant *increases* in risk *(9,11)*. Despite these inconsistencies, some studies suggest that whole-grain bread, pasta, and cereal intake may be related to a protective effect *(8,9,12,21,26–28)*. For example, in a Swiss case–control study, a high intake of whole-grain foods was associated with a 40% reduction in the risk of OPC *(28)*, whereas the cohort study of Iowan women revealed a 50% reduction *(21)*. However, the large Italian study found no relationship between consuming whole-grain bread at least weekly and OPC risk *(23)*. Clearly, further study is required in order to more fully understand the possible association between whole-grain foods and the risk of OPC.

3.1.3. MEATS

Whereas some studies have reported increased risks associated with a high, relative to low, consumption of meat in general *(9,18,20,22)*, other studies have reported protective or inconsistent patterns *(11,13,16,26,29)*. In a Brazilian investigation, charcoal-grilled meat was linked to an elevated risk of oral cancer *(10)*, but studies in the United States have found little evidence of such a relationship *(8,9,11)*. In a similar vein, some studies have suggested that salted meat and fish *(13,29)* or nitrite-containing *(9,11)* or processed meats *(23)* could be associated with increased risks of OPC in one or another population or subgroup; however, these potential associations have not been sufficiently corroborated and require further study. Although fish consumption has been identified as potentially protective in relation to OPC risk in a majority of studies *(9,11,14,16,18,23,25,30)*, other investigations have reported findings that do not support such a relationship *(8,13,20)*.

3.1.4. DAIRY FOODS

Dairy foods have not been consistently related to the risk of OPC. Whereas high milk intake has been linked to a reduced risk of cancer at these sites in some studies *(16,18,26)*, other investigations have not found a protective effect *(23,29)*. Conversely, high, relative to low, cheese intake has been associated with an increased risk in some *(12,20)* but not other *(23,26)* studies. The link between egg consumption has also varied by study, with some reports suggesting a positive relationship with OPC risk *(12,18,23)* and others suggesting the opposite *(16)*. Similar inconsistencies have been observed with regard to the use of butter *(12,15,23,26)*.

To date, in terms of food groups, fruits and vegetables are the best established dietary link to OPC risk. Moreover, the associations generally remain even after adjusting for smoking, drinking, and other potential confounders. In addition to studying specific food groups and items, researchers have also investigated potential relationships between OPC risk and specific components of the various foods consumed.

3.2. Fiber and Micronutrients

3.2.1. FIBER

There is evidence that fiber intake is inversely associated with OPC. Studies in the United States, Australia, China, and Italy have all reported decreases in oral and pharyngeal cancer risk of 40% or more in persons with a high, relative to low, intake of total fiber *(9,11,16,31–33)*. Whether the observed reductions in OPC risk are a function of the fiber per se; markers of a diet high in fruits, vegetables, and whole grains; or some other mechanism has not been entirely resolved.

3.2.2. MICRONUTRIENTS

3.2.2.1. Dietary Micronutrients

Various dietary micronutrients, including vitamins, provitamins, and minerals, have also been investigated for potential associations with OPC risk. Findings from studies reported in the early to mid-1980s suggested a possible inverse relationship between dietary vitamin A and OPC risk among men *(34,35)*, but not among women *(34)*. In those studies, however, the researchers were limited, both in terms of the food items included in the dietary questionnaire—which did not include, for example, liver—and by the US Department of Agriculture (USDA) food composition tables of the day— which did not differentiate between retinol (vitamin A from primarily animal sources) and provitamin A carotenoids, such as β-carotene, derived primarily from plants *(36)*. Subsequent studies, aided by more advanced food composition tables, have allowed for the partitioned evaluation of dietary retinol and carotene intake in relation to OPC risk.

In terms of retinol intake, findings have been inconsistent regarding the risk of OPC, with some evidence suggesting that a high intake is associated with an increased risk, but other evidence revealing little, if any, association. In the large US study, for example, patterns of increased risk were observed with increasing dietary retinol among black and white males and among white females *(9,11)*. For black females, however, no clear patterns of increasing or decreasing risk were observed with increasing retinol intake *(11)*. Similarly, retinol intake was not clearly associated with an increased or decreased risk of OPC in a case–control study conducted in Italy and Switzerland *(37)*.

With regard to dietary carotene, some studies *(16,37)* have suggested a protective association in relation to OPC while findings from other investigations have been more equivocal or suggested no effect *(9,11,13,22,31)*. On the basis of the large US study, McLaughlin et al. *(9)* reported a 60% reduction in cancer risk among high consumers of fruit carotene, but little risk reduction for persons with a high intake of carotene from vegetable sources. However, findings from a Chinese study conducted in Beijing revealed 40% and 50% reductions in oral cancer risk with high, relative to low, dietary intakes of carotene from fruits and vegetables, respectively *(16)*. A similar study in Shanghai, however, revealed no evidence of a protective relationship *(13)*. During the early 2000s, findings from two European case–control studies were reported. Although a Greek study found no relationship between carotene intake and OPC risk *(22)*, a large investigation conducted in Italy and Switzerland revealed strong protective effects that generally increased with the amount of carotene consumed *(37)*.

In addition to carotene, the dietary intake of various other antioxidants, primarily vitamins C and E, have been investigated in relation to OPC risk. With regard to vitamin C, a high, relative to low, dietary intake has generally been associated with a decreased risk of OPC in studies conducted in various regions of the world, including the US, China, Australia, Greece, Switzerland, and Italy *(9,11,16,22,32,35,37,38)*, although some studies have found only little *(31)* or no protective effect *(13)*. In the large US case–control study, for example, men and women who consumed a high level of dietary vitamin C had a 40% or more reduction in their risk of OPC compared to persons with a low intake *(9,11)*. On the other hand, evidence for an association between vitamin E and OPC is generally weak, although one large case–control study did report a moderate-to-strong inverse relationship *(37)*.

The dietary intake of various B vitamins—namely, thiamin, niacin, riboflavin, pyridoxine, and folic acid—has also been evaluated in terms of OPC risk *(9,11,22,31,37)*. Each of these vitamins has been identified as protective in one or more studies; however, conflicting findings have been reported as well, and more research is needed in order to further clarify these potential associations.

Likewise, some minerals, including calcium, iron, phosphorous, and potassium, have each been assessed in relation to OPC risk by at least two investigations *(9,11,16,22,31,37)*, but it is premature to conclude that any of these minerals is clearly related to OPC risk.

3.2.2.2. Vitamin Supplementation

The relationship between vitamin supplementation and OPC risk has received limited attention. In three studies carried out in the United States, there was little evidence of an association between cancer risk at these sites and the use of multivitamins per se *(38–40)*. On the other hand, in the largest and most comprehensive of the three studies, persons who reported taking one or more individual supplements for vitamins A, C, E, or B-complex for at least 6 mo had a 30% reduction in risk *(39)*. In that study, however, only vitamin E demonstrated a statistically significant risk reduction (OR = 0.5) after taking into account the fact that persons who use one vitamin supplement may also be using another (i.e., after adjusting for all other vitamins supplements). Moreover, the 50% reduction in risk with vitamin E supplementation was remarkably consistent across levels of tobacco and alcohol use, fruit and vegetable consumption, the use of other supplements, and level of dietary vitamin E intake. That is, for example, among persons with a high consumption of tobacco and alcohol, those who took vitamin E supplements had half the risk of those who did not. A protective effect with vitamin E supplementation was also evaluated and observed in one other study *(40)*, but additional research is necessary to determine whether the vitamin E supplementation per se or some other correlate, such as lifestyle, is responsible for the apparent risk reduction.

3.2.2.3. Serum Micronutrients

Apart from analyzing dietary and supplemental micronutrient intake, some researchers have compared serum micronutrient levels in persons with and without cancer as a way of further identifying and understanding relationships between specific nutrients and cancer. One approach has been to obtain blood from both OPC patients and individuals without cancer, measure specific serum micronutrient levels, and compare the levels in the two groups. Such an approach has merits, but cannot rule out the possibility that the disease might have modified the serum levels of micronutrients. Another study design has also been used that compares micronutrient levels in serum that was collected well in advance of a given individual's diagnosis of cancer. In one approach, blood is drawn from apparently healthy individuals and the serum is frozen and then stored for an extended period of time, often decades. The subjects are then followed to determine which individuals develop the disease of interest. Ultimately, the serum samples from identified cases and appropriate controls are analyzed to determine whether there are any notable differences in the various micronutrient levels being tested. The advantage of this approach is that the disease had not occurred at the time that the blood was drawn, and, therefore, the disease could not have influenced the serum levels being studied. Consequently, this design allows for the exploration of serum micronutrients that potentially impact the risk of future disease.

Three studies in the 1990s used the approach described above to evaluate possible associations between serum micronutrients and OPC *(41–43)*. Each of these investigations found an apparent protective relationship between high, relative to low, serum β-carotene levels and the subsequent development of OPC, although the findings were not always statistically significant. In addition, and although evaluated in only two of the three studies, serum levels of other carotenoids, including α-carotene and β-crytoxanthine, were also lower in cases than in their pair-matched controls *(42,43)*. However, findings regarding serum levels of vitamin E, including α- and γ-tocopherol, were inconsistent across studies.

Before leaving the topic of micronutrients, it is important to underscore the fact that although we are learning more about the manner in which various nutrients might influence the risk of various cancers, we are still far from our goal of understanding the apparent effects associated with diet, particularly those diets high in fruits and vegetables. We know, for example, that β-carotene and other carotenoids can quench singlet oxygen and capture free radicals, thereby helping to prevent the induction of genetic mutations and immune dysfunction. We also know that vitamin C can inhibit the formation of nitrosamine and act as an immune response enhancer. It is less clear, however, how various nutrients function together. For example, although there is evidence suggesting that certain antioxidants can act synergistically in some cancers, Negri et al. *(37)* found evidence of the opposite effect (antagonism) when the relationship between various antioxidants was evaluated in relation to OPC risk. Clearly, additional research and improved methodological tools are needed in order to further our understanding as to how nutritional factors influence the risk of OPC.

4. FINDINGS FROM STUDIES OF PRECANCEROUS ORAL LESIONS AND CONDITIONS IN RELATION TO DIET AND NUTRITION

One criticism of studies that investigate the relationship between diet and OPC risk is that symptoms associated with OPC could impact dietary intake and thereby influence the reporting of preillness diets by cases in case–control studies *(44)*. Such biased reporting could give rise to the identification of misleading associations between OPC risk and dietary and/or nutritional factors.

The study of some precancerous oral lesions such as leukoplakia (i.e., a predominantly white lesion of the oral mucosa that cannot be categorized as any other definable lesion *[45]*) is particularly useful in addressing this concern because such lesions are generally asymptomatic and therefore far less likely to initiate dietary changes. The same can be said for studying oral epithelial dysplasia (OED), a histopathologic diagnosis associated with an increased risk of oral cancer, particularly when the dysplasia is identified in asymptomatic oral lesions. Some investigations have also studied the relationship between diet and nutrition and oral submucous fibrosis (OSF), a precancerous condition characterized in its later stages by palpable fibrous bands in the mucosa of the upper digestive tract and seen most often in individuals living in or migrating from areas in Asia, particularly the Indian subcontinent. Unlike oral leukoplakia, however, OSF is often associated with a burning sensation when consuming spicy foods, a characteristic that could obviously lead to dietary alterations.

Some investigations focusing on oral precancer in relation to diet and nutrition have evaluated a possible link between the oral lesions or conditions and the intake of specific foods or food groups. For example, one study of male Indian tobacco users revealed marginally significant protective effects with the consumption of fruits (OSF) and vegetables (leukoplakia) as well as a significant inverse relationship between fiber intake and the risk of both leukoplakia and OSF *(46)*. Another Indian study of oral leukoplakia and OSF involving tobacco users and a US investigation of OED risk each reported findings consistent with a protective effect associated with fruit and/or vegetable consumption *(47,48)*.

Among those investigations studying the potential link between various precancerous lesions or conditions and selected dietary micronutrients, vitamin C *(46,47,49,50)* and β-carotene, iron, and zinc *(47,49)* have each been identified as having potentially protective effects by at least two studies, but further research is required to verify and ultimately understand the mechanisms through which such associations are manifest.

5. FINDINGS FROM STUDIES OF CANCER CHEMOPREVENTION

Cancer chemoprevention is the use of chemical agents to prevent cancer. Promising oral cancer chemopreventive agents have been evaluated in human intervention trials by assessing their effectiveness in reversing oral leukoplakia and, alternatively, in preventing second primary and recurrent cancers. Both synthetic and naturally occurring agents have been tested. The synthetic agents have included the vitamin A derivatives

13-*cis*-retinoic acid, fenretinide, and etretinate, but these will not be discussed further because they are outside the focus of this chapter. The naturally occurring agents have included vitamins A, C, and E, β-carotene, and selenium, which are generally administered as pills or capsules at high supplemental levels.

Most chemoprevention trials of oral premalignancy have focused on vitamin A and β-carotene, and both nutrients have been shown to reverse oral leukoplakia *(51–56)*. Many of these trials, however, were not placebo controlled and should be interpreted cautiously. In addition, vitamin A administered at high doses is often accompanied by toxic side effects.

One study has reported on the effectiveness of β-carotene in preventing second primary and recurrent cancers among persons diagnosed with a previous stage I or II carcinoma of the head and neck *(57)*. In that randomized clinical trial and after a mean follow-up of 51 mo, the β-carotene group experienced a 30% decrease in the risk of second or recurrent head and neck cancers, a 15% reduction in total mortality, but a 45% increase in the risk of lung cancer, although none of those findings were statistically significant. The increased risk of lung cancer associated with β-carotene supplementation has also been observed in earlier cancer chemoprevention trials focusing on endpoints other than OPC *(58,59)* and underscores the fact that there is still much to learn regarding the role of nutrients in cancer and cancer prevention.

6. CONCLUSIONS AND RECOMMENDATIONS FOR CLINICIANS

Around the world, OPC affects hundreds of thousands of individuals each year. In the United States and other Western countries, tobacco use and alcohol consumption are the primary causative agents, although at least some aspects of diet and nutrition also appear to play an important role. Most studies investigating a link between diet and OPC, and to a lesser extent precancer, have reported a protective effect associated with the consumption of fruits and vegetables. Some investigations also suggest that the consumption of whole-grain foods as well as a diet high in fiber intake may also be protective. Studies investigating specific dietary micronutrients in relation to OPC have most often identified vitamin C as being associated with a reduced risk. In addition, persons with high serum levels of β-carotene have been found to have reduced risks of OPC even when the blood was taken years before the diagnosis of OPC. It is not clear, however, whether these micronutrients are directly responsible for the risk reduction, or whether they are markers for some other responsible factor. Multivitamins have not emerged as protective in terms of OPC, and while two case–control studies have suggested that vitamin E supplementation could be protective, it is too early to recommend this supplement to patients. Finally, although various potential oral cancer chemopreventive agents have been and are being evaluated for their effectiveness and safety, the use of these agents remains experimental at this time.

7. SOURCES FOR ADDITIONAL INFORMATION

Further information regarding diet and nutrition in relation to OPC can be obtained by accessing the websites for the National Cancer Institute and the American Cancer Society (ACS).

Guidelines for Practice

	Oral Health Professional	Nutrition Professional

Prevention	• Encourage smoking cessation.
	
	• Discourage more than moderate alcohol consumption.
	
	• Conduct screening of all patients periodically for early signs of oral cancer and precancerous lesions and conditions.
	
	• Promote the National Cancer Institute's Five A Day of fruit and vegetable servings and the American Cancer Society (ACS) Diet for Cancer Prevention.
		• Encourage smoking cessation.
		
		• Discourage more than moderate alcohol consumption.
		
		• Promote the National Cancer Institute's Five A Day of fruit and vegetable servings and the ACS Diet for Cancer Prevention.
		
		• ACS Diet Guidelines (60):
		The following is reprinted from ref. 60.
		
		  ■ Eat a variety of healthful foods, with an emphasis on plant sources.
		
		    ◆ Eat five or more servings of a variety of vegetables and fruits each day.
		
		    ◆ Choose whole grains in preference to processed (refined) grains and sugars.
		
		    ◆ Limit consumption of red meats, especially those high in fat and processed.
		
		    ◆ Choose foods that maintain a healthful weight.
		
		  ■ Adopt a physically active lifestyle.
		
		    ◆ Adults: engage in at least moderate activity for 30 min or more on 5 or more days of the week.
		
		    ◆ Children and adolescents: engage in at least 60 min per day of moderate to vigorous physical activity at least 5 d per week.
		
		  ■ Maintain a healthful weight throughout life.
		
		    ◆ Balance caloric intake with physical activity.
		
		    ◆ Lose weight if currently overweight or obese.
		
		  ■ If you drink alcoholic beverages, limit consumption.

Intervention	• Provide dental care consistent with needs; make referrals as appropriate for medical nutrition therapy (MNT).	• Provide MNT consistent with treatment and posttreatment needs. • Recommendations of the ACS (61): ◆ Plan diet based on nutrient needs and individual side-effects experiences • Recommendations for after treatment ends (taken from ref 61).

Continued on next page

Guidelines for Practice

Oral Health Professional	Nutrition Professional
	• Ask your registered dietitian (RD) to work with you to develop a balanced eating plan. • Choose a variety of foods from all the food groups. Use the ACS Guidelines for Nutrition for Cancer Prevention. • Try to eat at least five to seven servings a day of fruits and vegetables, including citrus fruits and dark-green and deep-yellow vegetables. • Eat plenty of high-fiber foods, such as whole-grain breads and cereals. • Decrease the amount of fat in your meals by baking or broiling foods. • Choose low-fat milk and dairy products. • Avoid salt-cured, smoked, and pickled foods. • Drink alcohol only occasionally if you choose to drink. • If you are overweight, consider losing weight by reducing the amount of fat in your diet and increasing your activity. Choose activities that you enjoy. Check with your doctor before starting any exercise program.

REFERENCES

1. Parkin DM, Bray F, Ferlay J, Pisani P. Estimating the world cancer burden: Globocan 2000. Int J Cancer 2001; 94:153–156.
2. Blot WJ, McLaughlin JK, Winn DM, et al. Smoking and drinking in relation to oral and pharyngeal cancer. Cancer Res 1988; 48:3282–3287.
3. Rothman J, Greenland S. Modern Epidemiology. Philadelphia, PA: Lippencott-Raven Publishers, 1998.
4. Wynder EL, Hultberg S, Jacobson F, Bross IJ. Environmental factors in cancer of the upper alimentary tract: Swedish study with special reference to Plummer-Vinson (Paterson-Kelly) syndrome. Cancer 1957; 10:470–487.
5. Larsson LG, Sandstrom A, Westling P. Relationship of Plummer-Vinson disease to cancer of the upper alimentary tract in Sweden. Cancer Res 1975; 35:3308–3316.
6. Martinez I. Factors associated with cancer of the esophagus, mouth, and pharynx in Puerto Rico. J Natl Cancer Inst 1969; 42:1069–1094.
7. Graham S, Dayal H, Rohrer T, et al. Dentition, diet, tobacco, and alcohol in the epidemiology of oral cancer. J Natl Cancer Inst 1977; 59:1611–1618.

8. Winn DM, Ziegler RG, Pickle LW, Gridley G, Blot WJ, Hoover RN. Diet in the etiology of oral and pharyngeal cancer among women from the southern United States. Cancer Res 1984; 44:1216–1222.

9. McLaughlin JK, Gridley G, Block G, et al. Dietary factors in oral and pharyngeal cancer. J Natl Cancer Inst 1988; 80:1237–1243.

10. Franco EL, Kowalski LP, Oliveira BV, et al. Risk factors for oral cancer in Brazil: a case–control study. Int J Cancer 1989; 43:992–1000.

11. Gridley G, McLaughlin JK, Block G, et al. Diet and oral and pharyngeal cancer among blacks. Nutr Cancer 1990; 14:219–225.

12. Franceschi S, Bidoli E, Baron AE, et al. Nutrition and cancer of the oral cavity and pharynx in northeast Italy. Int J Cancer 1991; 47:20–25.

13. Zheng W, Blot WJ, Shu XO, et al. Risk factors for oral and pharyngeal cancer in Shanghai, with emphasis on diet. Cancer Epidemiol Biomarkers Prev 1992; 1:441–448.

14. Notani PN, Jayant K. Role of diet in upper aerodigestive tract cancers. Nutr Cancer 1987; 10:103–113.

15. Franceschi S, Barra S, La Vecchia C, Bidoli E, Negri E, Talamini R. Risk factors for cancer of the tongue and the mouth: a case–control study from northern Italy. Cancer 1992; 70:2227–2233.

16. Zheng T, Boyle P, Willett WC, et al. A case–control study of oral cancer in Beijing, People's Republic of China: associations with nutrient intakes, foods and food groups. Eur J Cancer B Oral Oncol 1993; 29B:45–55.

17. Franceschi S, Bidoli E, La Vecchia C, Talamini R, D'Avanzo B, Negri E. Tomatoes and risk of digestive-tract cancers. Int J Cancer 1994; 59:181–184.

18. Levi F, Pasche C, La Vecchia C, Lucchini F, Franceschi S, Monnier P. Food groups and risk of oral and pharyngeal cancer. Int J Cancer 1998; 77:705–709.

19. De Stefani E, Deneo-Pellegrini H, Mendilaharsu M, Ronco A. Diet and risk of cancer of the upper aerodigestive tract. 1. Foods. Oral Oncol 1999; 35:17–21.

20. Garrote LF, Herrero R, Reyes RM, et al. Risk factors for cancer of the oral cavity and oro-pharynx in Cuba. Br J Cancer 2001; 85:46–54.

21. Kasum CM, Jacobs DR Jr, Nicodemus K, Folsom AR. Dietary risk factors for upper aerodigestive tract cancers. Int J Cancer 2002; 99:267–272.

22. Petridou E, Zavras AI, Lefatzis D, et al. The role of diet and specific micronutrients in the etiology of oral carcinoma. Cancer 2002; 94:2981–2988.

23. Franceschi S, Favero A, Conti E, et al. Food groups, oils and butter, and cancer of the oral cavity and pharynx. Br J Cancer 1999; 80:614–620.

24. Sanchez MJ, Martinez C, Nieto A, et al. Oral and oropharyngeal cancer in Spain: influence of dietary patterns. Eur J Cancer Prev 2003; 12:49–56.

25. Tavani A, Gallus S, La Vecchia C, et al. Diet and risk of oral and pharyngeal cancer: an Italian case–control study. Eur J Cancer Prev 2001; 10:191–195.

26. La Vecchia C, Negri E, D'Avanzo B, Boyle P, Franceschi S. Dietary indicators of oral and pharyngeal cancer. Int J Epidemiol 1991; 20:39–44.

27. Chatenoud L, Tavani A, La Vecchia C, et al. Whole grain food intake and cancer risk. Int J Cancer 1998; 77:24–28.

28. Levi F, Pasche C, Lucchini F, Chatenoud L, Jacobs DR Jr, La Vecchia C. Refined and whole grain cereals and the risk of oral, oesophageal and laryngeal cancer. Eur J Clin Nutr 2000; 54:487–489.

29. De Stefani E, Oreggia F, Ronco A, Fierro L, Rivero S. Salted meat consumption as a risk factor for cancer of the oral cavity and pharynx: a case–control study from Uruguay. Cancer Epidemiol Biomarkers Prev 1994; 3:381–385.

30. Fernandez E, Chatenoud L, La Vecchia C, Negri E, Franceschi S. Fish consumption and cancer risk. Am J Clin Nutr 1999; 70:85–90.

31. Marshall JR, Graham S, Haughey BP, et al. Smoking, alcohol, dentition and diet in the epidemiology of oral cancer. Eur J Cancer B Oral Oncol 1992; 28B:9–15.

32. Kune GA, Kune S, Field B, et al. Oral and pharyngeal cancer, diet, smoking, alcohol, and serum vitamin A and beta-carotene levels: a case–control study in men. Nutr Cancer 1993; 20:61–70.

33. Soler M, Bosetti C, Franceschi S, et al. Fiber intake and the risk of oral, pharyngeal and esophageal cancer. Int J Cancer 2001; 91:283–287.

34. Middleton B, Byers T, Marshall J, Graham S. Dietary vitamin A and cancer: a multisite case–control study. Nutr Cancer 1986; 8:107–116.
35. Marshall J, Graham S, Mettlin C, Shedd D, Swanson M. Diet in the epidemiology of oral cancer. Nutr Cancer 1982; 3:145–149.
36. Mayne ST, Graham S, Zheng TZ. Dietary retinol: prevention or promotion of carcinogenesis in humans? Cancer Causes Control 1991; 2:443–450.
37. Negri E, Franceschi S, Bosetti C, et al. Selected micronutrients and oral and pharyngeal cancer. Int J Cancer 2000; 86:122–127.
38. Rossing MA, Vaughan TL, McKnight B. Diet and pharyngeal cancer. Int J Cancer 1989; 44:593–597.
39. Gridley G, McLaughlin JK, Block G, Blot WJ, Gluch M, Fraumeni JF Jr. Vitamin supplement use and reduced risk of oral and pharyngeal cancer. Am J Epidemiol 1992; 135:1083–1092.
40. Barone J, Taioli E, Hebert JR, Wynder EL. Vitamin supplement use and risk for oral and esophageal cancer. Nutr Cancer 1992; 18:31–41.
41. Knekt P, Aromaa A, Maatela J, et al. Serum micronutrients and risk of cancers of low incidence in Finland. Am J Epidemiol 1991; 134:356–361.
42. Nomura AM, Ziegler RG, Stemmermann GN, Chyou PH, Craft NE. Serum micronutrients and upper aerodigestive tract cancer. Cancer Epidemiol Biomarkers Prev 1997; 6:407–412.
43. Zheng W, Blot WJ, Diamond EL, et al. Serum micronutrients and the subsequent risk of oral and pharyngeal cancer. Cancer Res 1993; 53:795–798.
44. Marshall JR, Boyle P. Nutrition and oral cancer. Cancer Causes Control 1996; 7:101–111.
45. Axell T, Pindborg JJ, Smith CJ, van der Waal I for the International Collaborative Group on Oral White Lesions. Oral white lesions with special reference to precancerous and tobacco- related lesions: conclusions of an international symposium held in Uppsala, Sweden, May 18–21, 1994. J Oral Pathol Med 1996; 25:49–54.
46. Gupta PC, Hebert JR, Bhonsle RB, Sinor PN, Mehta H, Mehta FS. Dietary factors in oral leukoplakia and submucous fibrosis in a population-based case control study in Gujarat, India. Oral Dis 1998; 4:200–206.
47. Gupta PC, Hebert JR, Bhonsle RB, Murti PR, Mehta H, Mehta FS. Influence of dietary factors on oral precancerous lesions in a population-based case–control study in Kerala, India. Cancer 1999; 85: 1885–1893.
48. Morse DE, Pendrys DG, Katz RV, et al. Food group intake and the risk of oral epithelial dysplasia in a United States population. Cancer Causes Control 2000; 11:713–720.
49. Hebert JR, Gupta PC, Bhonsle RB, et al. Dietary exposures and oral precancerous lesions in Srikakulam District, Andhra Pradesh, India. Public Health Nutr 2002; 5:303–312.
50. Kaugars GE, Riley WT, Brandt RB, Burns JC, Svirsky JA. The prevalence of oral lesions in smokeless tobacco users and an evaluation of risk factors. Cancer 1992; 70:2579–2585.
51. Silverman S, Renstrup G, Pindberg JJ. Studies in oral leukoplakias. 3. Effects of vitamin A comparing clinical, histopathologic, cytologic and hematologic responses. Acta Odont Scandinav 1963; 21: 271–292.
52. Garewal HS, Meyskens FL Jr, Killen D, et al. Response of oral leukoplakia to beta-carotene. J Clin Oncol 1990; 8:1715–1720.
53. Garewal HS, Katz RV, Meyskens F, et al. Beta-carotene produces sustained remissions in patients with oral leukoplakia: results of a multicenter prospective trial. Arch Otolaryngol Head Neck Surg 1999; 125:1305–1310.
54. Stich HF, Hornby AP, Mathew B, Sankaranarayanan R, Nair MK. Response of oral leukoplakias to the administration of vitamin A. Cancer Lett 1988; 40:93–101.
55. Stich HF, Rosin MP, Hornby AP, Mathew B, Sankaranarayanan R, Nair MK. Remission of oral leukoplakias and micronuclei in tobacco/betel quid chewers treated with beta-carotene and with beta-carotene plus vitamin A. Int J Cancer 1988; 42:195–199.
56. Sankaranarayanan R, Mathew B, Varghese C, et al. Chemoprevention of oral leukoplakia with vitamin A and beta carotene: an assessment. Oral Oncol 1997; 33:231–236.
57. Mayne ST, Cartmel B, Baum M, et al. Randomized trial of supplemental beta-carotene to prevent second head and neck cancer. Cancer Res 2001; 61:1457–1463.
58. Omenn GS, Goodman GE, Thornquist MD, et al. Effects of a combination of beta carotene and vitamin A on lung cancer and cardiovascular disease. N Engl J Med 1996; 334:1150–1155.

59. The Alpha-Tocopherol, Beta Carotene Cancer Prevention Study Group. The effect of vitamin E and beta carotene on the incidence of lung cancer and other cancers in male smokers. N Engl J Med 1994; 330:1029–1035.
60. American Cancer Society. ACS Recommendations for Nutrition and Physical Activity for Cancer Prevention. American Cancer Society 2001 Nutrition and Physical Activity Guidelines Advisory Committee. Approved by the American Cancer Society National Board of Directors on November 1, 2001. Website: (http://www.cancer.org/docroot/PED/content/PED_3_2X_Recommendations.asp?sitearea= PED). Accessed January 2, 2004.
61. American Cancer Society. Nutrition for Cancer Patients .American Cancer Society. Website: (http:// www.cancer.org/docroot/MBC/MBC_6_1_things_to_think_about.asp). Accessed January 2, 2004.

13 Human Immunodeficiency Virus

Anita Patel and Michael Glick

1. INTRODUCTION

Oral health is an integral component of overall health and well-being in all patients. However, for an immunocompromised patient, many common oral conditions may have a significant impact on quality of life. Intraoral pain, which is a common complaint among patients with human immunodeficiency virus (HIV), will compromise patients' ability to maintain adequate and appropriate oral intake. Furthermore, the polypharmacopeia used to treat HIV and associated opportunistic infections may cause an increase in the incidence of caries. Changes in the levels of salivary flow caused by medications and the high sucrose content of nutritional supplements play a significant role in the progression of caries rate *(1)*.

Oral manifestations of HIV disease are frequently the initial signs of the disease and represent clinical signs of continuous immune suppression. Side effects of medications and underlying systemic and local opportunistic infections may also manifest by oral changes. Because there is a strong correlation with immune status and the manifestation of oral lesions, any abnormal oral finding may significantly influence clinical treatment decisions *(2)*. The use of oral lesions as clinical markers for immune suppression and disease progression is utilized for intervention therapy, as well as in different staging protocols *(3)*. Unfortunately, the majority of oral lesions are extremely painful and may also be refractory to conventional therapy. As a consequence, oral manifestations greatly hamper nutritional intake and influence general well-being. It is of vital importance that oral health care providers, physicians, and nutritionists work together during the management of HIV-infected patients.

2. HIV/ACQUIRED IMMUNODEFICIENCY SYNDROME

HIV, the known etiologic agent that causes acquired immunodeficiency syndrome (AIDS), is a lentivirus belonging to the larger family of retroviruses. This is a family of RNA viruses that is most notable for its possession of a viral reverse transcriptase (an RNA-dependent DNA polymerase) that transcribes viral RNA into proviral DNA, which is later incorporated into the host-cell genome. The T-helper lymphocytes, generally referred to as CD4 cells, are infected by HIV and are subsequently depleted during the progression of HIV disease. These cells are essential for the coordination of many critical immunological

From: *Nutrition and Oral Medicine*
Edited by: R. Touger-Decker, D. A. Sirois, and C. C. Mobley © Humana Press Inc., Totowa, NJ

functions. Consequently, the loss of these cells results in the progressive destruction of immune functions and is associated with worsening of the clinical course (4).

In 1981, the Centers for Disease Control and Prevention (CDC) noted a surprising increase in a rare form of cancer accompanied by progressive immune deterioration among homosexual and bisexual men in New York and San Francisco. The neoplastic growth was initially referred to as "gay cancer," and the condition causing immune deterioration, with its associated opportunistic infections, was named gay-related immune deficiency (GRID). Later it was recognized that "gay cancer" was a neoplasm, usually not seen in young males, called Kaposi's sarcoma (KS). Subsequent to discovering that nonhomosexual and nonbisexual men developed the same type of immune deterioration referred to as GRID, the name of this condition was changed to AIDS.

HIV is a disorder that is characterized by the development of opportunistic infections, malignancies, neurological dysfunction, and other conditions associated with immune deterioration. AIDS is defined as a clinical stage where individuals infected with HIV have developed specific diseases and conditions, according to a surveillance case definition put forth by the CDC, or have reached a level of immune deterioration determined by a specific level of remaining CD4 cells (3).

Transmission of HIV requires contact with body fluids containing free virions or infected cells. HIV may be present in any fluid or exudates that contain plasma or lymphocytes, blood, semen, vaginal secretions, breast milk, saliva, or wound exudates. This virus has not been known to be transmitted by casual contact.

HIV is actually caused by two similar retroviruses, HIV-1 and HIV-2. Both viruses are found primarily in different geographical areas, yet infection with either virus ultimately results in the development of AIDS. HIV-1 is known to cause most of the AIDS cases in the Western hemisphere; Europe; Asia; and central, south, and east Africa; whereas, HIV-2 is the primary agent of AIDS documented cases in west Africa.

The HIV/AIDS epidemic in the United States has entered its third decade with no cure in sight. Although there was an initial decline and later a plateau in the death rate, an increase in new infections was noted in 1999–2000. It is possible to estimate that 40,000 to 50,000 new infections occur annually in the United States, which projects to an estimated 850,000 to 950,000 individuals living with HIV in the United States in 2004 (5).

Oral manifestations during initial HIV infection are common and they have been reported among the earliest documented cases of the disease (6). Patients may present with nonspecific oral ulcerations, a sore throat, exudative pharyngitis, and oral candidiasis, which may be clinical presentations of the acute seroconversion syndrome (7–9). Signs of fever, fatigue, weight loss, and myalgia are also related to initial HIV infection (8). Occasionally, a macular erythematous nonpruritic rash may be found on the trunk and extremities (9). A thorough and comprehensive patient history, including sexual history, is one of the key factors in the differential diagnosis of HIV disease. An HIV antibody test is strongly recommended for patients engaging in high-risk sexual activity or sharing needles, or if there are reasons to assume that HIV infection has occurred. The duration of the acute phase of this nonspecific illness usually lasts from a few days to 14 d (8). The patient should be referred to an infectious disease clinic for a comprehensive evaluation and treatment.

In this chapter various oral lesions and conditions that may appear during the course of HIV disease and during treatment are described.

3. ORAL LESIONS

Numerous classification systems have been put forth describing and characterizing oral changes that occur in patients infected with HIV *(3,10,11)*. Most commonly, oral lesions are described according to etiology, and specific etiologic agents when possible.

3.1. Viral Etiology

Table 1 describes the viral sources of oral lesions common in HIV disease.

3.1.1. HERPES SIMPLEX VIRUS INFECTIONS

As of 2003, there are eight different types of herpes viruses that are known to infect humans; of these, at least six have been associated with lesions in the oral cavity *(12)*. Oral lesions caused by herpes simplex viruses are the most easily recognized in the spectrum of the manifestations associated with viruses *(13)*. Lesions associated with cytomegalovirus (CMV), varicella zoster virus (VZV), and human herpes virus 8 are more uncommon in non-HIV-infected individuals and pose more of challenge to recognize *(12,14)*.

Although both herpes simplex virus type 1 and type 2 (HSV-1 and HSV-2) can cause oral ulcerations, HSV-1 ulcers are generally found in and around the oral cavity, whereas HSV-2 ulcers are more commonly associated with genital manifestations. When, and if, HSV-2 produces oral ulcerations, the recurrence rate tends to be higher than those caused by HSV-1. Oral ulcerations produced by HSV-1 are more common than HSV-2 in HIV-infected individuals *(13)*.

The lesions may present as single or multiple, localized or generalized vesicles on intraoral surfaces and/or on the lips. The ulcers are usually small, oval, irregular, and shallow, with a diameter of 2 to 4 mm. In the immunocompromised patient, coalescent lesions may form large ulcers that can be hemorrhagic and covered by a pseudomembranous plaque. A raised white border may surround chronic ulcers that have persisted for more than 3 wk *(13)*.

In the immunocompromised patient, lesions may occur on any intraoral surface. However, in the immunocompetent individual the lesions are generally restricted to the more keratinized surfaces.

Ulcerations associated with HSV can be very painful and tend to make eating, swallowing, and speaking difficult. As a consequence, this may lead to dehydration, weight loss, and restricted oral intake, which could compromise or alter medication and nutritional regimens.

In the immunocompromised host, the healing time of HSV-associated ulcers may be delayed and may be misdiagnosed as aphthous ulcers or CMV-associated ulcers. A precise diagnosis is of great importance, as treatment, prognosis, and significance of the lesions may relate to a disseminated disease state of the herpes virus.

A diagnosis can be established by various methods: a cytologic staining for multinucleated giant cells, viral culture from the lesion, biopsy for detecting occurrence of viral intranuclear inclusions, or the use of monoclonal antibodies. As a rule, HSV-associated intraoral lesions are not used as markers for changes in immune states, although frequent or large confluent ulcers may indicate advanced HIV disease. To reduce the severity of lesions, the recommended treatment is either acyclovir 800 mg five times a day or valacyclovir 500 mg two to three times a day. Caution should be used when prescribing valacyclovir for immunocompromised patient, as this medication

Table 1
Viral Infections

Lesions	Clinical Presentation	Differential Diagnosis	Treatment	Significance	Marker for HIV	Nutritional Implications
HSV	Solitary, multiple, or confluentvesicles; keratinized mucosa; painful	Apthous ulcers, CMV	Acyclovir 800 mg five times a day or valacyclovir 500 mg BID for 14 d	Increases in frequency and severity based on progression of HIV	Not generally; indicates disease progression	Dehydration, restricted oral intake
CMV	Nonspecific >5 mm ulcers, nonkeratinized mucosa; painful	HSV, recurrent aphthous ulcers	Ganciclovir; acyclovir (solely for oral lesions)	CD4 cell count <200 mm^3	Not generally; indicates disease progression	Dehydration, restricted oral intake
VZV	Unilateral, generally on palate, along division of 5th cranial nerve; similar to HSV lesions; painful	HSV	Supportive and preventive; occasionally with oral or, if needed, intravenous acyclovir	No relation found	Not generally	Dehydration, restricted oral intake
EBV	Lateral borders of the tongue; a white, vertical, hyperkeratotic striae; cannot be wiped or rubbed off; asymptomatic	Hyperplastic or chronic candidiasis	Acyclovir 800 mg five times a day for 14 d	CD4 cell count <200 mm^3; viral load >20,000 copies/mL	Yes	None
HHV8	Red, purplish-blue macules or nodules; hard/soft palate, gingival; painful; caused by trauma	Bacillary (epithelioid) angiomatosis, lymphoma	Radiation, surgical intervention; vinblastine sulfate 0.1mg/mm^2 or sodium tetradecyl sulfate 0.1 mg/mm^2	CD4 cell count <100 mm^3	Yes	Difficulty eating with larger and/or traumatized lesions
HPV	Hyperplastic, papillomatous or verrucous	Fibroma	Topical podophyllum resin 25%; intralesional injections one to two times a wk with 1 million IU/cm^2 of the lesion, along with subcutaneous interferon-α injections of 3 million IU two to three times per wk	No relation found	No	Interference with chewing

HSV, herpes simplex virus; CMV, cytomegalovirus; VZV, varicella zoster virus; EBV, Epstein-Barr Virus; HHV8, human herpes virus 8; HPV, human papilloma virus.

may produce thrombotic thrombocytopenic purpura and hemolytic uremic syndrome in this patient population.

3.1.2. CMV

CMV, human herpes virus 5, can cause multiorgan dysfunction in an immunocompromised patient *(15,16)*. The intraoral presentation of CMV indicates severe immunosuppression, as measured by the CD4 cell count of less than 100 mm^3 and is usually linked with disseminated CMV infection *(2,17,18)*. The lesions are generally nonspecific ulcers that range from a few millimeters to 1 to 2 cm in diameter, primarily on the gingiva or the palate, but they can also be found on other mucosal surfaces. The ulcers may be shallow or deep with an eroded base and tend to be extremely painful *(19)*. Because of the ulcers, the nutritional status of the patient may be severely compromised. Pain added to prolonged healing of the ulcers may cause dehydration because of inadequate oral and nutritional intake.

The differential diagnoses should include recurrent aphthous ulcers and HSV lesions. To make a definitive diagnosis, a biopsy demonstrating perivascular inflammation and large basophilic intranuclear inclusions of CMV is required. An diagnosis of oral CMV requires additional workup to rule out ophthalmologic or other CMV-related disease and/ or lesions *(20)*. Intraoral manifestations of CMV can be treated with ganciclovir *(21)*.

3.1.3. VZV

VZV causes two well-defined diseases: chickenpox (varicella) and shingles (herpes zoster). After an initial infection, the virus remains latent in the dorsal root ganglia. Reactivation produces shingles in adult and immunocompromised patients. Shingles may commonly be seen during the progression of an individual's HIV disease. Although intraoral lesions have been noted, they are not common. If lesions do appear intraorally, they are typically found unilaterally along a division of the fifth cranial nerve, generally on the palate *(14)*. Lesions tend to resemble HSV-associated ulcers, but they are typically clustered unilaterally and are larger in size, and they too are painful. A significant correlation between intraoral VZV presentation and the immune status of an individual with HIV has yet to be shown *(22)*. Because of the painful nature of the lesions, especially in the acute phase, oral intake and consequently nutrition status may be affected. Treatment is usually supportive and preventive in nature. Although oral valacyclovir has been utilized, intravenous acyclovir may be indicated in severely immunocompromised patients *(14)*.

3.1.4. EPSTEIN-BARR VIRUS

Initially described in HIV-infected males, oral hairy leukoplakia (OHL), a lesion associated with Epstein-Barr virus (EBV), was initially thought to be an HIV-specific manifestation *(23,24)*. However, OHL is found not only among HIV-infected individuals, but has also been reported among other immunocompromised groups, and occasionally in immunocompetent individuals *(25,26)*. For an individual presenting with OHL and an unknown HIV status, an HIV test is strongly recommended, as the occurrence of OHL in individuals with HIV far exceeds the incidence of the lesion among other groups of patients.

OHL is commonly seen on the lateral borders of the tongue as white, vertical, hyperkeratotic striae sometimes extending onto the ventral or dorsal surfaces. The lesion cannot be wiped or rubbed off. As it is asymptomatic, the patient may not be aware of its presence, and it may be found incidentally during a routine intraoral examination. Occasionally, the lesion may appear as white patches on other intraoral surfaces. A definitive diagnosis of OHL must demonstrate the presence of EBV in the lesion *(10)*. A differential diagnosis of OHL includes hyperplastic or chronic candidiasis. *Candida albicans* has been shown to be present in over 50% of the lesions *(22)*. OHL is frequently found in patients with CD4 cells below 200 cells per mm^3 and is further associated with a viral load of 20,000 copies/mL or greater, irrespective of the CD4 cell count and the use of an antiretroviral regimen *(2,26–28)*.

Since OHL lesions are painless and not transmissible, treatment for OHL is generally initiated based on the patient's request when the lesion causes aesthetic problems or impairs masticatory functions. Therapy with acyclovir 800 mg five times a day for at least 10 to -14 d is usually successful. In some individuals, recurrence is common and prophylactic therapy of acyclovir 800 mg daily is recommended *(22)*.

3.1.5. HUMAN HERPES VIRUS 8

KS, traditionally known as an angiomatous tumor, was first described in 1872 by the Austrian dermatologist Moritz Kaposi. This form of tumor was known to predominantly affect men of Mediterranean decent in their sixth decade of life. However, since the onset of the HIV epidemic, the epidemiology of KS in the United States has changed dramatically. Today, KS is considered to be the most common neoplasm associated with HIV disease, mostly affecting homosexual and bisexual men. Because of its presence in men with multiple sexual contacts, it was hypothesized that KS may be caused by a transmissible pathogen. Studies have confirmed this suspicion, implicating the human herpes virus 8 (HHV8) as the etiologic agent for KS *(29,30)*. The presence of HHV8 in practically all KS lesions strongly suggests that this virus is associated with the development of the lesion *(31)*.

More than 90% of KS lesions are found either on the hard and/or soft palate, with the gingivae being the second most common site *(32)*. Lesions usually present as red, purplish, or blue macules, or nodules. In the early macular stage, the lesions are mostly asymptomatic and the patient may not be aware of their presence. Larger lesions may interfere with normal oral functions and become painful, mostly from secondary trauma or ulcerations. KS lesions may grow to such an extent that they may interfere with a patient's ability to eat, speak, and/or swallow.

Although lesions have been noted during all stages of HIV disease, intraoral KS generally presents when the patient's CD4 cell count drops below 100 cells per mm^3. Extrapalatal lesions and the change from a macular to a nodular presentation represent a progression and poorer prognosis. Similar to cutaneous lesions, intraoral KS is more frequently found in patients with increased incidence of sexually transmitted diseases.

A differential diagnosis must include physiologic pigmentation, bacillary (epithelioid) angiomatosis, and lymphoma. A biopsy is required for a definitive diagnosis of KS.

Therapies are aimed primarily at reducing the size and number of lesions. The most common treatments are systemic chemotherapy, radiation therapy, and surgical interventions. Smaller localized lesions can be treated by direct injection into the lesion with chemotherapeutic agent such as vinblastine sulfate 0.1 mg/mm^2 or sodium tetradecyl sulfate 0.1 mg/mm^2. Such local therapies are generally successful, although they may not be long lasting *(33–35)*.

3.1.6. Human Papilloma Virus

Human papilloma virus (HPV) is the known etiologic agent that causes warts in the oral cavity. Multiple lesions can occur in large areas of the mouth. The lesions are generally asymptomatic, unless traumatized. However, they frequently tend to interfere with mastication and may be disfiguring. HPV can present on all oral mucosal surfaces, although they have a predilection for the inside of the lips and the gingiva *(22,36)*. Various clinical forms have been described as hyperplastic, papillomatous, or verrucous. Oral squamous cell papillomas manifest as solitary or multiple, exophytic, pedunculated papules with a cauliflowerlike or pebbled surface. Condyloma acuminata are larger, white to pink nodules, with a cauliflowerlike or pebbled surface. The common wart, or verruca vulgaris, may appear as a firm and sessile, exophytic, white lesion. This lesion has a hyperkeratinized superficial epithelium with a slight invagination at the center of the lesion. Heck's disease, or focal epithelial hyperplasia, may appear as areas that are smooth, pebbled, or cauliflowerlike; large; solitary or multiple; whitish; hyperplastic; and slightly elevated. The differential diagnosis of oral HPV includes traumatic fibromas.

Although the incidence and prevalence of oral lesions have decreased since the institution of more effective anti-HIV medications, there has been a rise in the incidence of oral HPV *(28,37)*. It has been proposed that the increased incidence of HPV among patients with HIV who are taking highly active antiretroviral therapy (HAART) may be related not to immune suppression, but rather to immune reconstitution *(38)*.

Multiple successful treatment regimens have been reported *(36)*. Surgical removal with a scalpel, laser ablation, cryotherapy, topical application of keratinolytic agents, and intralesional injections of antiviral agents have been used. Podophyllum resin 25% may be used topically to reduce the size of the lesion and for removal of smaller lesions. Larger lesions can be treated using intralesional injections of interferon-α once or twice a week with 1 million IU per cm^2 of the lesion, accompanied with subcutaneous injections of 3 million IU two to three times a week for up to 3 mo *(36)*. Eradication of the lesions is possible over time using a combination of therapies, even though the recurrence rate is high.

3.2. Fungal Etiology

Table 2 describes the fungal sources of oral lesions common in HIV disease.

3.2.1. Candidiasis

C. albicans exists as a harmless inhabitant of the mucosal surfaces of the oral cavity in many immunocompetent individuals, generally without any signs of clinical manifestation. Candidiasis, or candidosis, has always been recognized as one of the most common and earliest intraoral manifestations of immune suppression *(39)*. In itself, candidiasis is not pathognomonic for HIV disease, but oral candidiasis may be an early sign of infection and a marker for disease progression, independent of CD4 lymphocyte count *(27)*. The clinical diagnosis should be verified by laboratory tests. Tests that may be used for a definitive diagnosis include cytological smear with potassium hydroxide, biopsy and staining for tissue infiltration of pathogenic agents (spores or hyphae), or routine culture. Four different clinical presentations of oral candidiasis have been described: pseudomembranous, erythematous, hyperplastic, and angular chelitis.

Table 2
Fungal Infections

Oral Manifestations	Clinical Presentation	Differential Diagnosis	Treatment	Significance	Marker for HIV	Nutritional Implications
Pseudomembranous candidiasis	White or yellowish, single or confluent plaques; easily rubbed off; any surface		Nystatin oral pastille, one to two pastilles dissolved slowly four to five times a day; clotrimazole oral troche 10 mg, 1 troche dissolved five times a day; nystatin oral suspension; fluconazole one to two 100 mg tablets QD: ketoconazole one to two 200 mg tablets QD taken with food; itraconazole two 100 mg capsules QD	CD4 cells below 400 cells/mm^3	Not generally, indicates early immune suppression	In severe cases, eating and swallowing can be uncomfortable
Erythematous candidiasis	Red or atrophic patches on any surface, however, greater on the tongue and hard palate		Same as pseudomembranous candidiasis	Any stage of HIV	Not generally, indicates early immune suppression	Longstanding lesions may produce a burning sensation
Hyperplastic candidiasis	White or discolored plaques; solitary or confluent; cannot be rubbed or wiped off	Leukoplakia, OHL	Fluconazole, one to two 100 mg tablets QD: ketoconazole one to two 200 mg tablets QD taken with food; itraconazole two 100 mg capsules QD	CD4 cell count below 100 cells per mm^3; high predilection for either having or developing esophageal candidiasis	Yes, severe immune suppression	Burning sensation and a feeling of having a "large ball of cotton in the mouth"; xerostomia; eating and swallowing may be uncomfortable
Angular chelitis	Radiating red fissures; commissures of the lips		Ketoconazole ointment 2%; apply to affected areas four times a day for 14 d; miconazole ointment 2%; apply to affected areas four times a day for 14 d		No	Difficulty opening the mouth because of pain
Histoplasmosis	Ulcerations to granulomas		Amphotericin B; ketoconazole; itraconazole	Severe immune suppression	Yes	Advanced stages, difficulty eating

3.2.1.1. Pseudomembranous Candidiasis

Commonly known as thrush, pseudomembranous candidiasis presents as white or yellowish, single or confluent plaques that can be easily rubbed off from the oral mucosa. The plaques may be found on any intraoral surface and leave an erythematous or bleeding surface when rubbed off. Patients are frequently not aware of the intraoral presentation. However, in more severe cases, eating and swallowing can be uncomfortable, which may have a negative impact on ability to eat and drink and, consequently, on nutritional status. The manifestation is an early indication of immune suppression, with CD4 cell counts below 400 cells per mm^3 (40).

3.2.1.2. Erythematous Candidiasis

Also known as atrophic candidiasis, erythematous candidiasis presents as red or atrophic patches. This lesion may affect any intraoral mucosal surfaces but has a predilection for the tongue and the hard palate. On the dorsal surface of the tongue, it manifests as areas of depapillation, sometimes creating smooth, erythematous patches. The erythematous form of candidiasis presents alone or in combination with the pseudomembranous form. Affected areas usually appear without a distinct border, thus making it difficult to mark the extent of the lesion. Long-standing lesions may be accompanied with a burning sensation or even ulcerations (14). The lesions can appear throughout the course of HIV disease, although they are generally seen during the earliest stages of immune suppression (22).

Treatment of both the pseudomembranous and erythematous forms of candidiasis is usually effective. Troches and mouth rinses are beneficial for patients with CD4 cell counts above 150 to 200 cells per mm^3. In patients with more severe immune suppression, systemic medications should be instituted.

Several different factors determine what medication is to be used. Troches are more convenient and practical than mouth rinses. However, decreased salivary flow makes it harder to dissolve the troches in the mouth. The type and use of systemic medications are dictated by patient's immune status, liver status, and compliance. Topical antifungal agents include nystatin oral pastille, one or two or pastilles dissolved slowly four or five times daily; clotrimazole oral troche 10 mg, one troche dissolved five times a day; and nystatin or itraconazole oral suspensions. Patients using topical antifungal agents need to be instructed in meticulous oral hygiene and home fluoride rinses as most of these formulations contain cariogenic sugars. Topical agents with low sugar content are vaginal preparations of clotrimazole or nystatin. One vaginal troche is dissolved in the mouth three times a day. The taste of the vaginal formulation is less agreeable to patients and may affect compliance.

The most frequently used systemic antifungal agents are fluconazole one or two 100 mg tablets daily; ketoconazole one or two 200 mg tablets daily to be taken with food; or itraconazole two 100 mg capsules daily. Unfortunately, oral *candidiasis* has a fairly high recurrence rate, and maintenance therapy may be indicated.

3.2.1.3. Hyperplastic Candidiasis

Frequently known as chronic candidiasis, hyperplastic candidiasis is an uncommon feature among ambulatory HIV-infected patients. This form of candidiasis is observed primarily in debilitated patients with severe immune suppression, represented by CD4 cell counts below 100 cells per mm^3. Patients with hyperplastic candidiasis have a high predilection for having, or developing, esophageal candidiasis, which is an AIDS-defining illness *(2)*.

Hyperplastic candidiasis presents as white or discolored plaques that may be solitary or confluent but, in contrast to pseudomembranous candidiasis, cannot be wiped or rubbed off the mucosa. Patients tend to complain of an oral burning sensation and a feeling of having a "large ball of cotton in mouth." The lesions may be found on any intraoral surface but have a high prevalence on the hard or soft palate.

Chronic candidiasis is often misdiagnosed as leukoplakia or, when it presents on the tongue, as OHL. Even though the clinical manifestation of the lesion is pathognomonic, the presence of hyphae and blastospores on a smear confirms a diagnosis. Treatment for this type of candidiasis involves systemic antifungal agents, which may include intravenous formulations.

3.2.1.4. Angular Chelitis

Angular chelitis presents as radiating red fissures, occasionally with a pseudomembranous cover, from the corner of the mouth. This condition is frequently observed in older individuals with ill-fitting complete dentures and is not pathognomonic for HIV disease. It is commonly found together with xerostomia and may worsen during the cold winter months.

Successful treatment of angular chelitis is accomplished by application of a topical antifungal agent such as clotrimazole, miconazole, ketoconazole cream, or nystatin ointment in combination with a topical antibacterial agent.

3.2.2. HISTOPLASMOSIS

Infections with histoplasmosis can be found in individuals who work near dust-producing activities in high endemic areas, such as the Ohio and Mississippi valleys. Histoplasmosis is caused by inhaling the spores of *Histoplasma capsulatum*, which is found in the soil throughout the world. Disturbances of contaminated soil can cause the spores to become airborne. Although rare in areas that are nonendemic, endemic areas have exhibited prevalence rates of approx 70% of the adult population having a positive histoplasmin test *(41)*. In the immunocompetent host, most infections by *H. capsulatum* are subclinical and self-limiting. However, in the immunocompromised patient, *H. capsulatum* can cause a serious opportunistic infection. Although not correlated with CD4 cell count, histoplasmosis was included in the AIDS-defining illnesses category in 1985 *(3)*. Many cases of histoplasmosis are disseminated by the time of oral manifestations *(42)*. The clinical presentations vary along a spectrum of ulcerations to granulomas. A definitive diagnosis is based on multiple factors, including clinical examination, serology, light microscopy, and culture *(42)*. The treatment modality of choice is intravenous amphotericin B, however itraconazole and ketoconazole have also been used successfully to treat disseminated histoplasmosis in immunocompromised patients *(42,43)*.

3.3. Bacterial Etiology

3.3.1. PERIODONTAL DISEASE

Periodontal disease is a common condition found in both HIV-positive and HIV-negative individuals. HIV-infected individuals may show signs of a more rapidly progressive type of conventional chronic periodontal disease, but this is not a consistent feature. Acute, rapidly progressive periodontal conditions may be early signs of immune suppression and HIV infection *(22)*. Studies have demonstrated an association between aggressive periodontal conditions in HIV-infected individuals and a progressive deterioration of individuals' immune status *(44,45)*. Even though different periodontal conditions in the HIV-infected individual are linked to the person's immune status, they are not associated with a change in the microflora *(22)*. There are three types of periodontal conditions that have been associated with HIV disease: linear gingival erythema (LGE), necrotizing ulcerative gingivitis (NUG), and necrotizing ulcerative periodontitis (NUP) *(11,46)*.

3.3.1.1. Linear Gingival Erythema

An erythematous 2–3 mm red band at the gingival margin, disproportional to plaque accretion, characterizes LGE with an equal distribution around the teeth. There is no ulceration, no increase in pocket depth with periodontal attachment loss, and minimal bleeding on probing *(22)*. Occasionally, punctuated or diffuse erythema is noted on the attached gingiva near the alveolar mucosa. The condition may be asymptomatic. This presentation does not have a strong correlation with HIV disease *(22)*. The differential diagnosis can be quite extensive and include localized effect secondary to dry mucosa associated with open-mouth breathing, localized candidiasis, oral lichen planus, mucous membrane pemphigoid, hypersensitivity reaction presenting as plasma cell gingivitis, *Geotrichum candidum* infection, and thrombocytopenia. The presentation of LGE may be caused by a subgingival candida infection *(22)*.

LGE will typically not respond to routine dental scaling and root planing. However, concomitant use of chlorhexidine gluconate (0.12%) mouth rinse twice a day for up to 3 mo generally produces a notable improvement. The patient should be advised to swish with 15 mL of the solution for 30 s and then expectorate. Addition of a topical antifungal agent may be advantageous. Meticulous oral hygiene is essential for both the treatment and maintenance.

3.3.1.2. NUG and NUP

Both NUG and NUP may represent different stages in a spectrum of the same severe periodontal condition. NUG is classically limited to the gingiva without related periodontal attachment loss, whereas NUP is recognized by the loss of periodontal attachment and ulceration of the adjacent alveolar mucosa. Both lesions manifest in the acute phase and may vary from initial lesions with restricted necrosis at the top of the papillae to involvement of the complete attached gingiva, accompanied by tooth mobility and bone sequestering *(44)*. Individuals with NUP generally complain of severe deep-seated jaw pain, spontaneous bleeding from the gingiva, and, in chronic cases, tooth movement *(47–49)*. Characteristically, foeter ex oris, or halitosis, is also present. Left untreated, NUP may progress with 1–2 mm of soft and hard tissue destruction per week. NUP has been linked with severe immune suppression and CD4 cell counts below 100 cells per mm^3 *(44)*. During the acute stage of these lesions, patient's oral intake may be severely limited.

Several conditions should be included in a differential diagnoses: benign mucous membrane pemphigoid, erythema multiforme, and acute forms of leukemia *(22)*.

The first step in the treatment of both NUG and NUP is debridement and antibiotic therapy with metronidazole 250–500 mg or tetracycline 250-500 mg four times a day for 7 d. Pain relief is rapid and tissue healing begins quickly after initial therapy. Concomitant antifungal therapy is recommended, as there is a greater chance of a secondary candidal infection. Chlorhexidine gluconate 0.12% mouth rinse, twice a day swish for 30 s and then expectorate, is recommended for both treatment and maintenance therapy *(22)*.

3.4. Conditions With Nonspecific Etiology

3.4.1. NECROTIZING STOMATITIS

Necrotizing stomatitis is a rapidly progressive localized ulceration that causes necrosis of the soft tissue overlying bone *(50)*. The lesion may be extremely painful and interfere with eating, speech, and swallowing. This presentation is generally seen in patients who are severely immunosuppressed, with the CD4 cell counts below 100 cells per mm^3 *(2)*.

Differential diagnosis should include aggressive forms of aphthous ulcers. It has been hypothesized that necrotizing stomatitis may be a more widespread type of NUP *(22)*.

Treatment includes thorough debridement of the necrotic areas. When possible, a stent should be fabricated and placed over the affected areas as protection against trauma and as a carrier for topical application of medication. Topical glucocorticosteroids such as clobetasole or fluocinonide gel, or dexamethasone elixir mouth rinse 0.5 mg/5 mL, for 10 to 14 d may be used. In more severe and resistant cases, systemic steroid formulation, such as prednisone up to 20 mg four times a day for 7 d may be indicated. The patient should be instructed to use chlorhexidine gluconate 0.12% rinse twice a day. Concurrent usage of a systemic antibiotic, metronidazole or tetracycline, can prevent bacterial superinfections and promote a faster healing phase *(22)*.

3.4.2. APHTHOUS ULCERS

Minor recurrent aphthous ulcers generally manifest as 2–5 mm diameter small ulcers and resolve within 5 to 7 d. Recurrent aphthous ulcers (RAUs) appear on less-keratinized tissue of the oral cavity, such as inside the lips or on the floor of the mouth or buccal mucosa. Minor RAUs are characterized by their frequent recurrence rate, often at the same site, and are generally associated with stressful events *(22)*. They can be slightly painful, yet heal without scarring. This type of ulcer is common in the general population and can be misdiagnosed as recurrent herpes virus infection. Swishing and expectorating with viscous lidocaine 2–4% solution, an analgesic mouth rinse, is recommended to decrease oral discomfort. This treatment greatly restores a patient's ability to eat, drink, chew, and swallow.

Recurrent ulcers that present as greater than 10 mm in diameter, with a crateriform and deeply eroded base, are known as major recurrent aphthous ulcers. These ulcers persist for more than 3 wk and tend to heal with scarring. Major RAUs severely hinder the patient's ability to eat, speak, and swallow *(51)*. Although no clear etiology has been established for these ulcers, several theories have been put forth: stress, vitamin deficiency, diet, hormonal changes, trauma, and immune dysfunction *(14,52)*. In patients with HIV disease, major RAUs have been correlated with severe immune suppression and CD4 cell count below 100 cells per mm^3 *(51)*.

Treatment of major RAU is crucial to restore masticatory function and reduce intraoral pain. Systemic or topical glucocorticosteroids may be administered as the first step in therapy. Prednisone 20 mg tablets three to four times a day for 7 d is the recommended systemic therapy regimen. Dexamethasone elixir 0.5 mg/5 mL, as a topical rinse, 15 mL four times a day for 7 d can also be used. Frequently, an antibiotic and an antifungal agent are prescribed to prevent superinfections. Topical medications may increase patient compliance for nutritional intake and maintaining treatment regimen. Thalidomide 100–200 mg/d has been used to treat oral and esophageal ulcerations with limited success *(53)*. There are some adverse reactions noted in people who use thalidomide, including somnolence, rash, and peripheral sensory neuropathy *(53)*.

3.5. Neoplastic Conditions

The association between HIV and non-Hodgkin's lymphomas (NHLs) was recognized early in the HIV epidemic and in 1985 it was added to the list of AIDS-defining diseases *(3)*. This neoplasm is rare, appearing in approx 3% of AIDS diagnoses worldwide *(54)*. The lesion may present as a large, painful, ulcerated or exophytic mass on any mucosal surface and may be accompanied with tooth mobility, dentoalveolar pain, widened periodontal ligament, and progressive paresthesia *(14,22)*. The average CD4 cell count in patients diagnosed with NHL is below 100 cells per mm^3 *(14)*.

Prior to HAART, NHL represented the second most common neoplasm associated with AIDS, after KS *(55)*. With the implementation of HAART, the incidence of KS cases has decreased, whereas patients developing NHL have remained relatively the same as prior to HAART *(55)*.

A biopsy is required for a definitive diagnosis, and an appropriate referral to an oncologist is indicated for initiation of treatment. Therapy may include surgical excision, chemotherapy, and/or radiation therapy *(14)*. Unfortunately, NHL is associated with an extremely poor prognosis, with an average survival rate of approx 6–9 mo after diagnosis *(56)*.

4. NUTRITIONAL MANAGEMENT OF ORAL MANIFESTATIONS OF HIV

Dental intervention in conjunction with nutrition management is an essential component of care at the earliest stage of HIV infection because of the magnitude and impact of HIV-associated oral diseases on dietary intake and nutritional status. Oropharyngeal fungal infections and viral diseases, including the accompanying painful ulcerations along with stomatitis and periodontitis, are associated with pain and can lead to reduced oral intake. Often esophagitis and oral and esophageal candidiasis can cause painful mastication, drinking, and swallowing, further compromising appetite and intake. KS, depending on the size and location in the oral cavity, has the combined effect of compromising oral intake and increasing nutrient needs.

Oropharyngeal fungal infections may cause a burning, painful mouth and dysphagia. Very hot and cold foods or beverages, spices, and sour or tart foods also may be painful and should be avoided. Consumption of temperate, moist foods without added spices should be encouraged. Small, frequent meals followed by rinsing with lukewarm water or brushing to reduce the risk of dental caries are helpful. Once the type and extent of oral manifestations are identified, a nutrition care plan can be developed.

Stomatitis can cause severe pain and ulceration of the gingiva, oral mucosa, and palate, which makes eating painful. Xerostomia, or dry mouth, secondary to medications or other concurrent disease can further compromise intake. Efforts to stimulate saliva production using pharmacologic agents and citrus-flavored, sugar-free candies may ease eating difficulty (*see* Appendix B). Dietary guidelines focus on the use of moist foods without added spices, increased fluid consumption with and between all meals and snacks, and judicious food choices. Problems with chewy (steak), crumbly (cake, crackers), dry (chips), and sticky (peanut butter) foods are common in individuals with severe xerostomia, and avoiding these foods may help a great deal with eating. Water with a lemon-lime twist, citrus-flavored seltzers, and sucking on frozen grapes may help. Good oral hygiene habits are important to reduce the risk of tooth decay and should be practiced after all meals and snacks. Xylitol-flavored gums and mints may help reduce the risk of associated decay.

5. CONCLUSIONS

Oral manifestations are commonly the first signs of an underlying systemic disease in a patient. This chapter discusses some of the more frequently found oral lesions associated with HIV disease, their clinical presentations, and current treatment modalities. The integration of dental management with nutrition care contributes to improved systemic, oral, and nutritional well-being and response to treatment. Collaboration across disciplines in detection, referral, and early intervention of oral and nutrition-diet-related problems are important for comprehensive care of the individual with HIV or AIDS.

Guidelines for Practice

	Oral Health Professional	*Nutrition Professional*
Prevention	• Conduct regular screening examinations for oral disease. • Assess nutrition risk and provide appropriate referrals for medical nutrition therapy (MNT) in all individuals with HIV and AIDS.	• Conduct oral screen as part of comprehensive nutrition assessment; refer nonnormal findings to a dentist. • Provide MNT to patients along with referrals for dental care on a routine basis.
Intervention	• Provide dental care and prophyaxis as needed. • Review appetite, weight change, intake, and oral factors affecting eating ability at all visits and refer as needed for MNT by a registered dietitian.	• Routinely conduct oral screen on all patients and refer for and reinforce importance of dental treatment. • Provide dietary guidelines consistent with symptoms to promote attaining and maintaining nutritional well-being.

REFERENCES

1. Sirois D. Oral manifestations of HIV disease. Mount Sinai J Med 1998; 65(Oct/Nov):322–332.
2. Glick M, Muzyka BC, Lurie D, Salkin LM. Oral manifestations associated with HIV-related disease as markers for immune suppression and AIDS. Oral Surg Oral Med Oral Pathol 1994; 77:344–349.
3. CDC. 1993 Revised classification system for HIV infection and expanded surveillance case definition for AIDS among adolescents and adults. MMWR 1992; 41:1–10.
4. Anker M, Schaaf D. WHO Report on global surveillance of epidemic-prone infectious diseases. Communicable Disease Surveillance and Response. WHO/CDS/CSR/ISR/2000.1. Available at

Website: (http://www.who.int/emc-documents/surveillance/whocdscsrisr20001c.html). Accessed September 3, 2002.

5. Fleming PL, Byers PA, Sweeney DD, Karon JM, Janssen RS. HIV prevalence in the United States, 2000. Seattle, WA: 9th Conference on Retroviruses and Opportunistic Infections, February 24–28, 2002. Abstract 11.

6. CDC. Pneumocystis pneumonia: Los Angeles. MMWR 1981; 30:250.

7. Roos MT, Lange JM, de Goode RE, et al. Viral phenotype and immune response in primary human immunodeficiency virus type 1 infection. J Inf Dis 1992; 165:427–432.

8. Schacker T, Collier AC, Hughes J, Shea T, Corey L. Clinical and epidemiologic features of primary HIV infection. Ann Int Med 1996; 124:257–264.

9. Kahn JO, Walder BD. Current concepts: acute human immunodeficiency virus type 1 infection. New Engl J Med 1998; 339:33–39.

10. Greenspan JS, Barr CE, Sciubba JJ, at al. Oral manifestations of HIV infection: definitions, diagnostic criteria and principles of therapy. Oral Surg Oral Med Oral Pathol 1992; 73:142–144.

11. EEC-Clearinghouse on oral problems related to HIV infection and WHO collaborating center on oral manifestations of the human immunodeficiency virus: an update of the classification and diagnostic criteria of oral lesions in HIV-infection. J Oral Pathol and Med 1991; 20:289–291.

12. Glick M, Siegel MA. Viral and fungal infections of the oral cavity in immunocompetent patients. Infect Dis Clin North Am 1999; 13:817–831.

13. Glick M. Recurrent oral herpes simplex virus infection: clinical aspects. Compend Contin Educ Dent 2002; 23(Suppl. 2):4–8.

14. Kademani D, Glick M. Oral ulcerations in individuals infected with human immunodeficiency virus: clinical presentations, diagnosis, management, and relevance to disease progression. Quintessence Int 1998; 29:523–534.

15. Mattes FM, McLauglin JA, Emery VC, Clark DA, Griffiths PD. Histopathological detection of owl's eye inclusions is still specific for cytomegalovirus in the era of human herpesviruses 6 and 7. J Clin Pathol 2000; 53:612–614.

16. Drew WL. Cytomegalovirus infection in patients with AIDS. J Infect Dis 1988; 158:449–456.

17. Spector SA, Hsia K, Grager M, et al. Cytomegalovirus (CMV) DNA load is an independent predictor of CMV disease and survival in advanced AIDS. J Virol 1999; 73:7027–7030.

18. Spector SA, Wong R, Hsia K, Pilcher M, Stempien MJ. Plasma cytomegalovirus (CMV) DNA predicts CMV disease and survival in AIDS patients. J Clin Invest. 1998; 101:497–502.

19. Syrjanes S, Leimola-Virtanen R, Schmidt-Westhausen A, Reichart PA. Oral ulcers in AIDS patients frequently associated with cytomegalovirus (CMV) and Epstein-Barr virus (EBV) infections. J Oral Pathol Med 1999; 28:204–209.

20. Schrier RD, Freeman WR, Wiley CA, McCutchan JA, the HNRC Group. Immune predispositions for cytomegalovirus retinitis in AIDS. J Clin Invest 1995; 95:1741–1746.

21. Spector SA, Hsia K, Grager M, et al. Cytomegalovirus (CMV) DNA load is an independent predictor of CMV disease and survival in advanced AIDS. J Virol 1999; 73:7027–7030.

22. Glick M, Berthold P. Oral manifestations of HIV infection. In Buckley RM, Gluckman SJ, eds. HIV infection in primary care. Philadelphia, PA: W.B. Saunders, 2002, 132–140.

23. Greenspan D, Greenspan JS, Conant M, et al. Oral "hairy" leukoplakia in male homosexuals: evidence of association with both papillomavirus and herpes-group virus. Lancet 1984; 2:831–834.

24. Greenspan JS, Greenspan D, Lennette ET, et al. Replication of Epstein-Barr virus within epithelial cells of oral hairy leukoplakia: an AIDS-associated lesion. N Engl J Med 1985; 313:1564–1571.

25. Felix DH, Watret K, Wray D, Southam JC. Hairy leukoplakia in an HIV-negative, nonimmunosuppressed patient. Oral Surg Oral Med Oral Pathol 1992; 74:563–566.

26. Greenspan D, Greenspan JS. HIV-related oral disease. Lancet 1996; 348:729–733.

27. Patton LL. Sensitivity, specificity, and positive predictive value of oral opportunistic infections in adults with HIV/AIDS as markers of immune suppression and viral burden. Oral Surg Oral Med Oral Pathol Oral Radiol Endod 2000; 90:182–188.

28. Patton LL, McKaig R, Strauss R, Rogers D, Eron JJ. Changing prevalence of oral manifestations of human immunodeficiency virus in the era of the protease inhibitor therapy. Oral Surg Oral Med Oral Pathol Oral Radiol Endod 2000; 89:299–304.

29. Chang Y, Cesarman E, Pessin MS, et al. Identification of herpes-like DNA sequences in AIDS-associated Kaposi's sarcoma. Science 1994; 266:1865–1869.

30. O'Neill E, Henson TH, Ghorbani AJ, Land MA, Webber BL, Garcia JV. Herpes virus-like sequences are specifically found in Kaposi's sarcoma lesions. J Clin Pathol; 49:306–308.

31. Leao JC, Porter S, Scully C. Human herpesvirus 8 and oral health care: an update. Oral Surg Oral Med Oral Pathol Oral Radiol Endod 2000; 90:694–704.

32. Gorsky M, Epstein JB. A case series of acquired immunodeficiency syndrome patients with initial neoplastic diagnoses on intraoral Kaposi's sarcoma. Oral Surg Oral Med Oral Pathol Oral Radiol Endod 2000; 90:612–617.

33. Muzyka BC, Glick M. Sclerotherapy for the treatment of nodular intraoral Kaposi's sarcoma in patients with AIDS. N Engl J Med 1993; 328:210–211.

34. Epstein JB, Scully C. HIV infection: clinical features and treatment of thirty-three homosexual men with Kaposi's sarcoma. Oral Surg Oral Med Oral Pathol Oral Radiol Endod 1991; 71:38–41.

35. Epstein JB, Lozado-Nur R, McLeod A, Spinelli J. Oral Kaposi's sarcoma in acquired immunodeficiency syndrome: review of management and report of the efficacy of intralesional vinblastine. Cancer 1989; 64:2424–2430.

36. Lozada-Nur F, Glick M, Schubert M, Silverberg I. Use of intralesional interferon-alpha for the treatment of recalcitrant oral warts in patients with AIDS: a report of 4 cases. Oral Surg Oral Med Oral Pathol Oral Radiol Endod 2001; 92:617–622.

37. Greenspan D, Cancola AJ, MacPhail LA, Cheikh B, Greenspan JS. Effect of highly active antiretroviral therapy on frequency of oral warts. Lancet 2001; 357:1411–1412.

38. King MD, Reznik DA, O'Daniels CM, et al. Human papillomavirus-associated oral warts among human immunodeficiency virus-seropositive patients in the era of highly active antiretroviral therapy: an emerging infection. Clin Infec Dis 2002; 34:641–648.

39. Campo J, Del Romero J, Castilla J, Garcia S, Rodriguez C, Basones A. Oral candidiasis as a clinical marker related to viral load, CD4 lymphocytes count and CD4 lymphocyte percentage in HIV-infected patients. J Oral Pathol Med 2002; 31:5–10.

40. Phelan JA, Begg MD, Lamster IB, et al. Oral candidiasis in HIV infection: predictive value and comparison of findings in injecting drug users and homosexual men. J Oral Pathol Med 1997; 26: 237–243.

41. Ng KH, Siar CH. Review of oral histoplasmosis in Malaysians. Oral Surg Oral Med Oral Pathol Oral Radiol Endod 1996; 81:303–307.

42. Warnakulasuriya KAAS, Harrison, JD, Johnson, NW, Edwards S, Taylor C, Pozniak, AL. Localized oral histoplasmosis lesions associated with HIV infection. J Oral Pathol Med 1997; 26:294–296.

43. Economopoulou P, Laskaris G, Kittas C. Oral histoplasmosis as an indicator of HIV infection. Oral Surg Oral Med Oral Pathol Oral Radiol Endod 1998; 86:1–6.

44. Glick M, Muzyka BC, Salkin LM, Lurie D. Necrotizing ulcerative periodontitis: a marker for immune deterioration and a predictor for the diagnosis of AIDS. J Periodontol 1994; 65:393–397.

45. Lucht E, Heimdahl A, Nord CE. Periodontal disease in HIV-infected patients in relation to lymphocyte subsets and specific micro-organisms. J Clin Periodontol 1991; 18:252–256.

46. Robinson PG. Which periodontal changes are associated with HIV infection? J Clin Periodontol 1998; 25:278–285.

47. Narani N, Epstein JB. Classifications of oral lesions in HIV infection. J Clinical Periodontol 2001; 28:137–145.

48. Winkler JR, Robertson PB. Periodontal disease associated with HIV infection. Oral Surg Oral Med Oral Pathol 1992; 73:145–150.

49. Greenspan JS, Barr CE, Sciubba JJ, Winkler JR, USA Oral AIDS Collaborative Group. Oral manifestations of HIV infection: definitions, diagnostic criteria, and principles of therapy. Oral Surg Oral Med Oral Pathol 1992; 73:142–144.

50. Muzyka BC, Glick M. HIV infection and necrotizing stomatitis. Gen Dent 1994:66–68.

51. Muzyka BC, Glick M. Major aphthous ulcers in patients with HIV disease. Oral Surg Oral Med Oral Pathol 1994; 77:116–120.

52. Ship JA. Recurrent apthous stomatitis: an update. Oral Surg Oral Med Oral Pathol Oral Radiol Endod 1996; 81:141–147.

53. Weidle PJ. Thalidomide for aphthous ulcers in patients infected with the human immunodeficiency virus. Am J Health Syst Pharm 1996; 53:368–378.
54. Tirelli U, Franceschi S, Carbone A. Current issues in cancer: malignant tumours in patients with HIV infection. Br Med J 1994; 308:1148–1153.
55. Tirelli U, Spina M, Gaidano G, Vaccher E, Franceschi S, Carbone A. Epidemiological, biological and clinical features of HIV-related lymphomas in the era of highly active antiretroviral therapy. AIDS 2000; 114:1675–1688.
56. Lozada-Nur F, de Sanz S, Silverman S Jr, et al. Intraoral non-Hodgkin's lymphoma in seven patients with acquired immunodeficiency syndrome. Oral Surg Oral Med Oral Pathol 1994; 82:173–178.

14 Autoimmune Diseases

David A. Sirois and Riva Touger-Decker

1. INTRODUCTION

Several autoimmune diseases are particularly important to oral health and nutrition because of their direct impact on the oral mucosa, masticatory apparatus, salivary glands, teeth and supporting structures, oral pain, or mechanical ability to chew. For some disorders, the earliest signs of systemic illness are found in the oral cavity, and these remain as significant manifestations of the primary immune disorder. Additionally, the medical management of autoimmune diseases can alter oral immune surveillance as well as introduce significant metabolic and nutritional complications. This chapter explores the impact on oral health and nutrition of the following autoimmune diseases: systemic lupus erythematosus (SLE), rheumatoid arthritis (RA), pernicious anemia (PA), and Sjögren's syndrome (SS), and the mucocutaneous disorders of pemphigus vulgaris and benign mucous membrane pemphigoid; type 1 diabetes mellitus, another important autoimmune disorder, is discussed separately in Chapter 11. The dentist may be the first to diagnose some of these conditions owing to their oral presentation, but he or she also has the responsibility to manage oral complications of the disease and its treatment as well as identify health promotion strategies to minimize long-term sequelae. Referral to a registered dietitian (RD) is an important aspect of total patient care and provides the best strategy for optimal disease management and health promotion. Likewise, the RD may see patients with these diseases for medical nutrition therapy (MNT); it is incumbent on the RD to ask patients about oral pain and dysfunction, conduct an oral screen, and refer patients appropriately to a dentist.

2. GENERAL FEATURES OF AUTOIMMUNE DISEASES AND THEIR TREATMENT

Autoimmune diseases share the feature of an immunologic disorder resulting in production of antibodies directed against normal tissue. The signs and symptoms of each disorder depend on the target tissue or tissues involved. In addition to the presence of an auto-antibody or evidence of other self-reactivity, criteria for autoimmune disease include the presence of the auto-antibody or lymphocytic infiltrate in the pathologic lesion and demonstration that the relevant auto-antibody or T cell can cause tissue pathology in laboratory models or by transplacental transmission. Although not exclusively,

From: *Nutrition and Oral Medicine*
Edited by: R. Touger-Decker, D. A. Sirois, and C. C. Mobley © Humana Press Inc., Totowa, NJ

Table 1
Target Antigens of Selected Autoimmune Disorders

| | Presence in autoimmune disease (% of cases) | | | | | |
| | Non-organ-specific autoimmune disorders | | | | Organ-specific disorders | |
Auto-antibody type	SLE	RA	SS	PA	PV	BMMP
Antinuclear	96–100	30–60	95			
Anti-native DNA	60	0–5	0			
Anti-rheumatoid factor	20	72–85	75			
Anti-Sm	10–30	0	0			
Anti-Ro	15–25	0–5	60–70			
Anti-La	5–20	0–2	60–70			
Anti-intrinsic factor				60		
Anti-gastric parietal cell				90		
Desmoglein 3					100	
Desmoglein 1					50	
Bullous pemphoid antigen 2						100

these disorders generally occur more frequently in women than in men and usually in individuals over age 40. Autoimmune diseases may be organ specific (pemphigus vulgaris, mucous membrane pemphigoid) or non-organ specific (i.e., multiple organ systems affected) (SLE, SS, RA). Individuals with one autoimmune disease are more likely to develop another; thus, it is not uncommon to find that patients have overlapping symptoms and multiple diagnoses (i.e., SLE and SS). Table 1 summarizes the target antigens of the autoimmune disorders discussed in this chapter, and each disorder is explored in greater detail in subsequent sections.

In general, autoimmune disorders are incurable and require continuous or periodic treatment to minimize disease-related sequelae. Treatment may be directed primarily at the immune system with the objective of reducing autoantibody production or immune activation, at protection or replacement of the affected target tissue or cell, at relieving symptoms, or a combination of the above. The common long-term use of immunosuppressant and immunomodulating medications presents significant risk for complications such as opportunistic infection, increased risk for cancer, and a myriad of potentially serious metabolic and biochemical problems. Progress in the development of gene therapy, tissue transplantation, and monoclonal antibody therapy provides the promise in the near future of more specific treatments with fewer side effects. Table 2 summarizes the spectrum of therapies for treating the autoimmune disorders discussed in this chapter, and Table 3 shows the related systemic, oral, and nutritional complications of these medications; details are discussed in subsequent sections.

3. ORGAN-SPECIFIC AUTOIMMUNE DISORDERS

PA, pemphigus vulgaris (PV) and benign mucous membrane pemphigoid (BMMP) represent autoimmune diseases with organ-specific antigen targets (see Table 1). Each has unique oral, systemic, and nutritional implications for the disease itself as well as for its therapy.

Table 2
Selected Systemic Therapies for Autoimmune Disorders

Drug	Class	Common indications					
		PA	PV	BMMP	SLE	SS	RA
Prednisone	Glucocorticoid		1	1	2	3	2
Mycophenolate mofentil	Immunosupp		1	2	2	3	3
Azathioprine	Immunosupp		2	2	2	3	3
Dapsone	Antileprosy/Disease modifying		2	1	2	3	2
Cyclophosphamide	Alkylating agent		2	2	2		3
Cyclosporin	Immunosupp		2	2	2		2
Methotrexate	Immunosupp; Antimetabolite		2	2	2		2
Gold	Disease modifying		4	3	3	3	2
NSAIDs	Anti inflammatory		4	3	1	2	1
IVIg	n/a		2	3		4	
Hydroxychloroqine	Antimalarial			3	2		2
Plasmapheresis	n/a		3	3	3		
Topical, injectable therapies	Immunosupp		2	1	2		2
Replacement therapy (B_{12})		1					3
Palliative therapy (e.g., artificial tears, sialagogue, analgesic)						1	3

1, first-line therapy; 2, second- or third-line therapy or in combination with 1; 3, on rare occasions; 4, not applicable.

3.1. Pernicious Anemia

3.1.1. Pathogenesis

Anemia is a decrease in oxygen-carrying capacity of red blood cells (RBC) and can result from RBC destruction, inadequate RBC production, or blood loss *(1,2)*. PA results from B_{12} (cobalamine) deficiency, most often caused by absorption deficiency rather than dietary deficiency *(1–3)*. Cobalamine is an essential compound in folate metabolism, and a lack of either folate or cobalamine results in a defect in DNA synthesis and the associated megaloblastic changes in cells with relatively high turnover such as hematopoietic precursors and gastrointestinal (GI) epithelium. Cytoplasmic development proceeds normally while cell division is slowed, resulting in large cells with an increased ratio of RNA to DNA. Megaloblastic anemia is certain when the mean corpuscular volume exceeds 100 fL. Other conditions that can lead to cobalamine deficiency and megaloblastic anemia include gastrectomy, small-intestine bacterial overgrowth, diverticulosis, scleroderma, tapeworm, tropical sprue, alcoholism, and medications such as neomycin and colchicine.

Cobalamine cannot be synthesized, and dietary sources are limited to animal protein foods (meat, fish, poultry, eggs, and dairy), although many enriched and fortified grain products have added B_{12} *(4)*. With a recommended daily allowance of only 2.5 μg and a storage of approx 4 mg in various body compartments, the onset of symptoms of anemia usually occurs after several years of inadequate consumption or absorption.

Table 3
Selected Adverse Effects of Therapies for Autoimmune Disorders

Drug	Class	Selected adverse effects		
		Oral	Systemic	Nutritional
Prednisone	Glucocorticoid	Candidiasis	Adrenal insufficiency Psychosis Mood swings Peptic ulcer Osteoporosis Edema Insomnia Hyperglycemia Hypertension	Appetite change Weight gain Dyspepsia Osteoporosis Hyperglycemia
Mycophenolate mofetil	Immunosupp	Candidiasis	Leukopenia Thrombocytopenia GI ulceration Hypertension Edema Anemia Headache Abdominal pain Constipation Insomnia	Dyspepsia Diarrhea GI ulceration Constipation Anemia
Azathioprine	Immunosupp	Candidiasis	Leukopenia Thrombocytopenia Anemia GI hypersensitivity Hepatotoxicity Malaise	Anorexia Vomiting Diarrhea Anemia

Drug	Classification			
Dapsone	Antileprosy/ Disease-modifying drug	Erythema multiforme	Hemolytic anemia Hepatotoxicity Fever Malaise Arthralgia	Anorexia Vomiting Nausea Albuminuria
Cyclophosphamide	Alkylating agent	Candidiasis Stomatitis	Cardiomyopathy Malignancy Heart failure Leukopenia Thrombocytopenia	Nausea Vomiting Anorexia Diarrhea
Cyclosporine	Immunosupp	Gingival hyperplasia Candidiasis	Seizures Leukopenia Thrombocytopenia Nephrotoxicity Hepatotoxicity Diabetes Hypertension	Diabetes Nausea Vomiting Diarrhea
Methotrexate	Immunosupp Antimetabolite	Candidiasis Erythema multiforme Stomatitis	Anemia Leukopenia Thrombocytopenia Hepatotoxicity Nephrotoxicity Seizures Encephalopathy Pulmonary fibrosis	Nausea Vomiting Diarrhea Anemia
Hydroxychloroquine	Antimalarial	Candidiasis	Anemia Agranulocytosis Thrombocytopenia Seizures	Nausea Vomiting Diarrhea Weight loss Anemia
Topical, injectable steroids	Immunosupp	Candidiasis Mucosal atrophy	Minimal glucocorticoid effects	

Intrinsic factor (IF) produced in gastric parietal cells binds to cobalamine and protects it from degradation until it can be absorbed in the ileum. Anti-IF antibodies and antibodies directed against gastric parietal cells result in a lack of IF and subsequent poor absorption of cobalamine and megaloblastic anemia. Correct identification of the underlying cause (i.e., folate vs cobalamine deficiency) is important, rather than empirical folate therapy, which will improve only the anemia and not the neurological symptoms of a cobalamine deficiency (paresthesia, impaired neurocognitve function).

3.1.2. CLINICAL FEATURES

3.1.2.1. General Features

Symptoms of anemia may include weakness, light-headedness, shortness of breath, palpitations, and angina. Physical findings in the patient with florid cobalamin deficiency include pale skin, with slightly icteric skin and eyes, and rapid pulse. There may be anorexia with varying degrees of weight loss. Megaloblastosis of the small intestine epithelium may result in diarrhea, resulting in malabsorption and contributing to weight loss. A hallmark feature of PA is the neurological symptoms of peripheral paresthesia, weakness, ataxia, and even dementia. Early demyelination can progress to axonal degeneration and neuronal death. These neurological symptoms are a direct result of the cobalamine deficiency (not the anemia) and can be permanent even after correction of both the cobalamine deficiency and the related anemia. Empirical treatment of undiagnosed PA using folate can correct the anemia but mask the underlying cobalamine deficiency, thus placing the patient at risk for worsening neurological symptoms.

3.1.2.2. Oral Features

Oral findings can occur quite early in PA and include atrophic glossitis (red and smooth tongue), burning mouth, and aphthous stomatitis. Any patient over age 40 with unexplained weakness and these oral findings should have a complete blood count with RBC indices and a B_{12} and folate level. A thorough diet, nutrition, and health history is also important to detect other contributing factors.

3.1.3. DIAGNOSIS

Diagnostic tests for pernicious anemia include the Shilling Test, which uses radio-labeled B_{12} to demonstrate inadequate absorption and urinary excretion of cobalamine, and anti-IF (60% of patients) or antiparietal cell (90% of patients) antibodies.

3.1.4. TREATMENT

There is no treatment directed at reducing the auto-antibody production. Once the diagnosis of PA is established, replacement therapy with monthly parenteral B_{12} or oral daily doses of B_{12} leads to rapid correction of symptoms (2,5,6). Prognosis is excellent, although established neurological symptoms may remain. Continuous evaluation and monitoring are necessary because of the increased prevalence of gastric polyps and possibility of gastric carcinoma in later years (7).

3.1.5. ORAL HEALTH AND NUTRITION COMPLICATIONS AND MANAGEMENT

3.1.5.1. Oral Complications and Management

The oral complications of PA (glossitis, burning mouth, aphthous stomatitis) generally improve with adequate cobalamine replacement. If burning persists and significantly impacts quality of life, adjuvant analgesic medications for neuropathic pain (low doses of tricyclic antidepressants and/or clonazepam) provide relief in the majority of patients. Periodic aphthous ulcerations can be managed by early and brief treatment with moderate to potent topical steroid ointments such as clobetesol or triamcinalone; patients with frequent or persistent lesions should be referred to a dentist oral medicine specialist for additional care.

3.1.5.2. Nutritional Management

MNT for the management of PA, like other diseases or disorders, begins with a comprehensive nutrition assessment (refer to Chapter 17 for a more detailed discussion) by an RD. Although the dentist may detect oral nutrition manifestations and difficulties eating, the level of nutrition intervention required for such individuals should be provided only by an RD. The dentist should provide baseline education relative to management of eating difficulties (*see* Appendix E) and refer patients to an RD.

Nutrition assessment of such individuals includes a thorough diet history including the use of any dietary supplements or special diets that may impact vitamin B_{12} absorption, metabolism, or excretion as well as overall nutrition and GI status. Signs and symptoms of oral dysfunction should be explored for impact on oral function (biting, chewing, and swallowing). Other concurrent diseases or surgical histories (e.g., gastrectomy) that may affect B_{12} status should also be explored. A clinical and physical assessment of nutrition status should be completed to determine overall nutritional well-being. Energy and nutrient needs should be based on goals for weight (gain, loss, and maintenance), prior intake, and estimated needs in light of current therapies. Use of dietary supplements and other forms of complementary and alternative medicine by individuals with autoimmune diseases is common and should be questioned in detail (*see* Chapter 9). Select supplements can impact oral health and function as well as interact with medications to affect nutritional well-being. Individuals should be cautioned against the use of any supplements that can affect vitamin B nutriture and immune function.

The tables at the end of this chapter and the diet education materials in Appendix E provide detailed instructions on diet management of oral sequellae. Nutritional management should be planned concurrently with the treating physician to complement pharmacologic therapies. Diet management must address oral dysfunction, side effects of any medications, concurrent diseases, and cultural and personal preferences. Constant monitoring by an RD is necessary to achieve goals. Oral function, appetite, side effects of medications, clinical parameters, level of fatigue, nutrient intake (via computerized assessment of energy and nutrient intake), and weight should be monitored regularly by the RD. The dentist in practice should monitor patient weights; question patients regarding oral function, appetite, and intake; and refer accordingly to an RD.

3.2. Pemphigus Vulgaris (PV)

3.2.1. Pathogenesis

PV is a mucocutaneous autoimmune bullous disease. Although there are several types of pemphigus (vulgaris, foliaceous, vegetans, and paraneoplastic), 80% of all patients with pemphigus have PV *(8,9)*. PV affects both sexes equally and is more common among Jews, particularly Ashkenazi Jews. Although rare pediatric cases have been reported, PV most commonly develops during the fourth to sixth decade of life *(8,9)*. PV is characterized by auto-antibodies directed against desmosome-associated protein antigens (desmoglein 3 in 100% of cases, desmoglein 1 in 50% of cases) found in epithelial and epidermal intercellular substance *(10)*. Because the desmosome is the primary attachment mechanism between keratinocytes, the inflammatory destruction of that attachment leads epithelial separation, formation of characteristic fluid-filled bullae, and subsequent ulceration. When the epithelial attachment is compromised or destroyed, even minor mucosal trauma may result in epithelial separation (acantholysis) and bullae formation. The bullae quickly rupture, leaving a relatively nonspecific, shallow ulceration with an irregular border.

3.2.2. CLINICAL FEATURES

3.2.2.1. General Features

The typical presentation of PV is multiple, chronic, shallow mucocutaneous ulcerations, preceded by bullae, occurring most often in patients over age 40. The lesions do not heal without treatment and often develop following minor trauma (referred to as the Nikolsky sign). Althogh the oral presentation of PV is by far the most common first site of lesions, and the exclusive site for approx 25% of patients, it is not well recognized in the mouth, and, unfortunately, the oral presentation is often associated with significant diagnostic delays *(11,12)*.

3.2.2.2. Oral Features

Multiple, shallow, chronic oral mucosal ulcerations are the typical presentation of PV. Generalized desquamative gingivitis is another common presentation of oral PV, appearing as generalized gingival erosion and erythema. Other diseases to be considered in the differential diagnosis include benign mucous membrane pemphigoid and erosive lichen planus; several other disorders may be considered but are exceptionally rare. The oral component of PV is the presenting sign in 80% of patients with PV, and the exclusive site in 24% of patients *(11,12)*. Despite this predominant oral presentation, the oral presentation is not well recognized and is associated with considerable diagnostic delays *(11,12)*. Oral complications of PV include painful gingival and mucosal lesions that can prevent adequate oral hygiene and intake of food, resulting in risks for significant dental and nutritional complications, and complications related to immunosuppressant medications used in the treatment of PV (see relevant sections below).

3.2.3. DIAGNOSIS

A perilesional biopsy must be performed and submitted for both routine (hematoxylin and eosin) and direct immunofluorescent (immunoglobulin G [IgG]) stains *(8–10)*. Additionally, circulating antibodies (IgG) are detectable in 80 to 90% of patients with PV; the titer is generally correlated with the level of clinical disease *(13)* and is a useful measure of treatment effectiveness and disease activity.

3.2.4. TREATMENT

PV is a serious, chronic, incurable disease that can lead to death. The goal of treatment is elimination of lesions by reduction in auto-antibody production using systemic therapy; local treatment is of limited value with the exception of topical or injection steroid medication to manage lesions recalcitrant to therapy. First-line therapy is usually prednisone in moderate to high doses (1–2 mg/kg) *(14,15)*. Doses of prednisone can be reduced while maintaining therapeutic benefit with the use of adjuvant medications such as azathiopine, cyclophosphamide, methotrexate, and dapsone (see Table 2). Mycophenolate mofetil is a newer immunosuppressant medication with a more desirable side effect profile compared to prednisone and can be effective as first-line and adjuvant (steroid-sparing) therapy (16). In addition to clinical improvement, monitoring of circulating auto-antibody using indirect immunofluorescence is useful for assessing treatment response (13). With aggressive treatment, a complete resolution of lesions is common, although many patients remain on lower maintenance doses of prednisone or the adjuvant medications owing to the chronic nature of the illness.

3.2.5. ORAL HEALTH AND NUTRITION COMPLICATIONS AND MANAGEMENT

3.2.5.1. Oral Complications and Management

The oral lesions of PV can be painful. Two-thirds of patients with PV find their oral lesions more problematic than the skin lesions (11). Especially when there is a gingival component, oral hygiene can be very difficult, and patients avoid cleaning their teeth near the gingivae. As a result, plaque accumulation can lead to significant caries and gingival and periodontal disease. Adequate management of the oral lesions of PV is essential so the patient can maintain a healthy oral environment; tooth loss can be very problematic because replacement by a removable prosthesis may not be possible in the presence of a blistering mucosal disease. Recalcitrant oral lesions can be managed with injectable and potent topical steroids; referral to a dentist oral medicine specialist is indicated. The patient with oral PV should be on an aggressive health-promotion and disease-prevention plan with frequent recall and dental prophylaxis. Diet evaluation and referral to an RD are essential.

Immunosuppressant medications prescribed to treat PV increase the risk for several oral disorders: candidiasis, stomatitis, and erythema multiforme (see Table 3). Systemic antifungal therapy (fluconazole) is indicated when there is oral candidiasis (Table 4). Oral lesions that are a result of medications such as methotrexate and cyclophasphamide may require substitution with an alternative medication.

3.2.5.2. Nutritional Management

PV increases nutrition risk by virtue of the medications used to manage the disease, the oral and systemic sequellae of the disease, and the patient's quality of life. There are no specific nutrient needs associated with the disease; in contrast, nutrient needs and diet modifications are varied and individual to every patient based on the manifestations of the PV and the treatment plan. Common symptoms to look for include anorexia secondary to the associated pain, significant weight loss during acute phases of the disease process, and risk for dehydration. Dehydration is not uncommon depending on the location and extent of oral lesions; at times a percutaneuous enteral gastrostomy feeding tube is needed to provide for energy, nutrient, and fluid needs. When diet alone cannot meet energy and nutrient needs, oral supplements can be used to augment diet. Efforts to control weight loss and combat the unpleasant systemic side effects of medications should be initiated early with a referral to an RD for MNT. When steroid therapy is initiated, serum glucose and lipid values should be monitored regularly, and individuals should be evaluated for risk for or presence of osteoporosis. Initiation of calcium supplementation early (see Chapter 15) can prevent problems with osteopenia or osteoporosis.

Table 4
Oral Candidiasis Treatment Regimens

Agent	Duration	Label
Treatment for Oral Candidiasis		
Topical		
Clotrimazole troches [a]	2 wk	Dissolve 1 10 mg troche in mouth 5 times/d
Nystatin vaginal suppositories [b]	2 wk	Dissolve 1 tablet (100,000 U) in mouth 6–8 times/d
Systemic		
Fluconazole	2 wk	100 mg/d
Ketoconazole [c]	2 wk	200 mg/d
Itraconazole [d]	2 wk	200 mg/d
Treatment for Angular Cheilitis		
Antifungal Cream	2 wk	Apply to affected area 4 times/d
Clotrimazole 1%		
Miconazole 2%		
Ketoconazole 2%		
Combination Creams [e]	2 wk	Apply to affected area 3 times/d
Hydrocortisone–iodoquinol cream		
Betamethasone–dipropionate–clotrimazole cream		
Triamcinolone–nystatin cream		

[a] Use with caution because of sugar content.

[b] Although this preparation is not designed for oral use, clinicians have found it useful for the treatment of oral candidiasis when the sugar content of other topical anticandidal medications is of concern. A sugarless flavored lozenge maybe dissolved simultaneously in the mouth to mask the taste of nystatin.

[c] Must use with caution; monitor for hepatotoxicity with liver function tests.

[d] Should be used for resistant strains of *C. albicans*.

[e] Some clinicians have found combinations creams more effective than antifungal medications alone in the treatment of angular cheilitis. These include combination preparations of topical hydrocortisone, antifungal agents, and hydrocortisone–iodoquinol cream, which combines an antifungal–antibacterial agent with an anti-inflammatory antipruritic.

Nutrition screening and assessment guidelines for dental and dietetics professionals are detailed in Chapter 17. Specific diet guidelines for xerostomia and oral dysfunction are provided in Appendix E. In the diet management of PV, topical anesthetics immediately prior to mealtime and use of a straw may help facilitate eating. Frequent and coordinated follow-up by the RD, dentist, and physician is critical to the management of patients with PV and other autoimmune diseases.

3.3. Benign Mucous Membrane Pemphigoid

3.3.1. PATHOGENESIS

BMMP, like PV, is an autoimmune disorder with auto-antibodies directed against the epithelium *(8,14,15)*. However, BMMP is limited to the mucosa, with the target antigen (bullous pemphigoid antigen) being found at the basement membrane zone, where the inflammation results in a separation from the underlying connective tissue, bullae formation, and then nonspecific ulceration. BMMP does not generally involve the skin surfaces, that variant of pemphigoid being termed bullous pemphigoid *(16)*. The clinical presentation is similar to that of a patient with PV: multiple, chronic oral ulcerations preceded by bullae. Only a biopsy with routine and direct immunofluorescence staining can definitively distinguish between the two disorders.

3.3.2. Clinical Features

3.3.2.1. General Features

The presentation of BMMP is nearly identical to that of PV, with the exception that it does not involve skin surfaces. However, it can involve extraoral mucosal surfaces such as the genital mucosa, conjunctivae, esophagus, and airway. Nikolsky sign (bulla and blister formation following minor trauma) occurs in BMMP, although not as reliably as in PV. Unlike PV, healing of BMMP lesions is often associated with cicatrix, or scar, formation, and a synonymous term for BMMP is cicatricial pemphigoid. The scars can be significant, leading to oral, pharyngeal, and esophageal strictures that limit motility and function. BMMP is a chronic, incurable disease that can be controlled with systemic, and at times local, potent anti-inflammatory medications.

3.3.2.2. Oral Features

Oral findings in BMMP include multiple, shallow, chronic ulcers that are preceded by bullae. Generalized desquamative gingivitis is a common presentation of BMMP. Cicatrix formation can limit oral opening and flexibility of oral mucosa. Differential diagnosis includes PV and erosive lichen planus. The oral cavity is the predominant site of BMMP. Oral complications of PV include painful gingival and mucosal lesions that can prevent adequate oral hygiene and intake of food, resulting in risks for significant dental and nutritional complications, and complications related to immunosuppressant medications used in the treatment of PV (*see* relevant subheadings below).

3.3.3. Diagnosis

Like PV, a definitive diagnosis of BMMP requires a perilesional biopsy and subsequent routine and DIF staining to confirm the presence of subepithelial antibody.

3.3.4. Treatment

Although prednisone is often a drug of first choice to rapidly control the disease, it is not typically used in large doses for prolonged periods (8,14,15). Dapsone, in addition to its antileprosy properties, is also very effective in controlling BMMP and has a more desirable side-effect profile than prednisone (17,18). It is important to determine whether the patient has a G6PD deficiency because these patients are at much greater risk for dapsone-induced hemolysis and methemoglobinemia. Adjuvant medications listed in Table 3 are helpful in refractory disease. Finally, BMMP is more responsive than PV to local treatment using potent topical (clobetesol, halbetesol) or injectable steroid medications.

3.3.5. Oral Health and Nutrition Complications and Management

3.3.5.1. Oral Complications and Management

The oral BMMP can be painful and can make it very difficult for patients to adequately clean their teeth near the gingivae. As a result, plaque accumulation can lead to significant caries and gingival and periodontal disease. Adequate management of the oral lesions of BMMP is essential so the patient can maintain a healthy oral environment; tooth loss can be very problematic because replacement by a removable prosthesis may not be possible in the presence of a blistering mucosal disease. Recalcitrant oral lesions can be managed with injectable and potent topical steroids, and referral to a dentist oral medicine specialist is indicated. The patient with BMMP should be on an aggressive heath-promotion and disease-prevention plan with frequent recall and dental prophylaxis. Diet evaluation and referral to an RD are essential when there is evidence that food choices are limited or inadequate.

Immunosuppressant medications prescribed to treat BMMP increase the risk for several oral disorders: candidiasis, stomatitis, and erythema multiforme (*see* Table 3). Systemic antifungal therapy (fluconazole) is indicated when there is oral candidiasis (Table 4). Oral lesions that are a result of medications such as methotrexate and cyclophasphamide may require substitution with an alternative medication.

3.3.5.2. Nutritional Management

Nutrition management is similar to that described for PV. Although guidelines for diet management are provided, it is important to recognize that the elevated energy and nutrient needs are challenged by compromised ability to consume adequate nutrition, pain, and altered quality of life. An RD should be consulted early for nutrition intervention. When diet alone cannot meet energy and nutrient needs, oral supplements will be used to augment diet. Likewise, when seeing patients with BMMP, it is incumbent on the RD to integrate oral hygiene instruction into counseling strategies and communicate regularly with the physician and dentist.

4. NON-ORGAN-SPECIFIC AUTOIMMUNE DISORDERS

4.1. Systemic Lupus Erythematosus

4.1.1. PATHOGENESIS

SLE is an autoimmune disease that affects multiple organ systems. Approximately 90% of patients are female, generally of childbearing age. Multiple auto-antibodies are found, the only disease-specific auto-antibody being anti-Sm, a small protein associated with RNA; antibody to double-stranded DNA is also highly suggestive *(19,20)*. The principal tissue damage in SLE comes from the deposition of immune complexes and small vessel vasculitis in multiple organs: heart, lungs, kidneys, joints, skin, nervous system, and GI tract. The manifestations of the disease depend on the organ system affected, and presentation can vary widely for the same reason.

4.1.2. CLINICAL FEATURES

4.1.2.1. General Features

Any young women presenting with multiorgan system symptoms should be evaluated for SLE. The clinical manifestations of SLE vary widely depending on the organ system affected. The more commonly encountered problems are briefly described here. The symptoms have periods of exacerbation and remission, and a patient may have periods of relatively inactive disease followed by a lupus "flare."

Arthralgia and myaglia are common and intense. Typical malar ("butterfly") rash is a fixed, erythematous rash over the nose and extending as far as the chin and ears. The rash is photosensitive, and damaging exposure to sun can also result in a generalized maculopapular rash. Immune complexes deposited in the glomeruli result in glomerulonephritis in about 50% of patients and can be rapidly progressive and result in renal failure. Neural involvement can lead to impaired cognition, headache, seizures, and a variety of other nonspecific neurological symptoms. Small-vessel vasculitis can result in thrombus formation and increased clotting. Libman-Sacks vegetations involving the heart valves can increase the risk for infective endocarditis. Hemolysis leading to anemia and thrombocytopenia can be severe. Pericarditis, pleurisy, and pneumonitis are not uncommon cardiopulmonary manifestations of SLE. Nausea, diarrhea, and vague abdominal discomfort are common GI symptoms, and intestinal vasulitis is a serious event that can lead to perforation.

4.1.2.2. Oral Features

SLE affects several areas of the orofacial region: oral mucosal ulceration, glossitis, salivary gland inflammation and fibrosis (similar to SS), and inflammation of the temporomandibular joints (TMJ) *(21,22)*. Thus, the patient with SLE can experience painful oral ulcers, xerostomia, burning tongue and mouth, and arthralgia. When taking immunosuppressive medications to control SLE symptoms, the patient may additionally develop oral candidasis and mucositis.

4.1.3. DIAGNOSIS

Four of eleven findings are sufficient to establish a diagnosis of SLE: malar rash, discoid rash, photosensitivity, oral ulcers, arthritis, serositis, renal disease, neurological disease, hematologic disorder, immunologic disorder, or anti-Sm and anti-ds-DNA antibodies *(19,20)*.

4.1.4. TREATMENT

SLE is incurable, and most patients experience continuous symptoms of varying intensity along with periods of disease flares. Mild disease activity is treated symptomatically, and those patients with life-threatening manifestations (renal, cardiopulmonary) require aggressive immunosuppressive therapy primarily with prednisone and in combination with adjuvant immunosuppressant and cytotoxic medications (Table 2). Symptomatic treatment includes the judicious use of nonsteroidal anti-inflammatory drugs (NSAIDs), antimalarial agents such as hydroxychloroquine, and adjuvant analgesics for neuropathic burning pain (tricyclic antidepressants).

4.1.5. ORAL HEALTH AND NUTRITION COMPLICATIONS AND MANAGEMENT

4.1.5.1. Oral Complications and Management

The oral complications of SLE include oral ulcers, xerostomia, glossitis, and arthritis *(21)*. There is no specific treatment for these disorders, and most improve with treatment of the SLE. Xerostomia and immunosuppressants place the patient at increased risk for oral candidiasis, periodontal disease, and caries; frequent recall is important to minimize the risk. Oral candidiasis should be treated with systemic antifungal therapy (fluconazole) or topical antifungal therapy (Table 4). Dental sealants and fluoride may reduce risk for caries. Topical steroid medications (clobetesol, triamcinolone) can be beneficial for focal oral ulcerations. Oral conditions that do not respond to therapy should be managed by referral to a dentist oral medicine specialist. Diet evaluation and referral to a registered dietitian can reduce risk for oral disease and are essential when there are GI symptoms or evidence of disease or treatment-related malabsorption.

Approximately 20% of patients with SLE have Libman-Sacks vegetations on cardiac valves, placing them at increased risk for infective endocarditis *(23)*. The dentist should consult with the physician to determine whether such lesions exist and follow the American Heart Association recommendations for endocarditis prophylaxis. Many patients with SLE may also have a coagulopathy (platelet and clotting factor antibodies) and should have a coagulation profile prior to extensive oral surgery, including management of the bleeding, following consultation with the physician.

Finally, it is possible that dental treatment or acute dental disease could trigger a lupus flare. Although there is little to reasonably be done to avoid this, patient education about the possibility is important so there is minimal delay in responding to the flare.

4.1.5.2. Nutritional Management

The recommendations for nutrition screening and assessment in Chapter 17 apply in cases of SLE as well. However, given its systemic nature, SLE can affect the GI tract from entry to exit. The manifestations of the disease, organ systems and joints affected, and presentation as well as the management of the disease all impact nutrition and diet needs and goals. Any individual presenting with SLE should receive MNT from an RD, including a comprehensive nutrition assessment from the outset. The RD will assess functional (oral motor, cranial nerve, integrity of the oral cavity), anthropometric (height, weight, body mass index, percent body fat), clinical (signs and symptoms of nutrient deficiencies), and biochemical parameters (serum albumin, prealbumin, glucose, and cholesterol as well as liver, renal, and immune function tests) parameters, and determine nutrient needs and route(s) of feeding. When diet alone cannot meet energy and nutrient needs, oral supplements will be used to augment diet. If needed, a tube feeding may be used for short- or long-term maintenance of nutritional well-being.

4.2. Rheumatoid Arthritis

4.2.1. PATHOGENESIS

RA is an autoimmune disease affecting multiple organ systems, although the principal characteristic is persistent inflammatory synovitis. The synovitis and subsequent joint pain and destruction can vary widely among patients. The disease affects women three times more frequently than men, and the majority of patients are in the fourth or fifth decades at the time of diagnosis (24). Although auto-antibodies are detected in the majority of patients with RA (about 50% antinuclear antibody and 80% rheumatoid factor), not all patients will demonstrate auto-antibodies. Although it is unknown what events initiate the inflammatory response, the hallmark synovial inflammation is characterized by infiltration of T-lymphocytes, macrophages, and fibroblasts (25).

4.2.2. CLINICAL FEATURES

4.2.2.1. General Features

The onset of painful peripheral joints in a symmetric fashion is the usual presentation of RA, often accompanied by nonspecific weakness and fatigue. Peripheral joint stiffness and swelling develop over time. The disease occurs more frequently in women than men, and generally between the ages of 35 and 50. The disease can be progressive and debilitating, leading to joint fibrosis and ankylosis.

4.2.2.2. Oral Features

Although oral signs of RA are not common, they do occur, and certainly there can be oral complications to RA treatment. Approximately 50% of patients with RA will have involvement of the TMJ determined by a variety of imaging techniques. However, probably less than half this number develop symptoms such as jaw stiffness, TMJ pain, and limited range of motion. Certainly, a small number of patients have aggressive and progressive destruction of the TMJ, leading to fibrosis, anklyosis, and anterior open bite because of condylar destruction. When SS occurs with RA (not uncommon), xerostomia can increase the risk for caries and periodontal disease. There is one report that suggests that alveolar bone loss may be a complication of RA independent of xerostomia (26).

4.2.3. DIAGNOSIS

The diagnosis of RA requires the presence of at least four out of seven criteria: morning stiffness, arthritis of three or more joints, arthritis of the hand joints, symmetric arthritis, rheumatoid nodules, serum rheumatoid factor, or radiographic changes consistent with RA (27,28). As discussed in the pathogenesis section, auto-antibodies are not found in all patients with RA (Table 1).

4.2.4. TREATMENT

The objectives of RA treatment are relief of pain, reduction of inflammation, protection of articular structures, maintenance of function, and control of systemic involvement. There is no cure for RA. Physical therapy is a major component of RA to minimize pain and maximize function. Medical management of RA generally first utilizes NSAIDs, although there is increasing evidence that low-dose glucocorticoids provide good disease control with minimal side effects (29,30). Intra-articular injection of anti-inflammatory medications is common. A class of medications referred to as disease-modifying anti-rheumatic drugs is used for patients not responding to other RA medications (Table 2) (31).

4.2.5. ORAL HEALTH AND NUTRITION COMPLICATIONS AND MANAGEMENT

4.2.5.1. Oral Complications and Management

If signs of TMJ involvement are found (condylar erosion, pain, limited opening), consultation with the physician and an oral medicine specialist is useful for considering medication adjustment or intra-articular injection; in rare instances, advanced TMJ destruction may require total joint replacement. When manual dexterity of the hands is affected, the patient's ability to clean the teeth can be significantly impaired. Individual assessment to identify strategies to improve the ability to clean the teeth is essential and includes customized toothbrush holders and irrigation and other devices to allow periodontal hygiene (i.e., floss holder). If xerostomia is present, caries prevention should include diet counseling, fluoride, and sealants where appropriate. If immunosuppressant medications are prescribed, there is increased risk for oral candidiasis and/or stomatitis (seen with some cytotoxic medications; see Table 3). Candidiasis treatment recommendations are summarized in Table 4. Severe TMJ ankylosis and/or destruction can significantly affect the ability to eat. Referral to an RD is essential to evaluate and manage nutritional deficiency.

4.2.5.2. Nutritional Management

Nutrition management of RA is similar to that cited for other autoimmune diseases, particularly SLE. However, the side effects of medications used to treat the disease may have severe side effects on appetite and intake, causing a significant impact on nutritional well-being. Diet management focuses on level of oral and joint function, dexterity, and range of motion of the head, arms, and hands. Nutrient and energy needs vary with the initial status of the individual, the organ systems affected, and the pharmacologic management of the patient. Early intervention is critical to successful management. The reader is referred to the other sections of this chapter and the Appendix for diet education materials and management strategies. Frequent follow-up is important as changes in medications and exacerbations of disease may impact diet and subsequently nutrition status.

4.3. Sjögren's Syndrome

4.3.1. PATHOGENESIS

SS is a chronic, multiorgan system autoimmune disease that affects most dramatically the exocrine lacrimal and salivary glands, resulting in profoundly dry eyes and mouth. It occurs in women about nine times more frequently than men, and most commonly begins between the ages of 30 and 40. It may occur alone (primary SS) or frequently in combination with another autoimmune or connective tissue disease (secondary SS) *(32,33)*. Auto-antibodies to Ro/SS-A and La/SS-B antigens are common and relatively disease specific but not necessary; ANA is very common but not disease specific (Table 1) *(34)*. The disease is characterized by a multifocal lymphocytic infiltration of the salivary and lacrimal glands, leading to acinar atrophy and parenchymal fibrosis; patients are left with decreased tear and saliva production. Extraglandular involvement also occurs primarily because of immune complex vasculitis. A small number of patients with auto-antibodies and multiorgan system manifestations are at risk for developing lymphoma *(35)*.

4.3.2. CLINICAL FEATURES

4.3.2.1. General Features

Symptoms of dry eyes and dry mouth are gradual in onset and slowly progressive. Eye irritability and photosensitivity are common eye complaints. Inability to swallow food or the need to wash it down with fluids is a common oral complaint. Some patients develop enlarged parotid salivary glands. The symptoms can become profound and lead to corneal injury, rampant caries and other oral diseases, and affect oral intake of nutrients.

4.3.2.2. Oral Features

Oral features of SS include diminished saliva pooling and dry oral mucosa. Smooth surface caries, dental erosion, candidiasis, and mucosal irritation or injury occur when the mouth is dry.

4.3.3. DIAGNOSIS

Diagnostic criteria for SS have been the subject of considerable debate, with as many as five varying criteria sets *(36–38)*. Most practitioners agree that there must exist evidence of decreased gland function, auto-antibodies, and a minor salivary gland biopsy demonstrating multifocal lymphocytic infiltration. Some have recommended diagnostic criteria based only on symptoms, although this is not widely accepted.

4.3.4. Treatment

There is no cure for SS, and treatment focuses largely on minimizing the symptoms. Artificial tears help protect the eyes. Saliva substitutes are available but are not easy to use or particularly effective. When there is evidence of remaining gland function, sialagogue medications (pilocarpine, cevimeline) can be very effective in producing more saliva. Steroid and NSAIDs have not shown any benefit in saliva or tear production.

4.3.5. Oral Health and Nutrition Complications and Management

4.3.5.1. Oral Complications and Management

The oral complications of SS can be serious and can dramatically affect quality of life *(39)*. Xerostomia leading to rampant caries can be very difficult to treat and result in infection, pain, loss of teeth, and inability to chew properly. Removable prostheses are not tolerated because of the dry mucosa, irritation, and lack of retention. Candidiasis can occur because of xerostomia (*see* Table 4 for treatment). Every effort should be made to prevent disease and promote health. Fluoride and frequent evaluation are essential. Diet evaluation and referral to an RD are critical elements of comprehensive care to minimize caries risk and optimize nutritional value of foods when eating ability is impaired.

4.3.5.2. Nutritional Management

Nutrition management of the patient with SS is challenged by insufficient or total lack of saliva, which serves to moisten food and facilitate mastication of foods, movement of foods in the oral cavity, and swallowing. Depending on the degree of salivary function remaining, eating ability is compromised. Dietary guidelines for xerostomia are provided in Appendix E. Patients should be instructed to always carry a water bottle, drink fluids with meals, increase fluidity of mealtime foods (gravies, sauces, soups), and avoid "coarse" foods that may irritate the mucosa such as hard bread crusts. Temperate foods with spices and seasonings adjusted to fit individual tolerances should be promoted. Small frequent meals are often preferable as eating time may be prolonged. When patients complain of altered taste, simple taste testing in the office to determine tolerable tastes (sweet, salt, bitter, sour) can be done, and those tastes that are better tolerated can be emphasized. If dairy products are not tolerated, alternative calcium sources should be identified or a calcium supplement should be recommended.

5. SUMMARY

Patients with autoimmune disorders present significant challenges to oral and nutritional health. Both the disease itself and its medical management can have profound impact on oral health and nutrition status, biting, chewing and swallowing ability, diet, and quality of life. Optimal patient management requires coordination and collaboration between medical, dental, and nutrition health care providers to minimize risk for disease, manage active disease, and improve quality of life.

Guidelines for Practice

	Nutrition and Diet	Oral Health
Assessment	• Comprehensive nutrition assessment of diet and supplement intake, anthropometrics (height, weight, body mass index), biochemical profile, clinical assessment. • Individualized diet based on symptoms, degree of oral compromise, other sequellae and chronic diseases. • Screen for osteoporosis risk. • As-needed multivitamin and mineral supplements. • Referral to physician and/or dentist as needed.	• Physical examination • Mucosal • Teeth • Periodontium • Saliva quantity and quality • Symptoms • Pain • Dry mouth • Oral burning • Impaired chewing
Prevention	• Frequent monitoring of above assessment parameters. • Referral to physician and/or dentist as needed.	• Frequent recall and dental prophylaxis. • Sialagogues, prescription fluoride, sealants for patients with xerostomia. • Modified techniques for improved oral hygiene. • Antibiotic prophylaxis based on immune status or cardiac risk. • Medical consult regarding health status and management strategies. • Referral to RD. • Avoid situations that may precipitate disease flare-up.
Intervention	• Frequent monitoring of above assessment parameters. • Referral to physician and/or dentist as needed. • Modify diet according to symptoms, changes in nutritional status, and oral pain and dysfunction. • Monitor drug–nutrient reactions or sequallae of drugs on diet and nutrition status, and adjust diet accordingly.	• Frequent recall and dental prophylaxis. • Sialagogues, prescription fluoride, sealants for patients with xerostomia. • Modified techniques for improved oral hygiene. • Medications that address specific oral components of autoimmune illness. • Referral to oral medicine specialist and/ or RD.

REFERENCES

1. Babior BM. The megaloblastic anemias. In Beutler E, Lichtman M, Coller B, Kipps T, Seligsohn U, eds. Williams' Hematology, 6th Ed. New York, NY: McGraw-Hill, 2000.
2. Toh BH. Pernicious anemia. N Engl J Med 1997; 337:1441–1448.
3. Carmel R. Malabsorption of cobalamin. Baillieres Clin Haematol 1995; 8:639–655.
4. Lee GR, Herbert V. Nutritional factors in the production and function of erythrocytes. In Lee GR, Foerster J, Paraskevas F, Greer JP, Rodgers GM, Lukens JN, eds. Wintrobe's Clinical Hematology. 10th Ed. Giza, Egypt: Mass Publishing, 1999, 228–266.
5. Kuzminski AM, Del Giacco EJ, Allen RH, et al. Effective treatment of cobalamin deficiency with oral cobalamin. Blood 1998; 92:1191–1196.
6. Lederle FA. Oral cobalamin for pernicious anemia: medicine's best kept secret? JAMA 1991; 265: 94–95.
7. Hsing AW. Pernicious anemia and subsequent cancer. Cancer 1993; 71:745.

8. Fine JD. Management of acquired bullous skin diseases. N Eng J Med 1995; 333:1475–1484.

9. Korman NJ. Pemphigus. J Am Acad Dermatol 1988; 18:1219–1238.

10. Eversole LR. Immunopathology of oral mucosal ulcerative, desquamative, and bullous disease. Oral Surg Oral Med Oral Pathol 1994; 77:555–571.

11. Sirois DA, Fatahzadeh M, Roth R, Ettlin D. Diagnostic patterns and delays in pemphigus vulgaris: experience with 99 patients. Arch Dermatol 2000;136(12):1569–1570.

12. Sirois D, Leigh JE, Sollecito TP. Oral pemphigus vulgaris preceding cutaneous lesions: recognition and diagnosis. J Am Dent Assoc 2000; 131(8):1156–1160.

13. Fitzpatrick RE, Newcomer VD. The correlation of disease activity and antibody titres in pemphigus. Arch Dermatol 1980; 116:285–290.

14. Chrysommlis F, Ioannides D, Teknetzis A, et al. Treatment of oral pemphigus vulgaris. Int J Dermatol 1994; 33:803–807.

15. Stanley JR. Therapy of pemphigus vulgaris. Arch Dermatol 1999; 135:76–77.

16. Enk AH. Mycophenolate is effective in the treatment pemphigus vulgaris. Arch Dermatol 1999; 135: 54–56.

14. Anhalt GJ. Pemphigoid: bullous and cicatricial. Dermatol Clin 1990; 8:701–712.

15. Korman NJ. Bullous pemphigoid: the latest in diagnosis, prognosis and therapy. Arch Dermatol 1998; 134:1137–1141.

16. Venning VA, Frith PA, Bron AJ, et al. Mucosal involvement in bullous and cicatricial pemphigoid: a clinical and immunopathological study. Br J Dermatol 1988; 118:7.

17. Rogers RS, Mehregan DA. Dapsone therapy of cicatricial pemphigoid. Sem Dermatol 1988; 7:201.

18. Ciarrocca KN, Greenberg MS. A retrospective study of the management of oral mucous membrane pemphigoid with dapsone. Oral Surg Oral Med Oral Pathol Oral Radiol Endod 1999; 88:159–163.

19. Boumpas DT, Fessler BJ, Austin, III HA, et al. Systemic lupus erythematosus: emerging concepts. 1. Renal, neuropsychiatric, cardiovascular, pulmonary and hematologic disease. 2. Dermatologic and joint disease, the antiphospholipid antibody syndrome, pregnancy and hormonal therapy, morbidity and mortality, and pathogenesis. Ann Intern Med 1995; 123:42, 940.

20. Arkachaisri T, Lehman TJ. Systemic lupus erythematosus and related disorders of childhood. Curr Opin Rheumatol 1999; 11:384–392.

21. De Rossi SS, Glick M. Lupus erythematosus: considerations for dentistry. J Am Dent Assoc 1998; 129:330–339.

22. Rhodus NL, Johnson DK. The prevalence of oral manifestations of systemic lupus erythematosus. Quintessence Int 1990; 21:461–465.

23. Miller CS, Egan RM, Falace DA, Rayens MK, Moore CR. Prevalence of infective endocarditis in patients with systemic lupus erythematosus. J Am Dent Assoc 1999; 130(3):387–392.

24. Michet C. Update on the epidemiology and of the rheumatic diseases. Curr Opin Rheumatol 1998; 10:129–135.

25. Lipsky PE, Davis LS. The central involvement of T cells in rheumatoid arthritis. Immunologist 1998; 6:121.

26. Kaber UR, Gleissner C, Dehne F, et al. Risk for periodontal disease in patient with longstanding rheumatoid arthritis. Arthritis Rheum 1997; 40:2248–2251.

27. Kwoh CK. American College of Rheumatology guidelines for the management of rheumatoid arthritis. Arthritis Rheum 1996; 39:713.

28. Harrison BJ. The performance of the 1987 ARA classification criteria for rheumatoid arthritis in a population-based cohort of patients with early inflammatory polyarthritis. J Rheumatol 1998; 25:2324.

29. Wolfe F, Hawley D. The long-term outcomes of rheumatoid arthritis: a prospective 18-year study of 823 patients. J Rheumatol 1998; 25:2108.

30. Abu-Shakra M. Clinical and radiographic outcomes of rheumatoid arthritis patients not treated with disease-modifying drugs. Arthritis Rheum 1998; 41:1190.

31. Rau R. Long-term combination therapy of refractory and destructive rheumatoid arthritis with methotrexate (MTX) and intramuscular gold or other disease-modifying antirheumatic drugs compared to MTX monotherapy. J Rheumatol 1998; 25:1485.

32. Tzioufas AG, Moutopoulos HM. Sjögren's syndrome. In JH Klippel, PA Dieppe eds. Rheumatology. London, UK: Mosby, 1998.

33. Fox RI, Kang HI. Pathogenesis of Sjögren's syndrome. Rheum Dis Clin North Am 1992; 18:517–538.
34. Fox RI, Howell FV, Bone RC, Michelson P. Primary Sjögren's syndrome and immunologic features. Sem Arthritis Rheum 1984; 14:77–105.
35. Kassan SS, Thomas TL, Moutosopoulos HM, et al. Increased risk of lymphoma in sicca syndrome. Ann Intern Med 1978; 89:888–892.
36. Fox RI, Saito I. Criteria for diagnosis of Sjögren's syndrome. Rheum Dis Clin North Am 1994; 20(2): 391–407.
37. Vitali C, Moutsopoulos HM, Bombardieri S, for the The European Community Study Group on diagnostic criteria for Sjögren's syndrome. Sensitivity and specificity of tests for ocular and oral involvement in Sjögren's syndrome. Ann Rheum Dis 1994; 53:637–647.
38. Fox R. Classification criteria for Sjögren's syndrome. Rheum Dis Clin North Am 1994; 20:391–407.
39. Atkinson JC. Sjögren's syndrome: oral and dental considerations. J Am Dent Assoc 1993; 124:74–86.

15 Osteoporosis

Elizabeth A. Krall

1. INTRODUCTION

Tooth loss and periodontal diseases become more prevalent with advancing age and result from the interaction of many factors, including local oral conditions, poor hygiene practices, lack of access to dental care, genetics, and systemic diseases. Osteoporosis is characterized by a decline in bone density and quality that predisposes to fracture and is one of several systemic diseases that has been hypothesized to increase the risks of periodontal disease and tooth loss *(1)*. Although the number of studies of these associations continues to grow as precise methods to measure both oral and systemic bone mineral density are developed, a physiological mechanism for the associations between osteoporosis and these oral conditions has yet to be clearly identified. The majority of human studies to date have not been able to distinguish between causation and mere association.

2. BONE LOSS IN ADULTS

Skeletal tissue exists in a dynamic state. Bone mineral at discrete sites throughout the skeleton is continuously being broken down (resorbed) by the osteoclasts and reformed by osteoblasts in a series of coordinated, or coupled, actions. The resorptive phase of this remodeling process is estimated to last 10 d, while replacement of lost bone continues for approx 3–4 mo *(2)*. In young, healthy adults, the two phases are balanced so that the amount of bone mineral remains fairly constant. In middle-aged and older adults and in disease states such as osteoporosis, the phases tend to be uncoupled and dominated by resorption. The result is a net loss of bone mineral over time.

The decline in bone mineral content and the structural deterioration in osteoporosis are evident microscopically. The compact cortical layer that forms the exterior shell becomes thin, and the normally dense network of calcified trabeculae in the bone interior also becomes thin and disconnected. On appearance, the bone is abnormally porous, which gives the disease its name. These changes result in bone that is fragile and susceptible to fracture even with a low amount of trauma.

This loss of mineral can be measured by dual or single x-ray absorptiometry to determine a person's bone mineral density (BMD) at specific skeletal sites. BMD is compared

From: *Nutrition and Oral Medicine*
Edited by: R. Touger-Decker, D. A. Sirois, and C. C. Mobley © Humana Press Inc., Totowa, NJ

Table 1
Common Risk Factors for Primary and Secondary Osteoporosis

Primary osteoporosis

- Advanced age
- Female sex
- Postmenopause
- White or Asian ethnicity
- Family history of osteoporosis or low-trauma fracture
- Low body weight
- Low dietary intakes of calcium and vitamin D
- Low physical activity level
- Cigarette smoking

Secondary osteoporosis

- Hypogonadism (male and female)
- Use of glucocorticoid or anticonvulsant medication
- Excess thyroid hormone
- Alcoholism

to values for a healthy, young, gender-specific reference population. The risk of fracture doubles for each 1 standard deviation increment below the reference value. The World Health Organization defines osteoporosis in women as BMD that is more than 2.5 standard deviations below the average value for a young healthy female, and osteopenia as BMD between 1 and 2.5 standard deviations below average *(3)*.

3. EPIDEMIOLOGY OF OSTEOPOROSIS

In the United States, it is estimated that at least 8 million women and 2 million men have osteoporosis, and another 34 million individuals have osteopenia *(4)*. After age 50, the lifetime risk of any fracture of the hip, spine, or distal forearm is nearly 40% for white women and 13% for white males *(5)*. Age and gender are two important risk factors for osteoporosis. A woman's risk is higher because on average, she will generally have achieved a lower peak bone mass as a young adult than a man, and her bone loss is accelerated during the 5 to 10 yr surrounding the menopause. A number of medical conditions and medications may also result in osteoporosis as a secondary outcome. Risk factors for primary and secondary osteoporosis are shown in Table 1. Known risk factors for periodontal disease also include age, smoking, race, socioeconomic status, diabetes, and genetic susceptibility *(6)*. Although osteoporosis and periodontal disease share some risk factors (age, smoking, and ethnicity), the relationships are not entirely consistent in both diseases. The prevalence of periodontal disease is greater with age and cigarette use, but lower in whites than in blacks *(6)*, whereas age, cigarette smoking, and white ethnicity all increase the risk of osteoporosis.

4. EFFECTS OF OSTEOPENIA
AND OSTEOPOROSIS ON THE ORAL CAVITY

Periodontal disease and tooth loss become more prevalent with increased age *(7,8)*, so it may be expected that a large proportion of the elderly population will exhibit these oral conditions concurrently with signs of osteoporosis or osteopenia. However, many epidemiologic studies find that individuals with poor bone status at systemic skeletal sites tend to have more oral bone loss, periodontal disease, and tooth loss than similarly aged individuals with good skeletal bone status *(1,9–14)*, which suggests that the relationship is more than coincidental. Other studies report no associations *(15–18)*. Each study has limitations. The strength of the evidence must be evaluated in the context of subject selection, sample size, and study design.

Given the complex causes of oral and systemic bone loss, associations between the two are likely to be moderate or weak, and large sample sizes are needed to ensure adequate statistical power. Randomized clinical trials offer the best evidence for a causal relationship, but none are available to date. The next best level of evidence consists of prospective studies that simultaneously follow changes in systemic bone and oral status over time. Finally, cross-sectional studies offer weak evidence for or against a causal relationship. Findings should be controlled for potential confounders such as age or years since menopause, smoking status, and hormone replacement status. The current state of the knowledge is such that most of the human studies of associations between systemic bone status and oral outcomes are cross-sectional and do not always control for multiple confounders. The prospective studies and more comprehensive cross-sectional studies are described in more detail below.

4.1. Periodontal Diseases: Alveolar Bone Loss

Periodontal disease involves the destruction of alveolar bone tissue by bacteria-induced inflammation. Although bacteria are necessary to initiate and continue the inflammatory response, osteopenia and osteoporosis might act as host characteristics that influence the initial bone quantity and quality. Few studies have included direct measurements of oral bone loss. Payne et al. *(9)* assessed changes in alveolar bone height over a period of 2 yr in 17 postmenopausal women with osteoporosis at the spine and 21 women with normal BMD. The osteoporotic women exhibited significantly more sites with alveolar bone loss than women with normal spine BMD. Moderate correlations between alveolar bone height and BMD of the hip, spine, and forearm have been reported in several small cross-sectional studies of women comprising a wide age range *(1,19–22)*. In contrast, Elders et al. (15) reported no association between spine BMD and loss of alveolar bone height on molars and premolars in healthy women between the ages of 46 and 55. Subjects in this latter study were all early postmenopausal with good periodontal health on average.

4.2. Clinical Measures of Periodontal Disease

Other studies *(10,15–17)* examined the relationship of systemic bone status to clinical measures of periodontal disease such as clinical attachment loss (CAL) and periodontal pocket depth (PPD). In a cross-sectional analysis of data from 11,655 participants in the third National Health and Nutrition Examination Survey (NHANES III), BMD of the total femur was associated with average CAL values and percent of sites with moderate to severe CAL in women *(10)*. The association appeared to depend on the level of calculus such that women with very high or extremely high calculus index scores had up to 2.5 times as many sites with CAL greater than 7 mm as women with comparable calculus but normal BMD. Similar trends were seen in men. Others found only weak or no associations between BMD and probing pocket depth or CAL *(15,16)*. CAL and PPD values were higher in women with low BMD at multiple sites in a study of elderly women, but the magnitude of the relationships was reduced when controlled for age, smoking, and number of teeth *(16)*. One group *(17)* reported an opposite relationship: scores of the Community Periodontal Index of Treatment Needs were higher among women with higher BMD, but these data were not adjusted for potential confounders. The findings from these studies do not offer strong support for an association between BMD and clinical periodontal indices.

4.3. Tooth Loss

The most consistent studies in support of a positive association are prospective and large cross-sectional studies of elderly subjects in which tooth loss is the dependent variable. In a prospective observational study of postmenopausal women, rates of bone loss at the hip, spine, and total body over a 7-yr period were higher in women who concurrently lost teeth than in women who retained teeth *(11)*. In women who lost teeth during that period, bone loss was three times faster at the hip and total body than in women who lost no teeth. The risk of tooth loss increased by at least 50% for each 1% per year increment in the rate of systemic bone loss. However, there was no information on other oral factors, such as caries burden, that cause tooth loss.

May et al. *(12)* reported that self-reported number of teeth remaining correlated with BMD of the hip and spine in more than 1400 men and women aged 65 and older. Average BMDs among edentate men were 5 to 9% lower than fully dentate men when adjusted for body mass index (BMI), age, and smoking status. A similar trend of smaller magnitude was seen in women, but the difference was not statistically significant. Krall et al. *(13)* reported significant correlations between number of teeth retained and BMD of the forearm, spine, and hip in a group of 329 postmenopausal women after having controlled for BMI, menopausal age, and smoking status. Daniell *(14)* studied 208 women aged 60–69 yr and found that those with low cortical bone area of the metacarpals were more likely to have become edentate after the start of menopause, a trend that was most striking in nonsmokers.

In contrast, Weyant et al. *(16)* saw no association between BMD at four skeletal sites and number of teeth remaining in a group of 292 elderly women using multivariate analyses. Two studies of early postmenopausal women also reported no associations of teeth remaining with spine *(15,18)* or hip BMD *(18)*.

4.4. Alveolar Bone Height in Edentate and Partially Dentate Subjects

Erosion of alveolar bone after tooth extraction is common and may cause denture fit to worsen over time. Findings from several *(22–25)* studies generally suggest a correlation between remaining bone height in the mandible and BMD at systemic sites, but not all studies agree *(26)*, and the strength of the relationship may not be consistent in all regions of the jawbone *(24)*. More studies are needed to determine how other factors such as age, mastication forces, and length of time since tooth extraction affect the relationship.

5. EFFECTS OF OSTEOPOROSIS PREVENTION AND TREATMENT STRATEGIES ON THE ORAL CAVITY

5.1. Medications for the Treatment of Osteoporosis

Approved treatments for osteoporosis include hormone replacement therapy (HRT), the hormone calcitonin, and antiresorptive medications. The *bis*-phosphonate class of antiresorptive medication has been shown to prevent alveolar bone resorption and preserve mandibular bone mass in animals *(27)*. In humans, the therapy that has been studied most extensively is HRT, either estrogen alone or a combination of estrogen and progestin. Three large population-based studies of postmenopausal women found that women who have ever used HRT retain more teeth than nonusers and have a lower likelihood of being edentate *(28–30)* independent of age, smoking, and other factors. Duration of use was also related to tooth retention. For each 4-yr increment in the duration of HRT use, the number of teeth retained increased by one and the risk of edentulism decreased by about 25% *(28,29)*. Payne, Reinhardt, and colleagues reported that estrogen sufficiency is associated with preservation of alveolar bone density and less frequent CAL *(9,31–33)*. HRT appears to also have beneficial effects on soft periodontal tissues, since it is associated with less bleeding on probing *(33,34)*.

5.2. Nutritional Approaches to Osteoporosis

5.2.1. CALCIUM AND VITAMIN D

A randomized, controlled trial in children demonstrated that increasing intake of calcium from an average of about 900 mg/d to 1600 mg/d enhanced the rate of increase in bone density during growth *(35)*. Several placebo-controlled studies in older adults of calcium and vitamin D supplements showed that higher intakes of these nutrients slow the rate of bone mineral loss *(36–38)* and reduce the risk of fracture *(39)*. The usual dietary intakes of calcium and vitamin D among subjects in these studies generally were below 800 mg and 200 IU/d, respectively, and the content of the supplements ranged from 500 to 1200 mg of calcium *(36,39)* and 200 to 800 IU of vitamin D *(38,39)*. Osteoporosis-like changes in oral bone of animals can be prevented by a diet containing an adequate amount of calcium *(40–42)*, but clinical signs of periodontal disease are not affected. A 1-yr controlled trial of calcium supplementation in humans did not find a difference in periodontal disease indices between the calcium and placebo groups *(43)*, but it is possible that a longer follow-up time is needed to observe an effect.

A prospective analysis in 552 older men suggested that higher calcium intake levels may be beneficial in slowing alveolar bone loss *(44)*. Progression of alveolar bone loss at each tooth was defined as a change from minimal bone loss (80% or more of alveolar bone remaining around the tooth) to bone loss (less than 80% of bone remaining), and the total number of teeth with progression was computed for each participant. Men whose calcium intakes were above 1000 mg/d had fewer teeth exhibiting progression of alveolar bone loss over an average 4-yr follow-up period (2.0 ± 2.5 teeth) compared to men with calcium intakes below this level (2.6 ± 2.0 teeth, $p = 0.04$), controlling for age, initial number of teeth, smoking status, vitamin D intake, caries status, and clinical periodontal disease status.

Nishida et al. *(45)* analyzed dietary intake surveys and periodontal data in more than 12,000 adults from NHANES III. After controlling for age and smoking status, there was

Table 2
Adult Dietary Reference Intake Values of Calcium
and Vitamin D in the United States *(49)*

Age	Calcium (mg/d)	Vitamin D (IU [μg]/d)	
0–6 mo	210	200	[5]
6–12 mo	270	200	[5]
1–3 yr	500	200	[5]
4–8 yr	800	200	[5]
9–13 yr	1300	200	[5]
14–18 yr	1300	200	[5]
19–30 yr	1000	200	[5]
31–50 yr	1000	200	[5]
51–70 yr	1200	400	[10]
70 yr and older	1200	600	[15]

an inverse association between calcium intake level (from diet only) and the odds of having periodontal disease (defined as mean periodontal attachment loss ≥1.5 mm) among younger adults. The odds were nearly double in both men and women whose calcium intake was below 800 mg/d relative to a higher intake. Although these findings support an association between low dietary calcium and increased risk of periodontal disease, the study was limited by its cross-sectional design and lack of data on calcium supplement use.

Calcium intake was associated with a reduction in the risk of tooth loss in a 5-yr study of elderly men and women *(46)*. During the first 3 yr of the study, when placebos and supplements containing 500 mg calcium and 700 IU vitamin D per day were randomly assigned, the odds of losing any teeth were reduced by more than half in the supplemented group. In a 2-yr follow-up of the same individuals, the odds of tooth loss were again about 50% lower in subjects whose total calcium intake was at least 1000 mg/d compared to those who consumed less than 1000 mg.

Calcium and vitamin D intakes have been associated with erosion of edentate regions of the alveolar ridge. In several small cross-sectional studies, subjects with low calcium or vitamin D intake tended to have more severe erosion *(22,47)*. Initiation of supplements containing 750 mg of calcium and 375 IU of vitamin D shortly after tooth extraction resulted in less alveolar bone loss 1 yr later *(48)*. Recommended intake levels for calcium and vitamin D in the United States *(49)* are shown in Table 2.

6. PROFESSIONAL AND PRACTICE ISSUES

The elderly are at increased risk of osteoporosis and osteopenia as well as tooth loss and periodontal disease. The available evidence supports the hypothesis that poor systemic bone status contributes to tooth loss and periodontal disease but is not conclusive. If such a relationship exists, the impact to an individual elderly patient is likely to be small. Good oral hygiene, professional prophylaxis, and avoidance of smoking play important roles in the preservation of alveolar bone and teeth. However, given the increasing number of elders in Western societies and the widespread presence of osteopenia and osteoporosis, instituting measures to prevent systemic bone loss could have a beneficial impact on oral health of the population as a whole. The dental practitioner can increase the patient's knowledge of risk factors, especially poor nutrition and smoking that affect both periodontal health and systemic bone health. It is important to stress good nutrition and lifestyle habits in childhood and early adulthood before the signs of osteoporosis become evident.

HRT used in the treatment and prevention of osteoporosis appears to reduce alveolar bone loss and the risk of tooth loss. Recent information on the adverse effects of estrogen-progestin combination therapy *(50)* will alter the pattern of HRT usage in the future. However, because many women have used HRT in the past, documentation of its use should be part of the patient records. Use of any osteoporosis drug should be recorded for male and female patients.

7. CONCLUSIONS AND RECOMMENDATIONS BASED ON EVIDENCE TO DATE

The existing studies generally support the hypothesis that osteoporosis and osteopenia are associated with oral health, particularly tooth loss in the elderly. However, the majority of the evidence to date comes from cross-sectional studies that cannot determine whether changes in the skeleton preceded the oral conditions or result from risk factors common to both conditions. Prospective studies are needed. Randomized clinical trials of agents for osteoporosis prevention could also provide useful information on the relationship if measurements of oral bone and teeth are integral parts of the study design. Even though the clinical relevance of the association between osteoporosis and oral health is not known, it remains prudent for dental patients to maintain good calcium and vitamin D nutrition for the benefit of systemic bone health at least, and possibly for oral health as well.

8. RESOURCES FOR THE PRACTITIONER

Knowledge of a dental patient's osteoporosis status is important, just as it is important to know whether the patient has heart disease or diabetes. But many people with osteoporosis are unaware that they have the disease. Accurate and cost-effective screening for osteoporosis requires equipment to measure bone densitometry of individuals at moderate and high risk, but that is beyond the scope of a dental or nutritional practice. However, several brief, self-administered osteoporosis risk questionnaires have been developed that can not only be employed as a first step in a multistage screening but also serve to increase osteoporosis awareness. For example, the Simple Calculated Osteoporosis Risk Estimation tool assigns scores for the presence or absence of major risk factors for osteoporosis such as age, race, underweight, estrogen therapy, rheumatoid arthritis, and previous fracture *(51)*. Total scores above a particular threshold indicate a possible increased risk for osteoporosis. Other questionnaires contain additional items such as smoking, alcohol use, and physical exercise.

It must be pointed out that although the risk assessment questionnaires by themselves have good sensitivity (individuals with osteoporosis will likely be correctly categorized as "high risk" by the questionnaires), specificity (healthy individuals are categorized as "low risk") is only moderate *(52)*, and there will be a large number of false-positives among those who complete the risk questionnaires. Dental providers and their patients need to understand that a follow-up examination with the primary care physician and a bone density scan are essential in order to make a diagnosis. Examples of osteoporosis risk questionnaires can be found at the following websites:

http://www.osteofound.org/osteoporosis/pdf/risk_test_e.pdf

http://www.askapharmacist.com/osteoform.htm

The following websites provide free information about osteoporosis: disease facts, risk factors and prevention, diagnosis, and treatments. Educational materials can also be ordered from the following organizations:

The National Osteoporosis Foundation, http://www.nof.org.

International Osteoporosis Foundation, http://www.osteofound.org

National Institutes of Health Bone Diseases Center, http://www.osteo.org

Guidelines for Practice

	Oral Health Professional	*Nutrition Professional*
Prevention	• Screen all patients for osteoporosis risk factors.	• Screen all patients for osteoporosis risk factors.
	• Refer high-risk patients to physician for evaluation.	• Refer high-risk patients to physician for evaluation.
	• Encourage calcium-rich diet and exercise.	• Encourage calcium-rich diet and exercise.
		• Review calcium-rich food sources and calcium supplements as needed.
Intervention	• Include an osteoporosis item on all medical history forms for new patients and when updating health status of current patients. Although osteoporosis is most common in postmenopausal women, approx 20% of cases of osteoporosis are older men *(4)*. Premenopausal women with a history of abnormal absence of menstrual periods can also be at increased risk *(4)*.	• Include an osteoporosis item on all medical history forms for new patients and when updating health status of current patients. Although osteoporosis is most common in postmenopausal women, approx 20% of cases of osteoporosis are older men *(4)*. Premenopausal women with a history of abnormal absence of menstrual periods can also be at increased risk *(4)*.
	• Document current and past use of osteoporosis drugs in the patient's medical and dental records. Currently approved medications include alendronate, risedronate, calcitonin, estrogen/hormone therapy, parathyroid hormone, and raloxifene.	• Document current and past use of osteoporosis drugs in the patient's medical and dental records. Currently approved medications include alendronate, risedronate, calcitonin, estrogen/hormone therapy, parathyroid hormone, and raloxifene.
	• Have a brief osteoporosis risk questionnaire available for the patient to complete or take home.	• Have a brief osteoporosis risk questionnaire available for the patient to complete or take home.
	• Encourage a balanced nutritional intake.	• Encourage a balanced nutritional intake.
	• Encourage smoking cessation.	• Encourage smoking cessation.

REFERENCES

1. Wactawski-Wende J, Grossi SG, Trevisan M, et al. The role of osteopenia in oral bone loss and periodontal disease. J Periodontol 1996; 67(Suppl.):1076–1084.
2. Mundy GR. Bone remodeling. In Favus MJ, ed. Primer on the Metabolic Bone Diseases and Disorders of Mineral Metabolism. Philadelphia, PA: Lippincott Williams & Wilkins, 1999, 30–38.
3. The WHO Study Group. Assessment of Fracture Risk and Its Application to Screening for Postmenopausal Osteoporosis. Geneva, Switzerland: World Health Organization, 1994.
4. National Osteoporosis Foundation. Fast facts on osteoporosis. Website: (http://www.nof.org/osteoporosis/stats.htm). Accessed July 31, 2003.
5. Melton LJ III, Chrischilles EA, Cooper C, Lane AW, Riggs BL. How many women have osteoporosis? J Bone Miner Res 1992; 7:1005–1010.
6. Pihlstrom BL. Periodontal risk assessment, diagnosis and treatment planning. Periodontology 2000 2001; 25:37–58.
7. Albandar JM, Brunelle JA, Kingman A. Destructive periodontal disease in adults 30 years of age and older in the United States, 1988–1994. J Periodontol 1999; 70:13–29.
8. Marcus SE, Drury TF, Brown LJ, Zion GR. Tooth retention and tooth loss in the permanent dentition of adults: United States, 1988–1991. J Dent Res 1996; 75(Spec Issue):684–695.
9. Payne JB, Reinhardt RA, Nummikoski PV, Patil KD. Longitudinal alveolar bone loss in postmenopausal osteoporotic/osteopenic women. Osteoporosis Int 1999; 10:34–40.
10. Ronderos M, Jacobs DR, Himes JH, Pihlstrom BL. Associations of periodontal disease with femoral bone mineral density and estrogen replacement therapy: cross-sectional evaluation of adults from NHANES III. J Clin Periodontol 2000; 27:778–786.
11. Krall EA, Garcia RI, Dawson-Hughes B. Increased risk of tooth loss is related to bone loss at the whole body, hip, and spine. Calc Tiss Int 1996; 9:433–437.
12. May H, Reader R, Murphy S, Khaw KT. Self-reported tooth loss and bone mineral density in older men and women. Age Ageing 1995; 24:217–221.
13. Krall EA, Dawson-Hughes B, Papas A, Garcia RI. Tooth loss and skeletal bone density in healthy postmenopausal women. Osteoporosis Int 1994; 4:104–109.
14. Daniell HW. Postmenopausal tooth loss: contributions to edentulism by osteoporosis and cigarette smoking. Arch Intern Med 1983; 143:1678–1682.
15. Elders PJ, Habets LL, Netelenbos JC, van der Linden LW, van der Stelt PF. The relation between periodontitis and systemic bone mass in women between 46 and 55 years of age. J Clin Periodontol 1992; 19:492–496.
16. Weyant RJ, Pearlstein ME, Churak AP, Forrest K, Famili P, Cauley JA. The association between osteopenia and periodontal attachment loss in older women. J Periodontol 1999; 70:982–991.
17. Klemetti E, Collin HL, Forss H, Markkanen H, Lassila V. Mineral status of skeleton and advanced periodontal disease. J Clin Periodontol 1994; 21:184–188.
18. Earnshaw SA, Keating N, Hosking DJ, et al., for the EPIC study group. Tooth counts do not predict bone mineral density in early postmenopausal Caucasian women. Int J Epidemiol 1998; 27:479–483.
19. Streckfus CF, Johnson RB, Nick T, Tsao A, Tucci M. Comparison of alveolar bone loss, alveolar bone density and second metacarpal bone density, salivary and gingival crevicular fluid interleukin-6 concentrations in healthy premenopausal and postmenopausal women on estrogen therapy. J Gerontol Series A: Biol Sci Med Sci 1997; 52:M343–M351.
20. Engel MB, Rosenberg HM, Jordan SL, Holm K. Radiological evaluation of bone status in the jaw and in the vertebral column in a group of women. Gerodontol 1994; 11:86–92.
21. Southard KA, Southard TE, Schlechte JA, Meis PA. The relationship between the density of the alveolar processes and that of post-cranial bone. J Dent Res 2000; 79:964–969.
22. Kribbs PJ, Smith DE, Chesnut CH III. Oral findings in osteoporosis. 2. Relationship between residual ridge and alveolar bone resorption and generalized skeletal osteopenia. J Prosthet Dent 1983; 50:719–724.
23. Kribbs PJ, Chesnut CH III, Ott SM, Kilcoyne RF. Relationships between mandibular and skeletal bone in an osteoporotic population. J Prosthet Dent 1989; 62:703–707.
24. Klemetti E, Vainio P. Effect of bone mineral density in skeleton and mandible on extraction of teeth and clinical alveolar height. J Prosthet Dent 1993; 70:21–25.

25. Klemetti E, Vainio P, Lassila V, Alhava E. Cortical bone mineral density in the mandible and osteoporosis status in postmenopausal women. Scand J Dent Res 1993; 101:219–223.

26. Mercier P, Inoue S. Bone density and serum minerals in cases of residual alveolar ridge atrophy. J Prosthet Dent 1981; 46:250–255.

27. Reddy MS, Weatherford TW III, Smith CA, West BD, Jeffcoat MK, Jacks TM. Alendronate treatment of naturally–occurring periodontitis in beagle dogs. J Periodontol 1995; 66:211–217.

28. Krall EA, Dawson-Hughes B, Hannan MT, Wilson PWF, Keil DP. Postmenopausal estrogen use and tooth retention. Am J Med 1997; 102:536–542.

29. Grodstein F, Colditz GA, Stampfer MJ. Post-menopausal hormone use and tooth loss: a prospective study. J Amer Dent Assoc 1996; 127:370–377.

30. Paganini-Hill A. The benefits of estrogen replacement therapy on oral health: the Leisure World cohort. Arch Intern Med 1995; 155:2325–2329.

31. Payne JB, Zachs NR, Reinhardt RA, Nummikoski PV, Patil K. The association between estrogen status and alveolar bone density changes in postmenopausal women with a history of periodontitis. J Periodontol 1997; 68:24–31.

32. Reinhardt RA, Payne JB, Maze C, Babbitt M, Nummikoski PV, Dunning D. Gingival fluid IL-1beta in postmenopausal females on supportive periodontal therapy: a longitudinal 2-year study. J Clin Periodontol 1998; 25:1029–1035.

33. Reinhardt RA, Payne JB, Maze CA, Patil KD, Gallagher SJ, Mattson JS. Influence of estrogen and osteopenia/osteoporosis on clinical periodontitis in postmenopausal women. J Periodontol 1999; 70: 823–828.

34. Norderyd OM, Grossi SG, Machtei EE, et al. Periodontal status of women taking postmenopausal estrogen supplementation. J Periodontol 1993; 64:957–962.

35. Johnston CC Jr, Miller JZ, Slemenda CW, et al. Calcium supplementation and increases in bone mineral density in children. N Engl J Med 1992; 327:82–87.

36. Dawson-Hughes B, Harris SS, Krall EA, Dallal GE. A controlled trial of calcium and vitamin D supplementation on bone density in men and women 65 years of age or older. N Engl J Med 1997; 337: 670–676.

37. Prince R, Devine A, Dick I, et al. The effects of calcium supplementation (milk powder or tablets) and exercise on bone density in postmenopausal women. J Bone Miner Res 1995; 10:1068–1075.

38. Peacock M, Liu G, Carey M, et al. Effect of calcium or 25OH vitamin D3 dietary supplementation on bone loss at the hip in men and women over the age of 60. J Clin Endocrinol Metab 2000; 85:3011–3019.

39. Chapuy MC, Arlot ME, Duboeuf F, et al. Vitamin D3 and calcium to prevent hip fractures in the elderly women. N Engl J Med 1992; 327:1637–1642.

40. Bissada NF, DeMarco TJ. The effect of a hypocalcemic diet on the periodontal structures of the adult rat. J Periodontol 1974; 45:739–745.

41. Oliver WM. The effect of deficiencies of calcium, vitamin D or calcium and vitamin D and of variations in the source of dietary protein on the supporting tissues of the rat molar. J Periodont Res 1969; 4:56–69.

42. Ferguson HW, Hartles RL. The effects of diets deficient in calcium or phosphorus in the presence and absence of supplements of vitamin D on the secondary cementum and alveolar bone of young rats. Arch Oral Biol 1964; 9:647–658.

43. Uhrbom E, Jacobson L. Calcium and periodontitis: clinical effect of calcium medication. J Clin Periodontol 1984; 11:230–241.

44. Krall EA. The periodontal-systemic connection: implications for treatment of patients with osteoporosis and periodontal disease. Ann Periodontol 2001; 6:209–213.

45. Nishida M, Grossi SG, Dunford RG, Ho AW, Trevisan M, Genco RJ. Calcium and the risk for periodontal disease. J Periodontol 2000; 71:1057–1066.

46. Krall EA, Wehler C, Harris SS, Garcia RI, Dawson-Hughes B. Calcium and vitamin D supplements reduce tooth loss in the elderly. Am J Med 2001; 111:452–456.

47. Wical KE, Swoope CC. Studies of residual ridge resorption. 2. The relationship of dietary calcium and phosphorus to residual ridge resorption. J Prosthet Dent 1974; 32:13–22.

48. Wical KE, Brussee P. Effects of a calcium and vitamin D supplement on alveolar ridge resorption in immediate denture patients. J Prosthet Dent 1979; 41:4–411.

49. Bloch AS, Shils ME. National and international recommended dietary reference values. In Shils, ME, Olson JA, Shike M, Ross AC, eds. Modern Nutrition in Health and Disease. Baltimore, MD: Williams & Wilkins, 1999, A19–A48.

50. Writing Group for the Women's Health Initiative Investigators. Risks and benefits of estrogen plus progestin in healthy postmenopausal women: principal results from the Women's Health Initiative randomized controlled trial. JAMA 2002; 288:321–333.

51. Lydick E, Cook K, Turpin J, Melton M, Stine R, Byrnes C. Development and validation of a simple questionnaire to facilitate identification of women likely to have low bone density. Am J Manag Care 1998; 4:37–48.

52. Geusens P, Hochberg MC, van der Voort DJ, et al. Performance of risk indices for identifying low bone density in postmenopausal women. Mayo Clin Proc 2002; 77:629–637.

16 Wound Healing

Marion F. Winkler and Suzanne Makowski

1. INTRODUCTION

A wound is defined as any physical break in tissue continuity. Wounds differ depending on the type and severity, mechanism of wounding, location, and desired outcome. The act of wounding or injury disrupts anatomical continuity, tissue function, and cellular integrity *(1)*. Alterations in wound healing may result in impaired or delayed healing. Impaired wound healing often occurs in the presence of concurrent injury or infection as in a patient who has diabetes or has received radiation therapy, and almost always leads to a poor wound outcome *(2)*. A delayed or poorly healing wound may have decreased tensile strength or low collagen accumulation but may eventually heal to normal *(3)*. Delayed wound healing, especially in the context of stress-induced immune suppression may result in increased infection, scarring, poor esthetic outcome, and poor regenerative potential *(4)*. Tissues in the oral cavity are capable of remarkable regeneration and repair. Depending on the severity and location of tissue damage and whether the source of injury or infection is eliminated, oral tissue will typically completely heal within 2 wk *(5)*. Healing results rapidly in the majority of instances because of the rich vascular nature of the oral cavity. Nutritional deficiencies and other factors such as smoking, chronic disease, and medications can make oral tissue more susceptible to injury and impact the healing process.

2. WOUND-HEALING PHYSIOLOGY

Oral tissues capable of repair include fibrous connective tissue, epithelium, and bone. Other tissue such as enamel does not have this capability. Cellular immune response plays a major role in wound healing by protecting against infection, preparing the wound for healing, and regulating repair *(4)*. Following injury to tissue, there is vasoconstriction and clot formation. The resulting increase in blood flow through the capillary beds is associated with increased permeability to leukocytes and plasma into the injured tissue. Cytokines (interleukin [IL]-1, IL-8) and tumor necrosis factor regulate phagocytic activity. Phagocytic cells clear away damaged tissue and regulate fibroblast and epithelial cell involvement in healing. Epithelialization begins at the edges of the wound and progresses in a sheet of cells toward its center. Clotting and epithelialization help maintain tissue hydration, strengthen the site of tissue injury, and provide a barrier limiting bacterial

From: *Nutrition and Oral Medicine*
Edited by: R. Touger-Decker, D. A. Sirois, and C. C. Mobley © Humana Press Inc., Totowa, NJ

Table 1
Role of Nutrients in the Wound-Healing Process

Nutrient	Role/function
Protein	Cell multiplication; enzyme synthesis; collagen and other connective tissue synthesis
Carbohydrate	Source of energy; part of ground substance
Fatty acids	Part of cell membrane; prostaglandin synthesis
Vitamin C	Cofactor in hydroxylation of proline and lysine; collagen synthesis
Vitamin A	Epithelial maintenance; glycoprotein and proteoglycan synthesis; stimulation of cellular differentiation in fibroblast and collagen formation
Vitamin D	Calcium homeostasis; calcium and phosphate absorption
Vitamin E	Maintenance of cell membrane
Calcium	Required by tissue collagenases; bone and tooth formation
Zinc	Transcription of RNA; cellular proliferation; protein synthesis
Iron	Involved in hydroxylation of proline and lysine
Copper	Component of lysyl oxidase; erythropoiesis

influx and foreign material contact, which may impede healing *(1)*. Connective tissue healing proceeds through three classical phases that can be summarized as follows:

1. Inflammatory phase: vascular and cellular response; hemostasis; cleaning of cellular debris and removal of infectious agents; secretion of factors that stimulate new epithelium; and migration of polymorphonuclear neutrophils, macrophages, and lympohocytes
2. Fibroblast phase: epithelial regeneration; new capillary formation; collagen synthesis; wound granulation; epithelialization and scar formation; vascularization
3. Remodeling phase: tissue repair; collagen synthesis and degradation; scar formation; wound strengthening.

Each step in the wound-healing process requires energy provided through carbohydrate and fat metabolism. Protein and amino acids contribute structurally to the wound as part of the ground substance in the form of proteoglycans and glycoproteins. Protein is also necessary for synthesis and cellular multiplication. Normal cellular function requires electrolytes, minerals, and vitamins that serve as enzymatic cofactors for many of the steps in the wound-healing process. Vitamin C, because of its function in collagen synthesis, plays a major role in wound healing. In the oral cavity, vitamin C is involved in maintenance of tissue including the periodontal ligament, formation of bone matrix and teeth, and maintenance of the integrity of blood vessel walls *(6)*. Table 1 summarizes the role of nutrients involved in normal wound healing. The reader is also encouraged to review Chapter 7 for a more detailed discussion on nutrients and the oral cavity.

3. INJURY TO THE ORAL CAVITY

Tissue damage in the oral cavity may be caused by physical (incision, crushing, extreme heat or cold), chemical (caustic materials applied to oral tissues, anti-cancer drugs), mechanical (trauma during mastication, mucosal tearing from dental appliances, unconscious biting), or infectious (microorganism invasion of oral tissue) disruption. Injury to tissue in the oral cavity results in inflammation. The extent and duration of the inflammatory response is related to the injury. This can range from local inflammation limited to the site of injury or to a systemic response characterized by fever, leukocytosis, and lymphadenopathy. Classical signs of inflammation include erythema, heat, edema, pain, and loss of normal tissue function. Serous or purulent exudate may be present.

The size of a wound in the oral cavity depends on the insult. Wounds are usually superficial, displaying a yellow center with a red margin. A severe ulcer becomes surrounded by a white margin, is deep and indurated, and may resemble a malignancy. Traumatic lesions occur most frequently on the tongue, labial mucosa, alveolar ridge, buccal mucosa, palate, and lips. Traumatic ulceration may become chronic if the underlying cause is not corrected—for example, repair of sharp-edged or fractured teeth or control of excessive tongue rubbing. Burns that may occur after ingestion of hot food or drink most frequently affect the palate and tongue. Pain, erythema, and mucosal sloughing are manifestations of mild burns, whereas vesicles and ulceration are characteristic of more severe burns. Burns caused by chewing on an electrical cord typically result in severe necrosis. The injured area is painless and blood-free and develops a black eschar. If the burn extends intraorally, the tongue and gingiva and developing tooth germs may be affected. Lesions on the hard palate may occur as a result of extensive smoking. Referred to as nicotine stomatitis, these lesions appear erythematous with increased keratinization and opacification and often are accompanied by inflamed salivary glands (5). Tobacco chewers may develop white lesions in the mucobuccal fold with atypical epithelialization. Acute necrotizing ulcerative gingivitis is an endogenous oral infection associated with poor oral hygiene, smoking, emotional stress, and systemic disorders such as leukemia, aplastic anemia, HIV infection, immunosuppressive states, and malnutrition. The interdental soft tissue has ulcerations that appear necrotic with excessive bleeding. In the oral cavity, infection, impaired healing, and overload are considered the major etiologic factors for the loss of oral implants (7). Nonnutritional factors such as correction of high muscle attachments and vestibular deficiencies creates a proper environment for soft tissue healing associated with implants (8). Nutritional deficiencies can adversely affect the outcome of implant surgery and rehabilitation, particularly in geriatric patients (9).

4. ORAL TISSUE REPAIR

Optimal oral tissue healing is a desired clinical outcome in oral mucosal disease, trauma, oral surgery, and periodontal disease and treatment. Healing occurs by primary intention when the edges of the wound are surgically approximated with sutures. Wounds usually have little tissue granulation formation, which results in minimal scarring. When there is large loss of tissue and clot formation, healing occurs by secondary intention. This often results in increased granulation tissue and increased scar formation. Wounds complicated by infection may require the wound site to be left open without surgically joining the edges until resolution or control of the infection. Healing of injury to bone involves the creation of bone tissue produced by osteoblasts. This process can be impaired by removal of osteoblast-producing tissue, increased movement, edema, or infection (5).

Scar formation can be minimized in the oral cavity by avoidance of bacterial contamination and excellent wound management including thorough irrigation to remove any foreign material within the wound, removal of all necrotic tissue, prevention of ischemia, and control of wound tension with proper suturing and well-positioned flaps *(1)*.

Surgical technique including hemostasis and adequate suturing and proper wound management have the greatest influence on healing of mucosal wounds. Occlusive dressings used alone or in combination with topical anesthestics and anti-inflammatory agents protect the suture line and help minimize trauma to the wound from normal activity and eating *(1)*. Strenuous activity and excessive exertion should be avoided to reduce stress on the wound margins and to prevent dehiscence for the first 24 h postoperatively. Gentle brushing with a soft nylon toothbrush rinsed in warm water is useful in minimizing trauma to oral and periodontal wounds. Oral rinses with chlorhexidine may be beneficial with routine oral hygiene; however, use of hydrogen peroxide is discouraged because this may delay healing or disrupt the normal flora in the oral cavity *(10)*. Alcohol should also be avoided.

5. PERIODONTAL DISEASE AND TREATMENT

An early form of periodontal disease is gingivitis, characterized by inflammation of the gingival tissue. The gingival tissue appears red and swollen and is prone to bleeding very easily. Local factors that promote the accumulation of bacterial plaque eventually leading to gingivitis include calculus, defective restorations, food impaction, and poor tooth alignment. With effective plaque removal and control, gingival tissue can often return to normal without permanent damage. However, as gingivitis progresses to early periodontitis, there is continued gingival inflammation with early bone loss and deep periodontal pockets. These pockets become deeper, tooth mobility increases, and tooth loss occurs as the destruction of the tissues in the periodontium and alveolar bone progress. Anaerobic bacterial plaque that colonizes the teeth and surrounding periodontal tissue and their by-products, including endotoxins, initiates gingival inflammation, which then promotes the inflammatory host response. As the inflammatory process continues, it can destroy surrounding cells, connective tissue, and bone *(11)*. Depending on the severity of the periodontal disease and the extent of tissue damage, various periodontal treatment procedures are available.

Effective plaque control is essential for optimal oral tissue repair. Personal oral hygiene in conjunction with periodic dental prophylaxis and, if necessary, antimicrobial agents to help destroy the pathogenic bacteria flora are essential. Often these techniques will be sufficient to resolve current gingivitis. If periodontal disease has progressed to periodontitis, scaling and root planing is often necessary to mechanically remove subgingival plaque, diseased tissue, and toxic substances *(12)*. Scaling and root planing combined with effective plaque control may be sufficient to promote periodontal healing in some cases of periodontitis *(13,14)*.

Periodontal surgery may be necessary in severe cases of periodontal disease. The goals of periodontal surgery are to reduce or eliminate periodontal pockets, improve access to root surfaces that require treatment, treat osseous defects, and attempt to create new attachment. Surgical methods routinely used include gingivectomy/gingivoplasty and apically positioned flap with or without osseous surgery. Techniques such as guided tissue regeneration using nonresorbable and bioresorbable membranes may be effective for the treatment of infrabony defects and furcation (15,16). In the immediate postoperative period, patients are advised to consume a "dental" soft diet (see Appendix) and to avoid foods that may irritate tissue such as popcorn and raw vegetables. In this respect a soft diet refers to the consumption of nonirritating (avoiding citrus, spicy, and coarse texture or seeded foods or beverages), cutting all foods into bite-size pieces, and avoiding very hot foods to avoid irritating an already inflamed oral mucosa. Patients are also instructed to eliminate alcohol, refrain from smoking, and avoid rigorous rinsing.

6. NUTRIENT DEFICIENCY AND ROLE OF SUPPLEMENTATION

Nutritional deficiencies may alter the host's resistance to disease, compromise the integrity of the tissues of the periodontium, and impair oral tissue repair and regeneration. The epithelial lining of the gingival sulcus has a very fast turnover rate of about 3–6 d (17). Because of the high turnover rate of epithelial and connective tissue cells of the periodontium, optimal nutrients are necessary for the synthesis of DNA and RNA and protein. Malnutrition, particularly protein-calorie malnutrition, causes marked changes in the oral microbial environment, resulting in increased pathogenic anaerobic organisms, enhanced binding of bacteria to oral mucosal cells, diminished acute phase protein responses, and an alteration in cytokine function that can augment the severity of oral infection and disease progression (18). Optimal nutritional status is therefore important in promoting wound healing and in mitigating the severity of oral inflammation and periodontal disease (19). It is prudent to encourage an adequate diet and sufficient nutrient intake. The role of specific nutrients in optimizing oral tissue wound healing is an active area of research.

Vitamin C, or ascorbic acid, is essential in the metabolism of the amino acids hydroxyproline and hydroxylysine, which form collagen in the periodontium. Histologically, a deficiency of vitamin C has been shown to decrease collagen formation by affecting the hydroxylation of proline and by increasing the permeability of the oral mucosa to bacterial endotoxins, thereby affecting the barrier function of the epithelium (20). In an experimental setting of vitamin C depletion, gingival bleeding significantly increased and then returned to baseline following repletion (21). These findings suggest that gingival bleeding may be improved with adequate vitamin C repletion, but gingivitis will continue until the bacterial plaque is effectively removed despite correction of any deficiency (21). Severe vitamin C deficiency may result in scorbutic gingivitis, characterized by ulceration, rapid development of periodontal pockets, and tooth exfoliation (6). Despite associations between vitamin C and dental health, there is little evidence to demonstrate a correlation between ascorbic acid deficiency and the prevalence of periodontal disease (22). There is no data to support the role of supplemental vitamin C in wound healing in the absence of deficiency.

Zinc serves as a cofactor for the enzymes responsible for cellular proliferation and is needed for the transcription of RNA, cellular replication, and collagen formation. Zinc deficiency impairs wound healing by reducing the rate of epithelialization, decreasing wound strength, and diminishing collagen synthesis. It has been shown in beagle dogs that oral zinc supplementation leads to increased healing in gingival tissue (23). Similarly, feline oral health is improved with the use of zinc ascorbate gel as an oral antiseptic

(24). In humans, zinc-containing dental materials are frequently used in clinical dentistry. Small quantities of zinc oxide-eugenol diffuse through the dentin to the pulp and exert anti-inflammatory and local anesthetic effects on the dental pulp. Temporary fillings with this compound may facilitate pulpal healing *(25,26)*. Clinical studies have shown that the administration of zinc may enhance wound healing in conditions of low zinc nutriture, but zinc supplementation in the presence of normal zinc status has not been shown to speed the healing process *(27)*.

Glutamine, an essential amino acid, is a principal nutrient for the gastrointestinal (GI) mucosa and helps maintain GI structure and function. The role of glutamine in the healing of oral mucositis is an emerging area of study. Oral mucositis is often a complication following chemotherapy with or without radiation. Some studies have demonstrated positive results when patients swish and swallow an oral glutamine suspension during and after chemotherapy. Results of these studies indicate a reduction in the incidence, duration, and severity of chemotherapy-induced mucositis *(28,29)*. Although the results are conflicting, adjunctive therapy utilizing oral glutamine suspension may benefit cancer patients undergoing chemotherapy in helping to minimize complications and discomfort from oral mucositis.

Antioxidants including vitamin C, β-carotene, selenium, and vitamin E also offer potential benefits to oral-tissue wound healing. It has long been hypothesized that tissue destruction in periodontal disease may be promoted by extended exposure to reactive oxygen species (ROS) that are created during the periodontal inflammatory process by polymorphonuclear leukocytes *(30)*. The free-radical scavenging capabilities of antioxidants may help to protect periodontium cell structures from tissue damage mediated by ROS. Investigators are currently studying the antioxidant activity of saliva in healthy individuals and in patients with periodontal diseases *(30–33)*. The possible therapeutic effects of antioxidants in preventing or treating periodontal disease is an active area of research *(34)*. The potential role of nutritional therapy in the treatment of periodontitis will likely follow *(35)*.

One interesting randomized, controlled clinical study compared the use of nutritional supplements and nutraceuticals in conjunction with routine oral hygiene for 60 d on the reduction of gingivitis, bleeding, probing depth, and attachment levels in patients with periodontal disease vs healthy individuals *(36)*. There were no significant changes for attachment levels with either the experimental or control group; however, in a subset of patients with deep pocket depths (>4 mm), there was significant improvement in the gingival index and periodontal pocket depth from baseline to 60 d in the experimental group. This concept merits further investigation but data at present are insufficient to support routine supplementation.

7. LIFESTYLE AND MEDICAL FACTORS

Smoking, chronic diseases, and medications can also affect oral tissue healing. Smoking negatively impacts wound healing and periodontal health. The deleterious effects on the periodontium include alterations of the periodontal tissue vasculature and bacterial microflora, inhibitory effects of immunoglobulin levels, and antibody responses to plaque bacteria *(37)*. Although the mechanism of how tobacco smoking influences periodontal disease is not completely understood, smoking is thought to interfere with protease inhibitors, thereby affecting the inflammatory response *(38)*. Smoking may also increase the risk of oral lesions such as nicotine stomatitis in heavy smokers, cause abnormal epithelium in tobacco chewers, and increase the risk of squamous cell carcinoma of the lips and skin.

Diabetes mellitus, because of the complications of peripheral neuropathy and microvascular disease, is associated with poor wound healing and alveolar bone loss. Elevated blood glucose levels may cause endothelial damage with potential occlusion of capillary vessels as well as hyperglycemia-induced leukocyte dysfunction, decreased chemotaxis, and phagocytosis resulting in impaired wound healing and increased risk of infection *(27,39)*. A model designed to study the combination of infection and advanced glycation end product-mediated cytokine up-regulation explains the increase in tissue destruction seen in diabetic periodontitis and how periodontal infection may complicate the severity of diabetes and the degree of metabolic control *(40)*. Defective collagen metabolism in diabetics is also thought to be a factor in delayed wound healing. Hyperglycemia in animal studies is associated with increased collagenase and protease activity in rat gingiva and impaired vascular wound healing *(41)*. Uncontrolled or poorly controlled diabetes mellitus is associated with increased frequency and severity of oral infections, including periodontal disease and dental caries *(42,43)*. Patients with diabetes who wear dentures also have an increased frequency of candida colonization and candida-associated denture stomatitis compared to denture wearers with normal blood glucose *(44)*.

Patients with renal failure or renal insufficiency may also be susceptible to impaired wound healing because of oral mucosal infections, dental caries, gingivitis, and periodontal disease *(45)*. Uremic stomatitis, characterized by erythemic thickening of the buccal mucosa, ulceration, gingival and mucosal hemorrhage, and ecchymoses may occur in dialysis patients *(46)*.

There are a variety of medications associated with impaired wound healing. Anticoagulation therapy may cause hemorrhage, petechiae, ecchymoses, or purpura of oral mucosal tissue *(47)*. Steroids, nonsteroidal anti-inflammatory drugs, and other immunosuppressive agents can also increase the risk of oral fungal and other opportunistic infections. Because the process of wound healing begins with inflammation, the use of anti-inflammatory agents may delay the healing process. Vitamin A given perioperatively may counteract the anti-inflammatory effects of steroids *(48)*. The surgical literature recommends 25,000 IU vitamin A supplementation perioperatively for patients with severe injuries and for those receiving steroids except for patients on immunosuppresive therapy following transplantation *(3,49)*. Because of direct irritation to skin or mucosal tissue, as well as the resultant immunosuppression, patients receiving radiation therapy and chemotherapy are also at high risk for impaired wound healing. Acute and chronic complications of the oral tissues following chemotherapy, bone marrow transplantation, and local radiation may include mucositis, stomatitis, salivary gland dysfunction, and gingival and oral mucosal hemorrhage. Mucosal lesions may become portals for the invasion of pathogens and increase susceptibility to oral microbial infection *(50,51)*. These complications may also increase the risk of dental caries and periodontal disease. Patients who have undergone radiation treatment to the head and neck are also at risk of development of osteonecrosis of the mandible or maxilla because of diminished blood supply to the bone.

8. SUMMARY AND CONCLUSIONS

Delayed or impaired oral wound healing can often be minimized or prevented by conducting a thorough comprehensive health history, medication review, and general nutrition risk assessment. Practitioners should focus especially on recent trauma or infection, increased nutrient requirements associated with physiologic states (pregnancy, lactation, growth), metabolic disorders and disease (diabetes, renal failure, malignancy), use of medications that may impact nutritional status or wound healing, and smoking. The physical exam of the oral cavity should focus on signs of nutritional deficiency, oral manifestations of disease or treatment, and other dental pathology including caries and physical condition of the teeth as well as oral conditions that may impact ability to use the oral cavity functionally for eating. Personal oral hygiene and plaque control are essential for oral health and wound healing. Prompt attention to oral trauma is imperative. For patients in whom there is a potential for increased risk of infection, maintenance of sutures for a longer period of time, excision of ragged wound edges to reduce vascularity, and antibiotic prophylaxis may be indicated *(52)*. Because of the relationship between nutrition and oral health, there is an ongoing need for practitioners to make recommendations about diet, nutrition, and lifestyle choices *(53,54)*. There is also an increasing role for nutrition assessment, evaluation, and intervention in patients with oral wound pathology and periodontal disease.

Severe oral pathology or recent oral surgery can often contribute to chewing and/or swallowing difficulties temporarily or permanently and may severely limit intake of nutritious foods. Without the appropriate adjustments in diet, individuals have the potential for excessive weight loss, dehydration, protein-energy malnutrition, vitamin/mineral deficiencies, and poor oral wound healing. The goal of nutrition therapy is to provide adequate calories, protein, vitamins, minerals, and fluids in a consistency best tolerated by the individual. Avoidance of foods with extreme temperatures and high acid, salt, or spice content, and dry coarse foods may be sufficient to limit discomfort when chewing or swallowing. Dietary texture modifications to mechanical soft or pureed may be necessary, and in some situations only liquids can be tolerated. Commercial nutritional supplements can be used as a meal replacement or to augment nutritional intake. Often individuals are encouraged to consume small, frequent meals and/or nutritional supplements as tolerated. A multivitamin with mineral supplement containing 100% of the recommended daily intake may be suggested. Individuals must also be encouraged to maintain good oral hygiene care and follow the recommendations of their oral health care practitioner. In some extreme cases, an oral analgesic may be prescribed. In most cases, these modifications will be temporary, and the individual can return to normal eating after oral healing is completed.

Guidelines for Practice

	Oral Health Professional	*Nutrition Professional*
Prevention	• Conduct thorough health history and medication review. • Screen patients for nutrition risk as part of oral exam.	• Conduct oral exam as part of nutrition assessment. • Provide guidelines for balanced nutrition and recommendations for supplements as needed. • Encourage daily oral hygiene.
Intervention	• Determine impact of planned surgery on oral function and provide guidelines accordingly. • Ask patients about alterations in intake and changes in weight on postoperative visits and refer as needed to a registered dietitian.	• Provide medical nutrition therapy tailored to individual nutrient needs and oral function. • Adjust diet as appropriate as wound healing progresses. • Monitor intake to ensure balanced nutrition to promote wound healing.

REFERENCES

1. Certosimo F, Nicoll B, Nelson R, Wolfgang M. Wound healing and repair: a review of the art and science. Gen Dent 1998; July/August:362–369.
2. Winkler M. Surgery and wound healing. In Skipper A, ed. Dietitian's Handbook of Enteral and Parenteral Nutrition. Gaithersburg, MD: Aspen Publishers, 1998.
3. Albina JE. Nutrition and wound healing. J Parenter Enteral Nutr 1994; 18:367–376.
4. Rozlog LA, Kiecolt-Glaser JK, Marucha PT, Sheridan JF, Glaser R. Stress and immunity: implications for viral disease and wound healing. J Periodontol 1999; 70:786–792.
5. Fehrenbach MJ, Lemborn UE, Phelan JA. Inflammation and repair. In Ibsen O, Phelan J, eds. Oral Pathology for the Dental Hygienist. 3rd Ed. Philadelphia, PA: W.B. Saunders, 2000, 43–101.
6. Nishida M, Grossi SG, Dunford RG, Ho AW, Trevisan M, Genco RJ. Dietary vitamin C and the risk for periodontal disease. J Periodontol 2000; 71:1215–1223.
7. Esposito M, Hirsch J, Lekholm U, Thomsen P. Differential diagnosis and treatment strategies for biologic complications and failing oral implants: a review of the literature. Int J Oral Maxillofac Implants 1999; 14:473–490.
8. Cranin AN. Implant surgery: the management of soft tissues. J Oral Implantol 2002; 28:230–237.
9. Winkler S, Mekayarajjananonth T, Garg AK, Tewari DS. Nutrition and the geriatric implant patient. Implant Dent 1997; 6:291–294.
10. Rees TD, Orth CF. Oral ulcerations with use of hydrogen peroxide. J Periodontal 1986; 57:689–692.
11. Kornman KS, Loe H. The role of local factors in the etiology of periodontal diseases. Periodontol 2000 1993; 2:83–97.
12. O'Leary TJ. The impact of research on scaling and root planing. J Periodontol 1986; 57:69–75.
13. Axelsson P, Lindhe J. The significance of maintenance care in the treatment of periodontal disease. J Clin Periodontol 1981; 8:281–294.
14. Badersten A, Nilveus R, Egelberg J. Four-year observations of basic periodontal therapy. J Clin Periodontol 1987; 14:438–444.
15. Heard RH, Mellonig JT. Regenerative materials: an overview. Alpha Omegan 2000 1993; 4: 51–58.
16. Eickholz P, Kim TS, Hausmann E, Holle R. Long-term results of guided tissue regeneration therapy with non-resorbable and bioabsorbable barriers. Infrabony defects. Abstract. IADR/AADR/CADR 80th General Session, March 6–9, 2002.
17. Alfano MC. Controversies, perspectives, and clinical implications of nutrition in periodontal disease. Dent Clin North Am 1976; 20:519–548.
18. Enwonwu CO, Phillips RS, Falkler WA. Nutrition and oral infectious diseases: state of the science. Compend Contin Educ Dent 2002; 23:431–438.
19. Enwonwu CO. Interface of malnutrition and periodontal diseases. Am J Clin Nutr 1995; 61:430S–436S.

20. Alfano MC, Miller SA, Drummond JF. Effect of ascorbic acid deficiency on the permeability and collagen biosynthesis of oral mucosal epithelium. Ann NY Acad Sci 1975; 258:253–363.
21. Leggott PJ, Robertson PB, Jacob RA, Zambon JJ, Walsh M, Armitage GC. Effects of ascorbic acid depletion and supplementation on periodontal health and subgingival microflora in humans. J Dent Res 1991; 70:1531–1536.
22. Ismail AI, Burt BA, Eklund SA. Relation between ascorbic acid intake and periodontal disease in the United States. J Am Dent Assoc 1983; 107:927–931.
23. Ehrlichman RJ, Seckel BR, Bryan DJ, Moschella CJ. Common complications of wound healing. Surg Clin North Am 1991; 71:1323–1351.
24. Williamson CE, Yukna RA, Gandor DW. Zinc concentration in normal and healing gingival tissue in beagle dogs. J Periodontol 1984; 55:170–174.
25. Clarke DE. Clinical and microbiological effects of oral zinc ascorbate gel in cats. J Vet Dent 2001; 18:177–183.
26. Markowitz K, Moynihan M, Liu M, Kim S. Biologic properties of eugenol and zinc oxide-eugenol: a clinically oriented review. Oral Surg Oral Med Oral Pathol 1992; 73:729–737.
27. Pitt Ford TR, Andreasen JO, Dorn SO, Kariyawasam SP. Effect of various zinc oxide materials as root-end fillings on healing after replantation. Int Endod J 1995; 28:273–278.
28. Anderson PM, Schroeder G, Skubitz KM. Oral glutamine reduces the duration and severity of stomatitis after cytotoxic cancer chemotherapy. Cancer 1998; 83:1433–1439.
29. Cockerham MB, Weinberger BB, Lerchie SB. Oral glutamine for the prevention of oral mucositis associated with high-dose paclitaxel and melphalan for autologous bone marrow transplantation. Ann Pharmacother 2002; 34:300–303.
30. Waddington RJ, Moseley R, Embery G. Reactive oxygen species: a potential role in the pathogenesis of periodontal diseases. Oral Dis 2000; 6:138–151.
31. Diab-Ladki R, Pellat B, Chahine R. Decrease in the total antioxidant activity of saliva in patients with periodontal diseases. Clin Oral Investig 2003; 7:103–107.
32. Sculley DV, Langley-Evans SC. Periodontal disease is associated with lower antioxidant capacity in whole saliva and evidence of increased protein oxidation. Clin Sci 2003; 105:167–172.
33. Brock GR, Matthews J, Butterworth C, Chapple ILC. Plasma and crevicular fluid antioxidant defense in periodontitis and health. Abstract. IADR/AADR/CADR 80th General Session, March 6–9, 2002.
34. Battino M, Bullon P, Wilson M, Newman H. Oxidative injury and inflammatory periodontal diseases: the challenge of anti-oxidants to free radicals and reactive oxygen species. Crit Rev Oral Biol Med 1999; 10:458–476.
35. Sculley DV, Langley-Evans SC. Salivary antioxidants and periodontal disease status. Proc Nutr Soc 2002; 61:137–143.
36. Munoz CA, Kiger RD, Stephens JA, Kim J, Wilson AC. Effects of a nutritional supplement on periodontal status. Compend Contin Educ Dent 2001; 22:425–432.
37. American Academy of Periodontology. The pathogenesis of periodontal diseases. J Periodontol 1999; 70:457–470.
38. Persson L, Bergstrom J, Ito H, Gustafsson A. Tobacco smoking and neutrophil activity in periodontal disease. J Periodontol 2001; 72:90–95.
39. Rudolph DM. Why won't this wound heal? Amer J Nurs 2002; 102:24DD–24HH.
40. Grossi SG, Genco RJ. Periodontal disease and diabetes mellitus: a two-way relationship. Ann Periodontol 1998; 3:51–61.
41. Grant-Theule DA. Periodontal disease, diabetes, and immune response: a review of current concepts. J West Soc Periodontol Periodontal Abstr 1996; 44:69–77.
42. Lin BP-J, Taylor GW, Allen DJ, Ship JA. Dental caries in older adults with diabetes mellitus. Spec Care Dent 1999; 19:8–14.
43. Taylor GW, Burt BA, Becker MP, Genco RJ, Shlossman M. Glycemic control and alveolar bone loss progression in type 2 diabetes. Ann Periodontol 1998; 3:30–39.
44. Dorocka-Bobkowska B, Budtz-Jorgensen E, Wloch S. Non–insulin-dependent diabetes mellitus as a risk factor for denture stomatitis. J Oral Pathol Med 1996; 25:411–415.
45. Naugle K, Darby ML, Bauman DM, Lineberger LT, Powers R. The oral health status of individuals on renal dialysis. Ann Periodontol 1998; 3:197–205.

46. DeRossi SS, Glick M. Dental considerations for the patient with renal disease receiving hemodialysis. J Am Dent Assoc 1996; 127:211–219.
47. Ghezzi EM, Ship JA. Systemic disease and their treatments in the elderly: impact on oral health. J Pub Health Dent 200; 60:289–296.
48. Anstead GM. Steroids, retinoids, and wound healing. Adv Wound Care 1998; 11:277–285.
49. Levenson SM, Demetriou AA. Metabolic factors. In Cohen IK, Diegelmann RF, Lindblad WJ, eds. Wound Healing: Biochemical and Clinical Aspects. Philadelphia, PA: W.B. Saunders, 1992, 248–273.
50. Peterson DE, D'Ambrosio JA. Diagnosis and management of acute and chronic oral complications of nonsurgical cancer therapies. Dent Clin North Am 1992; 36:945–966.
51. Carl W. Oral complications of local and systemic cancer treatment. Curr Opin Oncol 1995; 7:320–324.
52. Marciani RD. Critical systemic and psychosocial considerations in the management of trauma in the elderly. Oral Surg Oral Med Oral Pathol Oral Radiol Endod 1999; 87:272–280.
53. Position of the American Dietetic Association. Oral health and nutrition. J Am Diet Assoc 1996; 96: 184–189.
54. Dorsky R. Nutrition and oral health. Gen Dent 2001; November/December:576–582.

Selected Websites

A Comprehensive Color Photo Atlas of Dentistry: Wound Healing, Dental Images
   www.drdorfman.com/atlas/at204
American Academy of Periodontology
   www.perio.org
American Academy of Wound Management
   www.aawm.org
Association for the Advancement of Wound Care
   www.AAWC1.com
Center for Stress and Wound Healing
   www.med.ohio-state.edu/mindbody/
Comprehensive Training in Oral and Craniofacial Sciences (CTOC)
   www.ctoc.osu/edu/wound_healing.html
International Association for Dental Research and American Association for Dental Research
   www.iadr.com
Journal of Wound Care
   www.journalofwoundcare.com
National Institute of Dental and Craniofacial Research (NIDCR)
   www.nidr.nih.gov
The Wound Care Information Network
   www.medicaledu.com
The Wound Healing Society
   www.woundheal.org
UCLA Dental Research Unit: Wound Healing Research Center
   www.dent.ucla.edu/drl
Wound Healing Research Group, University of Wales College of Medicine, Wales, UK
   www.uwcm.ac.uk/study/dentistry/osmp/wound/wound.htm

V EDUCATION AND PRACTICE

Approaches to Oral Nutrition Health Risk Assessment

Riva Touger-Decker and David A. Sirois

1. INTRODUCTION

Oral health plays a significant role in overall and nutritional health. This role becomes increasingly important for patients with oral or medical illness, patients with physical limitations that affect chewing ability, and patients who take medications that affect immune surveillance, oral ecology, and oral physiology. The primary focus of this chapter is to describe approaches to oral nutrition and diet risk evaluation for both the dietetics and dental professional. It is the responsibility of dietetics and dental professionals to conduct baseline evaluation of oral and nutrition status, provide appropriate education, and refer patients accordingly to the appropriate health professional (1). The synergistic relationship between diet/nutrition and integrity of the oral cavity and its potential impact on general health support the need for oral nutrition risk assessment as a routine part of dental care (2,3). Nutrition and oral health can have a significant impact on general health (1,2,4,5). Compromised diet intake can lead to decreased intake of essential nutrients and subsequent malnutrition, which increases the risk for systemic and oral disease.

Table 1 outlines conditions associated with compromised nutrition and oral health. The list in Table 1 is by no means all inclusive-there are many oral and systemic diseases that are associated with oral and nutrition risk. The risk assessment process for dental and dietetics professionals differs somewhat in the approach; however, the outcomes and goals should be similar. Intervention needs may include referral to the appropriate provider, either the registered dietitian (RD) or dentist, provision of baseline education, and a plan for follow-up.

Table 2 outlines a model from the *American Dietetic Association Position on Oral Health and Nutrition (1)*. The goal of nutrition risk assessment is early detection and intervention to reduce the incidence and severity of nutrition risk and maximize response to treatment. Nutrition risk assessment, completed on the patient's initial and periodic reassessment appointments, takes approx 8–10 min; the amount of time that may be saved secondary to providing this assessment and subsequent care or referral is not quantifiable. The dental professional may refer a patient to an RD for medical nutrition therapy (MNT).

From: *Nutrition and Oral Medicine*
Edited by: R. Touger-Decker, D. A. Sirois, and C. C. Mobley © Humana Press Inc., Totowa, NJ

Table 1
Conditions Associated With Compromised Nutritional and Oral Health Status

Anorexia	Menopause
Autoimmune disorders	Multiple sclerosis
Bulimia	Musculoskeletal disorders
Cardiovascular disease	Neoplastic disease
Craniofacial anomalies	Osteoporosis
Developmental disorders	Physical/mental handicaps
Diabetes	Polypharmacy
Disorders of taste and smell	Poor dentition/edentulism
Early childhood caries	Protein-energy malnutrition/wasting
End-stage renal disease	Quadriplegia
Erosion	Radiation therapy
Fad dieting/nutrition quackery	Salivary dysfunction
Gastrointestinal disorders	Specific disease states
Hypertension	Substance abuse (alcohol and/or drugs)
Immunocompromising conditions	Transplant surgery
(e.g., cancer, HIV infection, AIDS)	Ulcers in the oral cavity
Infectious diseases	Von Willenbrandt's disease
Juvenile periodontitis	Weight status
Kaposi's sarcoma	Xerostomia
Lupus	Zinc deficiency

Table 2
Approaches to Oral Nutrition Management for the Dietetics and Dental Professional

Dietetics professional

- Conduct intra-/extraoral screening and cranial nerve exams.
- Include oral health screening in nutrition assessment protocols (i.e., cranial nerve function, occlusion, edentulism, masticatory ability, swallowing, salivary adequacy).
- Recognize oral manifestations of systemic diseases and provide patients with guidelines to maximize oral intake.
- Confer with and refer patients (via consults) to dental practitioners for management of oral diseases and/or risk factors for oral diseases.
- Consult with dental professionals in interpretation of oral nutrition assessment findings and planning in the long-term care setting.

Dental professional

- Include diet screening, education, and referral for oral infectious disease prevention/control, optimal masticatory function, and management of other oral diseases/treatments as a component of comprehensive dental care.
- Collaborate with dietetics professionals in delivery of MNT and provision of oral health care in long-term care settings.
- Provide diet and nutrition guidelines for health promotion and disease prevention to patients and provide guidelines for diet to maximize oral intake.
- Consult with and refer patients (via consult) to dietetics professionals for management of nutrition risk caused by compromised oral health (e.g., caries, immunosuppressive disorders, xerostomia, diabetes, oral surgery, cancer).

Adapted with permission from ref. *1* .

Table 3
Oral Nutrition Risk Factors

Acute/Chronic disease(s)	Inadequate diet
(see Table 1)	Altered taste
Masticatory compromise	Poverty
(biting/chewing /swallowing difficulty)	Substance abuse
Unintentional weight change	Polypharmacy
Extensive caries	Acute oral pain
Dental procedures altering ability	Oral infections
to eat a usual diet	Oral surgery
Ulcerations/lesions	Xerostomia
Cranial nerve disorders	Chronic orofacial pain

MNT is defined as "nutritional diagnostic, therapy, and counseling services for the purpose of disease management which are furnished by a registered dietitian or nutrition professional" *(6)*.

2. DETERMINING NUTRITION RISK: THE ROLE OF THE DENTAL PROFESSIONAL

Nutrition risk evaluation at a minimum includes subjective statements relative to diet, oral health, biting and chewing ability, and weight history as well as objective assessment of height, weight, and the condition of the oral cavity. The extent to which laboratory data and other components are used depends, in part, on the type of dental practice and the overall health and disease history of the patient. Patients with complex medical histories who take multiple medications may require a more extensive physical and laboratory assessment.

Nutrition risk factors are defined as "characteristics that are associated with an increased likelihood of poor nutritional status" *(7)*. Oral health nutrition risk factors are outlined in Table 3. Nutrition risk is based on the type and extent of risk factors present. The elderly patient who lives alone, has lost more than 10 lbs in 6 mo and has difficulty chewing is at significant risk, as is the 35-yr-old woman who tests positive for human immunodeficiency virus (HIV) and presents with candidiasis. It is always prudent to refer any patient for whom you suspect nutrition or diet concerns to an RD for MNT.

The outcomes of nutrition risk assessment are based on individual needs and may include the following:

- basic diet evaluation and education by the dental professional to meet oral and nutritional health needs; this service both promotes health and prevents disease by focusing on risk identification and risk reduction;
- basic oral health screening by the RD and referral to a dentist;
- MNT by an RD;
- referral to social services for food and supplement resources in the community; and
- referral to an RD for a nutrition consult and MNT; this service is both interventional and preventive, identifying strategies to minimize nutrition-related disease as well as interventions to improve oral and systemic health.

Table 4
Nutrition Risk Questions to Ask Patients About Common Symptoms

Weight

Has your weight changed at all in the past 6 months?
    If yes, how?
    If weight loss, was it intentional?
    If weight loss was intentional, what type of diet were you following and for how long?
    If weight gain, what are possible reasons you can attribute to weight gain?
Do your clothes fit differently now than they did 6 months ago (1 clothing size = ~10 lbs)?

Diabetes

How do you manage your diabetes in terms of any special diet, medications, monitoring?
    If you take insulin, what is the type, quantity, and dose schedule?
Do you follow any special diet?

Xerostomia

Do you have any difficulty chewing or swallowing?
    If yes, with liquids, thin or thick solids, semisolids, or both?
Has this difficulty been progressive: in degree of difficulty and types of foods?
Is swallowing painful? If yes, when?
Can you eat a meal or snack without needing liquids?
    If no, how many cups of liquids do you need to consume?
Have there been any changes in your medications or nutrient/herbal supplement use?
    If yes, describe changes.

Taste

Describe any changes in taste that have occurred; what types of food, beverage?
    Has medication (Rx or OTC) changed at all during this time?
Is your sense of taste different or missing or does everything taste bad/metallic? How does it taste?
Do you have any difficulties chewing or swallowing food?
    If yes, what?
Do you take any vitamin, mineral, herbal, or other nutrition supplements?
    If yes, what, how much, what form, what frequency?
Do you follow any special diet?

Activities of daily living

Do you do your own food shopping and preparation?
    If no, what help do you have/need?
Do you ever run out of money for food during the month?

Oral risk factors

Do you have any difficulty biting, chewing, or swallowing foods or fluids (swallowing)?
    If yes, detail what foods/fluids cause difficulty and how.
    How often during the day do you eat, including meals and snacks?
How many times a day do you drink sweetened coffees, teas, soda, juices, or other sweet beverages?
When in the course of the day do you brush your teeth?

Questions to ask about osteoporosis risk

How many servings of dairy products do you have on a typical day?
    (1 serving = 1 oz cheese or 1 c yogurt or milk)
Do you take a calcium supplement?
    If yes, what is the name and how much do you take in 1 d?
Do you get any exercise in the course of a day or week?
    If yes, how many times a week and for how long?
If a woman, are you peri- or postmenopausal?
Have you or a first-degree relative broken one or more bones?

Table 5

Formulas for Weight and Body Mass Index and Other Anthropometric Calculations

Wt change is calculated based on usual body wt:

$$\frac{\text{today's wt}}{\text{usual wt}} \times 100 = \% \text{ wt change} \qquad \text{Ex:} \frac{\text{today's wt} = 50 \text{ lbs}}{\text{usual wt} = 100 \text{ lbs}} \times 100 = \% \text{ wt change}$$

Current (today's) wt < usual wt = negative wt change
Current wt > usual wt = positive weight change

Ranges of desirable height and weight for adults: rule of thumb

Men   = 106 lbs for first 5 ft + 6 lbs/in
         Ex: 5'6" man = 106 + (6 inches × 6 lbs/inch) = 106 + 36 = 142 lbs ± 10% desirable wt
Women = 100 lbs for first 5 ft + 5 lbs/in
         Ex: 5'2" woman = 100 lbs + (2 inches × 5 lbs/inch) = 100 lbs + 10 = 110 lbs ± 10%
Note: ±10% = based on frame size; weight range may be 10% greater or less than the calculated wt

Body mass index

$$\frac{\text{Body wt in kilograms (kg)}}{(\text{ht in meters})^2} \quad \text{or} \quad \text{Wt (in lbs)} \times 703 \text{ divided by (height in inches)}^2$$

If patient does not know his or usual weight, desirable weight can be used to calculate % desirable weight. This will also give an indication of body stores. Weight alone does not differentiate between body fat vs muscle mass.

2.1. History

Patient history is an important component of nutrition evaluation. Medical history will reveal information about acute, chronic, and terminal diseases that may impact on oral and nutritional well-being. There are more than 100 systemic diseases with oral manifestations (7). In addition to asking patients about their medical, surgical, and drug history, diet and nutrition risk evaluation questions may also be asked. It is likely that the dental and dietetics professional will take a complete patient history as part of routine care. Supplemental questions relative to oral health and nutrition are in Table 4.

Unintentional weight change may signal potential nutrition deficits, lack of money for food, or systemic disease. A weight change of more than 10 lbs in less than 6 mo is considered a significant risk factor in any individual (8). Weight loss is characterized by loss of body-fat stores and lean body mass. Patients should be weighed during initial visits and subsequent check-ups. The initial-visit weight provides a baseline for comparison for future reference and self-reported weight. Reliance on self-reported weights does not provide the professional with a baseline from which to monitor weight status. Weight change typically is associated with either a change in eating habits or systemic disease. Eating habit changes may be intentional with a goal of weight loss or gain or caused by oral or systemic health issues influencing appetite or functional ability to eat. In either case, the result is a change in nutrient intake.

There are several web-based programs available to calculate weight change and body mass index. Table 5 includes some easy-to-use formulas for calculating weight statistics. Some provide access to computerized nutrient analysis programs, including the US Department of Agriculture's Interactive Healthy Eating Index (9).

2.1.1. MEDICAL HISTORY

Medical history will reveal individual information about acute or chronic diseases or immunologic disorders that are risk factors for individuals with concurrent oral or dental problems that affect their ability to consume their usual diet. Acute or chronic diseases or immunologic disorders are risk factors in patients with concurrent oral and dental problems that affect their ability to consume their usual diet. The 65-yr-old woman whose chief complaint is, "I can't chew my food," is at risk if she has type 2 diabetes mellitus. Diabetes is associated with oral manifestations, particularly when blood sugars are elevated and other disease sequelae are evident. These manifestations, including periodontal disease, dysgeusia, increased caries risk, candidiasis, burning tongue, and poor wound healing, particularly when blood sugars are elevated, may in turn impact appetite, eating ability, and, finally, oral intake *(10)*. Neuropathies and opportunistic microbial infections in the oral cavity affect oral health, nutrition status, and inevitably diabetes control. Complications including burning tongue, gingivitis, and periodontal diseases, along with xerostomia, are common in individuals with diabetes.

Autoimmune diseases such as pemphigus vulgaris increase nutrition risk by virtue of the oral and facial sequelae of the disease and the medications used to manage the disease *(2,3)*. Inflammatory arthritides have associated medication side effects, and joint pain or mechanical limitation may compromise eating ability. Steriod medications used to manage these diseases increase risk of diabetes and nitrogen (protein) and calcium losses, thus increasing protein and calcium needs. The xerostomia associated with Sjögren's syndrome increases risk for dental caries, periodontitis, and oral mucosal injury or pain, which may make eating difficult or painful *(2)*. Temporomandibular joint pain may result in limited opening of the mouth and compromised masticatory ability.

Head and neck and oral cancers affect nutrition and oral health status. Surgery to remove tumors in the oral cavity may have severe functional effects on eating ability. Radiation to the oral cavity can destroy taste as well as the quality and quantity of saliva. Chemotherapy can cause anorexia, stomatitis, nausea, and vomiting, ultimately compromising nutrition status.

Individuals with HIV infection or acquired immunodeficiency syndrome (AIDS) are at increased risk of oral infections and disease manifestations that alter functional and sensory functions of the oral cavity *(11)*. Oral complications and malnutrition may occur secondary to the disease process and associated gastrointestinal, metabolic, immune, pharmacological, and psychosocial sequellae. Altered micronutrient metabolism may contribute to oral manifestations and subsequent malnutrition, further compromising oral integrity and the ability to combat infections. Nutrition screening by the dental professional with a particular focus on the integrity of the oral cavity and medications and their combined impact on oral function is important. A referral to an RD for MNT is routine in this population.

2.1.2. MEDICATIONS AND OTHER OVER-THE-COUNTER PRODUCTS

Adults in the United States are using increasing amounts of over-the-counter (OTC) and prescription medications *(12)*. Drug use tends to be greatest in the elderly *(12)*. Medications used to treat the oral and systemic manifestations of HIV infection, cancer, autoimmune diseases, and cardiovascular diseases, as well as local oral diseases, may also affect a person's ability to ingest, digest, and absorb an adequate diet. Common consequences of several classes of medications—including antiretroviral, antiviral, antifungal, antiparasitic, antihypertensive, antidepressant, antihistamine, narcotic, sedative, and antineoplastic agents—include xerostomia, stomatitis, reduced salivary flow, altered taste, and/or oral ulcers. All of these factors impact food choices, quality and quantity of foods consumed, and the local effect of foods on the oral cavity, leading to compromised nutrient intake *(13)*. Patients should be carefully questioned about use of prescription and OTC drugs, as well as use of herbs, minerals, vitamins, and other dietary supplements. It is up to the provider to review the potential drug–drug, drug–nutrient, drug–symptom, and drug–supplement interactions with patients and guide them appropriately.

2.1.3. DIETARY SUPPLEMENTS

Chapter 6 in this text is dedicated to this topic. Select dietary supplements may alter the integrity of the oral cavity, interfere with action of prescription or OTC medications, and/or alter response to a select therapy. Supplements impacting the immune system such as echinacea may interfere with the actions of immunosuppressing medications secondary to its immune enhancing effects. Other supplements such as ma huang, or ephedra, may have systemic side effects. The principal alkaloids of ephedra are ephedrine and pseudoephedrine. When epinephrine- and ephedrine-containing supplements are taken simultaneously, the resultant stimulatory effects, including increased blood pressure and heart rate and central nervous system stimulation, may be additive (P. Gregory, personal communication, April 2002). The impact of the combination is difficult to estimate because it depends on how much of each agent is taken and the actual ephedrine content of the ephedra-containing supplement consumed. According to the Natural Medicines Comprehensive Database, ephedrine has a short half-life (2.5–3.6 h); it would therefore be prudent to recommend that consumption of ephedrine-containing supplements be withheld for 24 h prior to a dental procedure in which a local anesthetic with epinephrine would be administered.

Part of a routine history and even follow-up appointments should include questions about use of dietary supplements, form, dosage, and frequency. The *Physician's Desk Reference for Herbal Supplements (14)*, the *Natural Medicines Database (15)*, or the *Commission E Monographs (16)* can be used to evaluate potential symptoms and side effects of these dietary supplements.

2.1.4. ORAL EXAM FINDINGS

Although the oral exam is a routine component of the initial workup in the dental office, the diet and nutrition implications are often not considered. Whereas dental professionals may do a comprehensive oral exam, their role is to detect nonnormal findings or symptoms relative to diet and nutrition, provide basic education, and refer patients to the RD. Dietetics professionals can readily add these parameters to their initial physical exam with the caveat that their role is to detect non-normal findings and refer patients to the dentist. The RD can provide baseline guidance relative to oral health and nutrition. Table 6 provides guidelines for dietetics professionals conducting a nutrition-focused oral examination.

Patients with biting, chewing, or swallowing difficulties may be at risk depending on the presence of other risk factors and length and severity of the problem. Simple guidelines on modification of food form and consistency may be adequate for individuals

Table 6
Functional Oral Nutrition Risk Evaluation

Structure	Patient-focused exam	Management
Lips	• Dryness; sensation; cracking or fissuring, swelling; history of blisters or ulcers	• Alter diet texture and consistency
Gingiva and oral mucosa	• Soreness/pain; bleeding spontaneously, change in appearance; swelling, growths, discharge; bad taste; halitosis • Red or white patches/lesions • Erosion/ulceration; focal pigmentation; erythema	• Alter diet texture, temperature, and consistency • Screen for oral cancer, nutrient deficiencies
Teeth	• Toothache/pain; looseness and mobility; dental prosthesis (removable or fixed); edentulism	• Adjust diet, consistency; evaluate caries risk; consider altered taste/smell
Tongue	• Soreness/pain; burning; rough patches; dryness; cracking or fissuring; growths; change in taste; ulcers	• Screen for systemic disease, nutrient deficiencies; alter diet texture
Temporomandibular	• Difficulty or painful opening; grinding sounds on joint opening/chewing with limited range or pain; weakness of chewing muscles	• Change diet consistency, food "hardness"; limit "chewy" foods
Salivary glands	• Mucosal dryness; too little or too much saliva; drooling; change in color, consistency, difficulty swallowing dry food, altered taste, dry	• Increase fluids; evaluate for dysgeusia, dysphagia; limit spices, "hard" foods; review changes in Rx; evaluate zinc
status	eyes; gland pain or swelling	
Neck	• Tender/swollen lymph nodes, other swellings	• Medical consult
Skin	• Change in appearance; rashes, sores, lumps; itching	• Medical consult

Note: For each section, ask about patient complaints, duration of symptom(s), and any changes in appearance, size, acuity, frequency, and pain.

without other nutrition risk factors. Denture wearers or individuals who will be getting dentures for the first time need education on diet modification during the initial fitting and adjustment phases. However, if other risk factors are present, individualized counseling may be indicated.

Individuals with moderate to extensive caries (based on American Dental Association criteria) are at risk and should have their treatment planned for diet and nutrition evaluation and counseling. Individuals with soft-tissue lesions, oral pathologies, orofacial pain or disorders that interfere with the ability to eat, or exam findings suggestive of nutrition deficits should be referred to the RD for MNT.

2.1.5. Eating Disorders

The dental professional has a distinct role in detecting eating disorders, including anorexia and bulimia, given some of the changes that are evident on head, neck, and oral exams. Bitemporal wasting, thinning hair, and boney prominences are symptomatic of anorexia nervosa. Swollen salivary glands, redness in the back of the throat, lingual erosion, and symptoms of frequent regurgitation, sometimes tinged with blood, are common in bulimia. Individuals with eating disorders are at oral and nutrition risk. Such patients should be referred to the RD for evaluation and possible referral to an eating disorder program. Diet evaluation for cariogenic risk and nutritional adequacy and individualized counseling focused on oral health should be completed. Referrals for comprehensive medical care should be provided.

Questions regarding self-imposed diet modifications, "fad" diets, provide insight into abnormal eating patterns that may precipitate nutrient deficits. Any questions on appropriateness or potential risk of the diet should be referred to the RD. Patient questioning should refer to the types, quantity, and duration of supplement use and rationale for use.

2.1.6. OSTEOPOROSIS

Osteoporosis is increasingly common in women (one in two women) and men (one in eight men) *(17)*. The relationship between osteoporosis and oral health is increasingly evident *(18,19)*, particularly in reference to periodontal disease and implant surgery. Chapter 15 provides a detailed insight into oral and nutrition health and osteoporosis. The dental and dietetics professionals should be familiar with high-risk individuals and question them about any history of osteoporosis and whether they have undergone a screening or diagnostic evaluation. Risk factors for osteoporosis *(17)* include the following:

- long-term (more than 1 mo) steroid use;
- hyperparathyroidism, hyperthyroidism, end-stage renal disease;
- history of organ transplants treated with cyclosporine and steroids;
- spinal cord injury;
- women who are perimenopausal or of small stature;
- family history of osteoporosis;
- prolonged low calcium intake combined with inactivity; and
- prolonged lack of exposure to sunlight.

2.1.7. DIETARY HABITS

Questions regarding previous and current diet habits should focus on dietary patterns, nutritional adequacy, and factors influencing eating and fluid intake. Table 4 *(20)* provides suggested questions on factors influencing xerostomia, masticatory function, occlusion, and other risk factors. Responses to these questions will help the dental and dietetics professional identify the impact of oral disease and symptoms on ability to consume foods and fluids. It is assumed that the RD will approach this section of patient assessment in a more detailed manner than the dental professional and provide more targeted nutrition and diet recommendations. However, it is incumbent on the dental professional to ask questions regarding oral function and diet as well as specific questions about diet intake. The following paragraph provides a strategy that is time sensitive and perhaps more reasonable for the dental office setting. It is the strategy used in several dental schools as part of routine patient care.

Dietary habit assessment should include general questions about food habits (*see* the Appendix for nutrition risk evaluation and diet evaluation forms for use in dental practices). The dietary habit assessment will provide insight into caries risk of the diet as well as specific questions about typical daily diet routines. A 24-h recall, or recall of a typical day's diet, will provide a "snapshot" of the patient's diet pattern and a global assessment of nutrient intake. Simply asking a patient to recall everything he or she had to eat and drink on a previous or typical day and recording approximate times, specific foods, and portion sizes is all that is needed. This intake can then be analyzed in one of two ways. For a general assessment of dietary adequacy, the foods and fluids can be quantified into where they fit in the food guide pyramid. Once that is done, one has a general picture of the individual's ability to meet the food group recommendations for the food guide pyramid and any missing or excessive intakes by food group. For a more specific assessment of nutrient adequacy, the diet may be analyzed using one of many computerized nutrient analysis packages. The Interactive Healthy Eating Index *(9)*, available free on the internet, may be used. This provides an assessment of actual calories and macro- and micronutrient intake according to the individual's gender, age, and body size.

Although a thorough diet and nutrition history and analysis are routine for the dietetics professional as a component of MNT, questions regarding oral dysfunction and a clinical exam of the oral cavity are not necessarily routine practice. The RD is encouraged to integrate the components of oral nutrition risk assessment in the tables included in this chapter, along with a brief intra- and extraoral examination *(1)*, into nutrition assessment protocols.

2.1.8. FINAL STEPS

Once the health professional has completed the assessment of risk factors, the determination of nutrition and oral health risk and needs for intervention must occur. In respect to the dental professional, this may include a brief discussion with the patient about recommendations to improve diet and suggestions for diet modification based on identified oral dysfunction or disease, as well as referral to an RD for MNT. In contrast, the dietetics professional will be able to provide comprehensive nutrition care and a diet modified to meet oral disease or dysfunction, along with a referral to a dental professional for dental care.

3. CONCLUSIONS

There are no hard and fast rules to determine nutrition risk levels in dental practice. Nutrition risk is more accurately based on the type and extent of risk factors and their impact on oral function. Examples of conditions or diseases associated with nutrition risk are in each of the chapters of this text.

REFERENCES

1. American Dietetic Association. Oral health and nutrition: position of the American Dietetic Association. J Amer Dietet Assoc 2003; 103:615–625.
2. DePaola DP, Mobley C, Touger-Decker R. Nutrition and oral medicine. In Handbook of Nutrition and Food. New York, NY: CRC Press, 2001, 1113–1134.
3. National Institute of Dental and Craniofacial Research. Spectrum Series. The Oral-Systemic Health Connection. May 1999. Website: (http://www.nidcr.nih.gov/spectrum/NIDCR2/2menu.htm). Accessed April 19, 2002.
4. Papas AS, Palmer CA, Rounds MC, Russell RM. The effects of denture status on nutrition. Special Care in Dentistry 1998; 18:17–25.

5. Ritchie CS, Joshipura K, Silliman RA, Miller B, Douglas CW. Oral health problems and significant weight loss among community-dwelling older adults. J Gerontol Series A Biol Sci Med Sci 2000; 55:M366–371.

6. H.R.5661 Medicare, Medicaid, and SCHIP Benefits Improvement and Protection Act of 2000. Sec. 105. Coverage of Medical Nutrition Therapy Services for Beneficiaries with Diabetes or a Renal Disease. Website: (http://thomas.loc.gov/cgi-bin/query/D?c106:1:./temp/~c106Wgp2IQ:e29796). Accessed August 21, 2002.

7. American Academy of Family Practice. Nutrition Screening Initiative. Website: (http://www.aafp.org/nsi/). Accessed April 19, 2002.

8. Saltzman E, Mogensen K. Physical assessment. In Coulston AM, Rock CL, Monsen ER eds. Nutrition in the Prevention and Treatment of Disease. New York, NY: Academic Press, 2001, 43–55.

9. Anonymous. Interactive Healthy Eating Index. Website: (http://147.208.9.133/Default.asp). Accessed April 19, 2002.

10. Slavkin HC, Baum BJ. Relationship of dental and oral pathology to systemic illness. JAMA 2000; 284: 1215–1217.

11. Sirois DA. Oral manifestations of HIV disease. Mt Sinai J Med 1998; 65:322–332.

12. Kaufman D, Kelly J, Rosenberg L, et al. Recent patterns of medication use in the ambulatory adult population of the United States. JAMA 2002; 287(3):337-344.

13. Position of the American Dietetic Association and the Canadian Dietetic Association: nutrition intervention in the care of persons with human immunodeficiency virus infection. J Am Diet Assoc 2000; 100: 708–717.

14. Greenwald J, Brendler T, Jaenicke C, eds. PDR for Herbal Medicines, 1st ed. Montvale, NJ: Medical Economics, 1998.

15. Jellin JM, ed. Natural Medicines Comprehensive Database. Stockton, CA: Therapeutic Research Faculty, 2002.

16. American Botanical Council. The Complete German Commission E Monographs: Therapeutic Guide to Herbal Medicines. Newton, MA: Integrative Medicine Communications, 1998.

17. National Osteoporosis Foundation. Disease Statistics: Fast Facts. Website: (http://www.nof.org/osteoporosis/stats.htm). Accessed July 2, 2002.

18. Krall EA, Wehler C, Garcia RI, Harris SS, Dawson-Hughes B. Calcium and vitamin D supplements reduce tooth loss in the elderly. Am J Med 2001; 111:452–456.

19. Wactawski-Wende J. Periodontal diseases and osteoporosis: association and mechanisms. Ann Periodontol 2001; 6:197–208.

20. Touger-Decker R. New Jersey Dental School Oral Medicine Clinic Nutrition Manual. 7th Ed. Newark, NJ: New Jersey Dental School, unpublished manual, 2002.

18 Oral Medicine and Nutrition Education

Riva Touger-Decker and David A. Sirois

1. INTRODUCTION

In order to ensure the integration of nutrition and oral health education (and vice versa), it is essential that a body of knowledge for both dietetics and dentistry be delineated *(1)*. A clear understanding of the synergy between oral health and nutrition should be promoted in all health professions' education programs. Nutrition education as a component of pre- and postdoctoral dental education and continuing dental education is important in order to translate theory into practice. Likewise, oral health and disease education as a component of preprofessional and graduate dietetic education and continuing professional education is necessary. This chapter addresses both dental and dietetics professional education and consumer education. Consumer education is critical to ensure the integration of oral and diet/nutrition health behaviors into lifestyles.

2. NUTRITION AND ORAL HEALTH EDUCATION OF HEALTH PROFESSIONALS

In the practice setting, collaborative efforts between dental and dietetics professionals to promote interdisciplinary health care teams will foster successful strategies related to oral health and nutrition. Table 1 *(1)* represents a paradigm for collaboration and referral between dietetics and dental professionals to address oral health and nutrition issues in practice.

To achieve this paradigm, it is essential to foster core knowledge development starting on the preprofessional level. Basic levels of care skills, including risk identification and referral for intervention, are becoming essential for health professionals *(2)* as clients seek comprehensive health care. The Institute of Medicine (IOM) study supports comprehensive training of dental professionals to ensure that they can "assess and treat the whole patient, not just the mouth" *(2)*. The need for preventive health, including institution of improved feeding practices *(2)*, is clearly supported in this report. The 1998 Pew Health Professions Commission Report recommends that relationships between dentists and allied health professionals be developed and expanded and that interdisciplinary competence be required of all health professionals *(3)*.

From: *Nutrition and Oral Medicine*
Edited by: R. Touger-Decker, D. A. Sirois, and C. C. Mobley © Humana Press Inc., Totowa, NJ

Table 1
Dietetics and Dental Professional Role Modeling to Achieve Effective Integration of Oral Health and Nutrition Service in Health Promotion and Disease Prevention and Intervention

1. Dietetics professional

Clinical Setting

- Conduct intra-/extraoral screening and cranial nerve exams.
- Integrate oral health screening as a component of nutrition assessment protocols (i.e., cranial nerve function, occlusion, edentulism, masticatory ability, swallowing, salivary adequacy).
- Recognize oral manifestations of systemic diseases and provide patients with guidelines to maximize oral intake.
- Confer with and refer patients (via consults) to dentists for management of oral symptoms of diseases and/ or risk factors for oral diseases.
- Consult with dental professionals in interpretation of oral nutrition assessment findings and planning in the long-term care setting.

Community Setting

- Establish partnerships with dental professionals in community and private practice settings.
- Develop and implement collaborative oral health and nutrition screening/education programs in schools, worksites, and health maintenance organizations.
- Promote collaborative education on nutrition and oral health among dietetics and dental professionals.
- Develop nutrition education messages that encourage oral health.
- Promote oral health in school and community nutrition programs.

Research Setting

- Promote collaborative nutrition and oral health research initiatives.
- Design and conduct nutrition/diet components of oral health research initiatives.
- Identify and support integration of oral health issues (e.g., screening, disease, management, education) as a component of nutrition research.

2. Dental professional

Clinical Setting

- Include diet screening, education, and referral for oral infectious disease prevention/control, optimal masticatory function, and management of other oral diseases/treatments as a component of comprehensive dental care.
- Collaborate with dietetics professionals in delivery of MNT and provision of oral health care in long-term care settings.
- Provide diet and nutrition guidelines for health promotion and disease prevention to patients and provide guidelines for diet to maximize oral intake.
- Consult with and refer patients (via consult) to dietetics professionals for management of nutrition risk caused by compromised oral health (e.g., caries, immunosuppressive disorders, xerostomia, diabetes, oral surgery, cancer).

Community Setting

- Establish partnerships with dietetics professionals in community and private practice settings to promote nutrition/diet screening and education in dental practice.
- Develop and implement collaborative oral health and nutrition screening/education initiatives in schools, worksites, and health care organizations.
- Promote collaborative education on nutrition and oral health among dietetics and dental professionals.
- Develop oral health messages that integrate nutrition and diet education.
- Promote diet and nutrition as a component of school and community oral health programs.

Research Setting

- Promote collaborative oral health and nutrition research initiatives.
- Design and conduct oral health component of nutrition /diet research initiatives.
- Identify and support integration of nutrition topics as a component of oral health research as appropriate.

Adapted from ref. *1.*

2.1. Nutrition in Dental Education

Dental accreditation standards and the *2000 Competencies for the New Dentist (4,5)* do not specify predoctoral nutrition education competencies. Although the 1990 standards for nutrition in dental education specifically addressed knowledge of basic nutrition, the role of diet and nutrients in health and oral diseases, and nutrition counseling as it relates to oral health, the 1998 standards focus on broad-based competency statements. Nutrition as a component of oral health education is not explicitly stated; it is implied, however, throughout several areas of the competencies and standards. The biomedical sciences standards do not address specific sciences; rather, they must "ensure an in-depth understanding of basic biological principles, consisting of a core of information on fundamental structures, functions and interrelationships of the body systems" *(5)*. Similarly, "in-depth information" must be provided to develop understanding of oral health, oral disease, oral epidemiology, and the role of diet and nutrition in the etiology, diagnosis, prevention, and treatment of oral disease. Knowledge of principles of nutrition and diet and their clinical application in practice is implied throughout the document *(5)* because it provides the underpinning for achievement of several of the competencies. The accreditation standards for the majority of advanced specialty postdoctoral education programs vary in the specificity with which they address nutrition. The specialty postdoctoral program in periodontics does address knowledge of "principles of nutrition, especially as they relate to patient evaluation, disease processes, and wound healing" *(6)*. Other postdoctoral programs include competencies focusing on management of medically compromised patients, those with chronic and terminal diseases, and those who have undergone surgical interventions. Implied in these required competencies is knowledge of diet and nutrition as they relate to comprehensive dental management *(7)*.

In the last decade of the 20th century, several national surveys documented that curriculum hours devoted to nutrition are low compared to time dedicated to other curriculum areas *(8–12)*. These surveys and more recent papers *(1)* have, as the core of their recommendations, the integration of nutrition in the dental curriculum *(10–12)* throughout the 4 yr of didactic and clinical coursework.

Development of a core curriculum on nutrition and oral health for medical, dental, and allied health education has been suggested *(13)*, along with the need to survey the state of the art of nutrition in dental education and vice versa *(13)*. Similarly, neither the standards nor the competencies state the need for demonstration of clinical competence in dental school; however, the need for this is clear in order to translate knowledge into practice. These recommendations are supported by the original Healthy People (HP) 2000 *(14)*, the more recent HP 2010 *(15)*, and the Competencies for Health Care Practitioners for 2005 *(3)*. They highlight the need for expanded access to care by health providers in coordinated teams. Consistent with professional needs and federal and private association recommendations, suggested nutrition curriculum topics in undergraduate dental education include diet and nutrition screening, intervention, and referral; formulation of diet orders; and education strategies *(1–13,15,16)* (*see* Table 2). Historically, the focus of nutrition education in dental schools has been on oral infectious disease management. However, consistent with the rest of health care, the focus has shifted to health promotion, disease prevention, and intervention in oral and systemic diseases *(4,10–12)*. There is sufficient evidence to support the need for competency in

Table 2

Didactic and Practice Components of a Curriculum Model for Dietetics and Dental Education Programs to Promote Collaboration and Multiskilling in Nutrition and Oral Health

Dietetics education (ADA competencies)

1. Baccalaureate Program
   a. Didactic topics
   - Oral anatomy and physiology
   - Oral manifestations of acute, chronic, terminal, and systemic diseases
   - Oral sequellae of medications, chemo-, and radiation therapies
   - Primary diseases of the oral cavity and their effects on taste, smell, and mastication
   b. Clinical Experiences
   - Field visits to dental schools/clinics
   - Work with dental students in clinical/community settings
   - Oral health screening questions as a component of nutrition assessment activities

2. Dietetic Internship/Coordinated Program Competencies
   - Conduct nutrition screening and diet counseling in dental school and community dental clinic rotations
   - Integrate oral health screening questions in diet/nutrition assessment activities
   - Integrate appropriate oral health guidelines into the conduct of diet counseling and education
   - Participate in oral health and nutrition research
   - Perform basic physical assessment including oral and cranial nerve screening exams
   - Design nutrition care plans for patients with compromised oral health

3. Graduate Education
   - Design oral health and nutrition research
   - Perform oral physical assessment exams including intra-/extraoral screening and cranial nerve examinations

4. Continuing Professional Education
   - Collaboration between dietetics and dental professionals in case presentations, multidisciplinary care meetings, conferences about diseases and the lifespan, multidisciplinary seminars
   - Training opportunities using different media; for example, distance learning, CD-ROMs, videotapes

Dental education

1. Doctoral Program
   a. Didactic topics
   - Nutritional biochemistry
   - Nutrition and oral health throughout the life span
   - Diet education and intervention relative to oral health/disease
   - Effect(s) of oral disease(s), symptomatology and their treatment(s) on diet and nutrition status
   - Diet/nutrition screening, education, and referral in dental practice
   - Diet/nutrition concerns and management strategies of high-risk patients
   b. Clinical experiences
   - Self-evaluation of diet
   - Training techniques for diet evaluation and education
   - Nutrition risk screening and diet education relative to oral health of patients
   - Consultation and supervised practice with registered dietitians and/or dietetic technicians

2. Graduate Programs
   - Oral health and nutrition research
   - Integration of nutrition screening and diet education into dental and oral disease specialties
   - Collaborative education endeavors on related topics with dietetics programs

3. Continuing Professional Education
   - Collaboration between dietetics and dental professionals in case presentations, multidisciplinary care meetings, conferences about diseases and the life span, multidisciplinary seminars
   - Multiskilling training opportunities using different media; for example, distance learning, CD-ROMs, videotapes

From ref. *1*.

basic nutrition care by dentists *(1,15)*. Dental visits provide a unique opportunity for dental professionals to integrate lifestyle management (diet and smoking cessation) into treatment and long-term care plans.

Nutrition is clearly delineated in the Accreditation Standards for Dental Hygiene Education Programs *(17)*. The biomedical science component of the curriculum must include nutrition. Clinical instruction competencies indirectly address competency in the ability to evaluate an individual's diet and provide diet education relative to oral health. In the practice setting, it may be the dental hygienist who completes the patient health assessment and any diet or nutrition evaluation, subsequently providing oral hygiene and health promotion instruction including diet.

2.2. Oral Health in Dietetics Education

In a similar venue to dental education and nutrition, oral health education is not outlined as a specific competency or criterion in the standards of education for dietetics education *(18)*. However, the standards do require that entry-level dietetic education programs with a nutrition therapy emphasis include competency in the performance of basic physical assessment. This should include novice-level competency in the performance of a head, neck, and oral screening exam. Because a healthy, functional oral cavity is a necessary part of mastication and digestion, oral health concepts should be incorporated into didactic and clinical training in baccalaureate, preprofessional, and graduate levels of dietetics education (Table 2) *(19)*.

The clinical training of dietetics professionals during dietetic internship or coordinated program clinical experiences should include opportunities for clinical experiences in dental school clinic or dental office settings *(1)*. Students in these programs should be given opportunities to work side by side with dental students or residents in the clinical setting to provide nutrition and diet intervention as a component of oral health management. Competencies in oral screening (head and neck exams, intra- and extraoral assessment, and cranial nerve exams) should be taught to students in the preprofessional setting *(19)*.

At the graduate and professional level, academic and continuing education programs should include research and applications as they relate to medical and nutrition management of orally compromised patients. The conduct of oral assessments and identification of dental risk should be included *(3,19)*.

The educational outcomes of such training include competencies in the identification of nonnormal conditions of the oral cavity; oral dysfunction factors affecting biting, chewing, drinking, and swallowing; and potential nutrient deficiencies. As individuals progress from entry-level to beyond entry-level and advanced-level training, so will their competency in the performance of these outcome competencies. The value of these competencies in nutrition assessment, monitoring, and evaluation across the life span in health and disease will significantly impact development of nutrition care plans and diet protocols.

3. A MODEL FOR COLLABORATION IN NUTRITION AND ORAL HEALTH EDUCATION

The continual shifting of the social and economic realities of today's health care system have had a dramatic effect on the preparation and training of health professionals, including dietetics professionals, dentists, and allied dental personnel. The American

Dietetics Association position on nutrition education of health professionals advocates "that nutrition education is an essential component of the curricula for the majority of health care professionals. Curricula should include nutrition principles and identification of nutrition risk factors" *(15)*.

The need for the recognition of nutrition as an essential part of training for dental professionals and as an important component of educational programs for dietetic and other health professionals *(20)* is clearly delineated in the joint World Health Organization (WHO)/Food and Agricultural Organization expert consultants' recommendation that encouraged this joint approach by international organizations including the WHO and the Food and Agricultural Organization *(20)*. In order to be successful, educators and leaders in oral health and nutrition must promote this dual-content area in the curriculums of other allied health professions. Dental and dietetics professionals need to form networks with other health professionals (e.g., physicians, physician assistants, speech and language pathologists, nurses) to advance health promotion and preventive and community health initiatives that promote oral health and nutrition as they relate to general health. These new models of health care provider cross-training and collaboration will require innovative approaches to new models of health care delivery if training is to successfully carry over to practice. Recommendation 5 of the IOM study states: "To prepare future practitioners for more medically based modes of oral health care and more medically complicated patients, dental educators should work with their colleagues in medical schools and academic health centers" *(2)*.

4. SUMMARY AND NEXT STEPS

This chapter has provided a historical perspective on nutrition and dental education along with 21st-century initiatives and recommendations for nutrition education of dental professionals and oral health education of dietetics professionals (Tables 1 and 2). A collaborative effort of members of both disciplines including academicians, clinicians, and administrators is needed to actualize the recommendations into practice. The practical model envisioned as an outcome of the recommendations within this chapter includes teams of registered dietitian nutrition experts in dental schools and dental faculty in dietetics programs, with both disciplines represented on accreditation boards for dietetics and dentistry. Professional initiatives and federal grants to build such curriculum models and a forum for creating and sharing model curricula would provide the infrastructure to grow and develop these models. Opportunities for collaboration across disciplines exist.

REFERENCES

1. American Dietetic Association. Position of the American Dietetic Association: Oral health and nutrition. J Am Diet Assoc 2003; 103:615–625.
2. Institute of Medicine. Dental education at the crossroads: summary. J Dent Educ 1995; 59(1):7–15.
3. Pew Health Professions Commission. Recreating Health Professional Practice for a New Century: The Fourth Report of the Pew Health Professions Commission. Center for the Health Professions, December 1998.
4. Commission on Dental Accreditation. Accreditation Standards for Dental Education Programs. Chicago: American Dental Association, 1998.
5. American Dental Education Association. The 2000 competencies for the new dentist. Website: (www.adea.org). Accessed January 5, 2004.

6. Commission on Dental Education. Accreditation Standards for Advanced Specialty Education Programs in Periodontics. American Dental Association, 2001.

7. Commission on Dental Accreditation. Accreditation Standards for Advanced Education Programs in General Practice Residency. Chicago, IL: American Dental Association, 1998.

8. DePaola DP, Jacobs JHH, Slim LH. Nutrition education in United States and Canadian schools of dentistry. J Am Diet Assoc 1982; 81:580–583.

9. Faine MP. Nutrition in the dental curriculum: Seattle model. J Dent Educ 1990; 54:510–512.

10. Palmer CA. Applied nutrition dental education: issues and challenges. J Dent Educ 1990; 54:513–518.

11. Touger-Decker R, Gilbride JA. Nutrition education of dental students and professionals. Top Clin Nutr 1997; 12(3)23–32.

12. DePaola D. Nutrition and oral infectious disease workshop recommendations. Boston, MA: The Forsyth Institute, 2000. Website: (www.forsyth.org/nutrition/recommendations.htm). Accessed on May 10, 2002.

13. National Center for Health Statistics. Healthy People 2000 Final Review. Hyattsville, MD: Public Health Service, 2000.

14. U.S. Department of Health and Human Services. Healthy People 2010. 2nd Ed. With Understanding and Improving Health and Objectives for Improving Health. 2 vols. Washington, DC: U.S. Government Printing Office, 2000.

15. Commission on Dental Education. Accreditation Standards for Dental Hygiene Education Programs. Chicago: American Dental Association, 2000.

16. Position of the American Dietetic Association: nutrition education of health professionals. J Am Diet Assoc 1998; 98:343–346.

17. Unpublished draft report of the Joint WHO/FAO expert consultation: Diet, nutrition and the prevention of chronic diseases. April 2002.

18. American Dietetic Association. Knowledge, skills and competencies for entry level dietitian education programs. In Commission on Accreditation for Dietetics Education Accreditation Handbook. Chicago, IL: The American Dietetic Association, 2002. Website: (http://www.eatright.org/Member/Files/CADEHandbook.pdf). Accessed January 5, 2004.

19. Mackle T, Touger-Decker R, O'Sullivan Maillet J, Holland B. Registered dietitians' use of physical assessment parameters in practice. J Am Diet Assoc 2003; 103(12); 1632–1638.

20. Unpublished draft report of the Joint WHO/FAO expert consultation: Diet, nutrition and the prevention of chronic diseases. April 2002.

Appendix A

Oral Nutrition Risk Assessment Tools

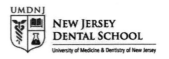

New Jersey Dental School – Diet and Nutrition Risk Evaluation

	YES	NO
Does the patient use any tobacco products? What kind? _____ How much?_____ per day / week For how long? _____		
Does the patient suffer from an immuno-suppressive disorder? If Yes, which one:		
Does the patient have diabetes? Type 1 or Type 2 (circle one). If yes, How is it controlled? Diet, OHA, insulin (circle all that apply). If insulin, list regimen		
Does the patient have high blood pressure?		
Does the patient have new carious lesions? (since last screening evaluation)		
Has the patient had carious lesions in the last three (3) years?		
Does the patient consume sugar-containing drinks, gum or candy > 4 times per day?		
Does the patient perceive to have dry mouth?		
Is the patient > 65 years old?		
Does the patient live alone?		
Height: _____ Weight: _____ BMI: (use BMI chart on reverse side) _____	▓	▓
Has the patient had an unintentional weight change of > 10% in the past 6 months?		
How many teeth does the patient have (maximum 32) _____	▓	▓
Does the patient have RPD? Mandibular or Maxillary (circle one or both)		
Does the patient use it while eating? Mandibular or Maxillary (circle one or both)		
Does the patient complain of poor fit or irritation? Mandibular or Maxillary (circle one or both)		
Does the patient have full denture? Mandibular or Maxillary (circle one or both)		
Does the patient use it while eating? Mandibular or Maxillary (circle one or both)		
Does the patient complain of poor fit or irritation? Mandibular or Maxillary (circle one or both)		
Does the patient have difficulty or pain in biting or chewing foods? (circle all that apply)		
Does the patient have difficulty or pain in swallowing (circle all that apply)		
Does the patient have soft tissue lesions or oral infections that interfere with eating? (e.g. ulcers, angular cheilitis, candidiasis)		
Does the patient have difficulty shopping for, or preparing food?		
Does the patient run out of money for food during the month?		
Does the patient take vitamin, mineral, or other dietary supplements? If yes, list type and dosage:		
Does the patient follow a special diet? If yes, type of diet:		
Does the patient present with an eating disorder? Anorexia Bulimia Obesity (circle all that apply)		

DATE COMPLETED: _____

DATE REVISED:_____

University of Texas at San Antonio Dental School

Patient Name ——————————————— **Age** ——————— **Patient Number** ————

Oral Health Evaluation

Note: Use a ballpoint pen, press firmly, you are making 4 copies. For edentulous patients, complete items 1-5, 13-16, and 19-21.

CARIES RISK ASSESSMENT

Dietary Screening for caries risk		Date →	/ /
1	Do you eat food or drink beverages five or more times a day?	1 pt if yes	
2	Do you chew regular (non-sugar-free) gum?	1 pt if yes	
3	Do you drink any sweetened beverages between meals?	2 pts if yes	
4	Do you eat mints, candies, pastries, chips, crackers, etc., between meals?	2 pts if yes	
5	Do you drink milk or eat cheese every day?	1 pt if no	
Dietary Screening Total			

Caries Activity – consider clinical findings, radiographic interpretation and other findings incorporated into caries charting approved by faculty. Use caries assessment and management decision trees.

6	Are carious lesions present? (cavitated)	3 pts if yes	
7	Number of carious lesions (include coronal and root caries): (cavitated)	1 pt each	
8	Number of carious lesions limited to enamel (incipient, uncavitated) and incipient of root	1 pt each	
9	Five or more filled surfaces (amalgams, composites, crowns)?	2 pts if yes	
10	One or more teeth missing due to caries?	2 pts if yes	
Caries Activity Total			

Fluoride Exposure			
11	No fluoride from water, tablets or drops?	1 pt	
12	No fluoride from regular personal use of toothpaste, rinse or gel?	1 pt	

Caries Risk Assessment (Total of # 1-12)

Very High – CRA Score > 15, or > 4 cavitated lesions	Caries Risk Category at Left	
High – CRA Score 10-15, or 3-4 cavitated lesions	Caries Risk Category after indicated Saliva Tests (See Below*)	
Mod – CRA Score 5-9		
Low – CRA Score 4 or less		

XEROSTOMIA SCREENING (JADA 115; 581, 1987)

13	Does your mouth feel dry when eating a meal?	Y/N	
14	Do you have difficulty swallowing food?	Y/N	
15	Do you have to sip liquids needed to aid in swallowing?	Y/N	
16	Is the amount of saliva in your mouth "too little" most of the time?	Y/N	

Indications for Additional Testing:

Diet

If Caries Risk Assessment is Very High or High, or Dietary Screening Total > 3:
- ☐ Complete 24 hour recall diet diary
- ☐ Otherwise - these additional dietary assessments are not indicated for caries.

The analysis of this dietary data and the dietary screening will lead to specific desirable dietary changes to be entered in the daily treatment record, and acted on through patient counseling and reinforcement.
- ☐ A 3 day prospective diet diary may be required in consultation with faculty

Saliva Tests

If Caries Activity Total is > 5, or Dietary Screening Total > 3, or Xerostomia Screening includes >1 'YES':
- ☐ a) Determine unstimulated saliva flow rate AND
- ☐ b) Collect stimulated whole saliva for M. Strep count for lab OR
- ☐ Otherwise - additional saliva tests are not indicated

  a)_____ml/min
  b)_____cfu/ml

* Revised Caries Risk Assessment
If (a) is < 0.2 ml/min. or (b) > 5.5 x 10⁵ cfu/ml, raise caries risk category by one and enter new or unchanged category above, at "Caries Risk Category after indicated Saliva Tests".

OTHER ORAL HEALTH RISK FACTORS

1 7	PSR or full perio. evaluation indicates periodontal prevention will be required?	Y/N	
1 8	Poor oral hygiene? (Plaque index >20%)	Y/N	
1 9	Presence of any systemic disease which compromises oral health?	Y/N	
2 0	Oral cancer risk factors? (alcohol, tobacco, sunlight, history of oral cancer)	Y/N	
2 1	Risk of oral injury? (contact sport, no seatbelt use, physical abuse)	Y/N	
2 2	Evidence of tooth erosion?	Y/N	

White – Community Dentistry   Yellow – Chart Copy   Pink – Chart Copy   Gold – Community Dentistry

Faculty signature_____ Faculty ID_____ Date_____

University of Texas at San Antonio Dental School

Patient Name _____ Age _____ Patient Number _____

Student Name _____ Student Number _____

Oral Health Reevaluation _____

Note: If patient is edentulous, reevaluation does not apply.

CARIES RISK ASSESSMENT			
Dietary Screening for caries risk at Re-evaluation	Date →	/ /	/ /
1 Do you eat food or drink beverages five or more times a day?	1 pt if yes		
2 Do you chew regular (non-sugar-free) gum?	1 pt if yes		
3 Do you drink any sweetened beverages between meals?	2 pts if yes		
4 Do you eat mints, candies, pastries, chips, crackers, etc., between meals?	2 pts if yes		
5 Do you drink milk or eat cheese every day?	1 pt if no		
Dietary Screening Total			
Caries Activity at Re-evaluation – consider clinical findings, radiographic interpretation and other findings incorporated into caries charting approved by faculty. Use caries assessment and management decision trees.			
6 Are carious lesions present? (cavitated)	3 pts if yes		
7 Number of carious lesions (include coronal and root caries): (cavitated)	1 pt each		
8 Number of carious lesions limited to enamel (incipient, uncavitated) and incipient of root	1 pt each		
9 Five or more filled surfaces (amalgams, composites, crowns)?	2 pts if yes		
10 One or more teeth missing due to caries?	2 pts if yes		
Caries Activity Total			
Fluoride Exposure at Re-Evaluation			
11 No fluoride from water, tablets or drops?	1 pt		
12 No fluoride from regular personal use of toothpaste, rinse or gel?	1 pt		
Caries Risk Assessment (Total of # 1-12) at Re-evaluation			

Very High – CRA Score > 15, or > 4 cavitated lesions High – CRA Score 10-15, or 3-4 cavitated lesions Moderate – CRA Score 5-9 Low – CRA Score 4 or less	**Caries Risk Category at Re-evaluation** **Re-evaluated Caries Risk** – raised one category if indicated by retest 18 or 19 - See Below †		

Prior Dietary Evaluation ☐ 24-hour ☐ 3-day ☐ Dietary Screen Only		
13 Was diet found to be caries-promoting?	Y/N	
14 What were the most prevailing caries-promoting factors? ☐ Soda or other sweetened beverages ☐ Starchy processed snack foods ☐ Sweet processed snack foods ☐ Patterns of eating ☐ Absence of cariostatic foods (dairy products, sugar substitute products) ☐ Others_____		
15 Is patient compliant with dietary recommendations?	Y/N	
16 Are further dietary recommendations needed? If yes, make a chart note.	Y/N	

OTHER ORAL HEALTH RISK FACTORS AT RE-EVALUATION		
17 Poor oral hygiene? Rescore if originally >20%	Y/N	
18 **Retest** saliva flow rate - if originally <0.2ml/min. (unstim)† ____ml/min	Y/N	
19 **Retest** Mutans strep count - if originally >5.5x10⁵ cfu/ml† ____cfu/ml	Y/N	
20 Oral cancer risk factors? (alcohol, tobacco, sunlight, history of oral cancer)	Y/N	
21 Risk of oral injury? (contact sport, no seatbelt use, physical abuse)	Y/N	

If prevention is to be changed or Preventive Behaviors reinforced, refer to the original Preventive Plan Guide and enter changes on the Prevention and Treatment Plan Additions Form, and below.   Add (+)   Delete (-)   Substitute (=)

Change Code (+ /- / =)	Phase	ADA Code	Tooth/Surface	Description

Faculty sig. (Eval.)_____ Faculty ID_____ Date_____

Faculty sig. (Reeval.)_____ Faculty ID_____ Date_____ REV 6/01

Appendix B
Body Mass Index Table

The following table shows Body Weight (pounds) by Height (inches) and BMI. BMI categories: Normal (BMI 19–24), Overweight (BMI 25–29), Obese (BMI 30–39), Extreme Obesity (BMI 40–54).

BMI → Height (inches) ↓	19	20	21	22	23	24	25	26	27	28	29	30	31	32	33	34	35	36	37	38	39	40	41	42	43	44	45	46	47	48	49	50	51	52	53	54
58	91	96	100	105	110	115	119	124	129	134	138	143	148	153	158	162	167	172	177	181	186	191	196	201	205	210	215	220	224	229	234	239	244	248	253	258
59	94	99	104	109	114	119	124	128	133	138	143	148	153	158	163	168	173	178	183	188	193	198	203	208	212	217	222	227	232	237	242	247	252	257	262	267
60	97	102	107	112	118	123	128	133	138	143	148	153	158	163	168	174	179	184	189	194	199	204	209	215	220	225	230	235	240	245	250	255	261	266	271	276
61	100	106	111	116	122	127	132	137	143	148	153	158	164	169	174	180	185	190	195	201	206	211	217	222	227	232	238	243	248	254	259	264	269	275	280	285
62	104	109	115	120	126	131	136	142	147	153	158	164	169	175	180	186	191	196	202	207	213	218	224	229	235	240	246	251	256	262	267	273	278	284	289	295
63	107	113	118	124	130	135	141	146	152	158	163	169	175	180	186	191	197	203	208	214	220	225	231	237	242	248	254	259	265	270	278	282	287	293	299	304
64	110	116	122	128	134	140	145	151	156	162	168	174	180	186	192	197	204	209	215	221	227	232	238	244	250	256	262	267	273	279	285	291	296	302	308	314
65	114	120	126	132	138	144	150	156	162	168	174	180	186	192	198	204	210	216	222	228	234	240	246	252	258	264	270	276	282	288	294	300	306	312	318	324
66	118	124	130	136	142	148	155	161	167	173	179	186	192	198	204	210	216	223	229	235	241	247	253	260	266	272	278	284	291	297	303	309	315	322	328	334
67	121	127	134	140	146	153	159	166	172	178	185	191	198	204	211	217	223	230	236	242	249	255	261	268	274	280	287	293	299	306	312	319	325	331	338	344
68	125	131	138	144	151	158	164	171	177	184	190	197	203	210	216	223	230	236	243	249	256	262	269	276	282	289	295	302	308	315	322	328	335	341	348	354
69	128	135	142	149	155	162	169	176	182	189	196	203	209	216	223	230	236	243	250	257	263	270	277	284	291	297	304	311	318	324	331	338	345	351	358	365
70	132	139	146	153	160	167	174	181	188	195	202	209	216	222	229	236	243	250	257	264	271	278	285	292	299	306	313	320	327	334	341	348	355	362	369	376
71	136	143	150	157	165	172	179	186	193	200	208	215	222	229	236	243	250	257	265	272	279	286	293	301	308	315	322	329	338	343	351	358	365	372	379	386
72	140	147	154	162	169	177	184	191	199	206	213	221	228	235	242	250	258	265	272	279	287	294	302	309	316	324	331	338	346	353	361	368	375	383	390	397
73	144	151	159	166	174	182	189	197	204	212	219	227	235	242	250	257	265	272	280	288	295	302	310	318	325	333	340	348	355	363	371	378	386	393	401	408
74	148	155	163	171	179	186	194	202	210	218	225	233	241	249	256	264	272	280	287	295	303	311	319	326	334	342	350	358	365	373	381	389	396	404	412	420
75	152	160	168	176	184	192	200	208	216	224	232	240	248	256	264	272	279	287	295	303	311	319	327	335	343	351	359	367	375	383	391	399	407	415	423	431
76	156	164	172	180	189	197	205	213	221	230	238	246	254	263	271	279	287	295	304	312	320	328	336	344	353	361	369	377	385	394	402	410	418	426	435	443

Source: Adapted from *Clinical Guidelines on the Identification, Evaluation, and Treatment of Overweight and Obesity in Adults: The Evidence Report.*

From National Institutes of Health, National Heart, Lung and Blood Institute, Website: http://www.nhlbi.nih.gov/guidelines/obesity/bmi_tbl.htm

Appendix C

Dietary Reference Intake Charts

Dietary Reference Intakes: Vitamins

Nutrient	Function	Life Stage Group	RDA/AI*	UL[a]	Selected Food Sources	Adverse effects of excessive consumption	Special Considerations
Biotin	Coenzyme in synthesis of fat, glycogen, and amino acids		(μg/d)		Liver and smaller amounts in fruits and meats	No adverse effects of biotin in humans or animals were found. This does not mean that there is no potential for adverse effects resulting from high intakes. Because data on the adverse effects of biotin are limited, caution may be warranted.	None
		Infants					
		0–6 mo	5*	ND[b]			
		7–12 mo	6*	ND			
		Children					
		1–3 y	8*	ND			
		4–8 y	12*	ND			
		Males					
		9–13 y	20*	ND			
		14–18 y	25*	ND			
		19–30 y	30*	ND			
		31–50 y	30*	ND			
		50–70 y	30*	ND			
		> 70 y	30*	ND			
		Females					
		9–13 y	20*	ND			
		14–18 y	25*	ND			
		19–30 y	30*	ND			
		31–50 y	30*	ND			
		50–70 y	30*	ND			
		> 70 y	30*	ND			
		Pregnancy					
		≤ 18 y	30*	ND			
		19–30y	30*	ND			
		31–50 y	30*	ND			
		Lactation					
		≤ 18 y	35*	ND			
		19–30y	35*	ND			
		31–50 y	35*	ND			

Choline		AI (mg/d)	UL (mg/d)	Selected Food Sources	Adverse Effects of Excessive Consumption	Special Considerations
Precursor for acetylcholine, phospholipids and betaine				Milk, liver, eggs, peanuts	Fishy body odor, sweating, salivation, hypotension, hepatotoxicity	Individuals with trimethylaminuria, renal disease, liver disease, depression and Parkinson's disease, may be at risk of adverse effects with choline intakes at the UL.
Infants	0–6 mo	125*	ND			Although AIs have been set for choline, there are few data to assess whether a dietary supply of choline is needed at all stages of the life cycle, and it may be that the choline requirement can be met by endogenous synthesis at some of these stages.
	7–12 mo	150*	ND			
Children	1–3 y	200*	1000			
	4–8 y	250*	1000			
Males	9–13 y	375*	2000			
	14–18 y	550*	3000			
	19–30 y	550*	3500			
	31–50 y	550*	3500			
	50–70 y	550*	3500			
	>70 y	550*	3500			
Females	9–13 y	375*	2000			
	14–18 y	400*	3000			
	19–30 y	425*	3500			
	31–50 y	425*	3500			
	50–70 y	425*	3500			
	>70 y	425*	3500			
Pregnancy	≤ 18 y	450*	3000			
	19-30y	450*	3500			
	31-50 y	450*	3500			
Lactation	≤ 18 y	550*	3000			
	19-30y	550*	3500			
	31–50 y	550*	3500			

NOTE: The table is adapted from the DRI reports, see www.nap.edu. It represents Recommended Dietary Allowances (RDAs) in **bold type**. Adequate Intakes (AIs) in ordinary type followed by an asterisk (*), and Tolerable Upper Intake Levels (ULs)[a]. RDAs and AIs may both be used as goals for individual intake. RDAs are set to meet the needs of almost all (97 to 98 percent) individuals in a group. For healthy breastfed infants, the AI is the mean intake. The AI for other life stage and gender groups is believed to cover the needs of all individuals in the group, but lack of data prevent being able to specify with confidence the percentage of individuals covered by this intake.

[a]UL = The maximum level of daily nutrient intake that is likely to pose no risk of adverse effects. Unless otherwise specified, the UL represents total intake from food, water, and supplements. Due to lack of suitable data, ULs could not be established for vitamin K, thiamin, riboflavin, vitamin B12, pantothenic acid, biotin, or carotenoids. In the absence of ULs, extra caution may be warranted in consuming levels above recommended intakes.

[b]ND = Not determinable due to lack of data of adverse effects in this age group and concern with regard to lack of ability to handle excess amounts. Source of intake should be from food only to prevent high levels of intake.

SOURCES: *Dietary Reference Intakes for Calcium, Phosphorous, Magnesium, Vitamin D, and Fluoride* (1997); *Dietary Reference Intakes for Thiamin, Riboflavin, Niacin, Vitamin B6, Folate, Vitamin B12, Pantothenic Acid, Biotin, and Choline* (1998); *Dietary Reference Intakes for Vitamin C, Vitamin E, Selenium, and Carotenoids* (2000); and *Dietary Reference Intakes for Vitamin A, Vitamin K, Arsenic, Boron, Chromium, Copper, Iodine, Iron, Manganese, Molybdenum, Nickel, Silicon, Vanadium, and Zinc* (2001). These reports may be accessed via www.nap.edu.

Dietary Reference Intakes: Vitamins

Nutrient	Function	Life Stage Group	RDA/AI*	UL[a]	Selected Food Sources	Adverse effects of excessive consumption	Special Considerations
Folate Also known as: Folic acid Folacin Pteroylpolyglutamates Note: Given as dietary folate equivalents (DFE). 1 DFE = 1 µg food folate = 0.6 µg of folate from fortified food or as a supplement consumed with food = 0.5 µg of a supplement taken on an empty stomach.	Coenzyme in the metabolism of nucleic and amino acids; prevents megaloblastic anemia	Infants 0–6 mo 7–12 mo	(µg/d) 65* 80*	(µg/d) ND[b] ND	Enriched cereal grains, dark leafy vegetables, enriched and whole-grain breads and bread products, fortified ready-to-eat cereals	Masks neurological complication in people with vitamin B_{12} deficiency. No adverse effects associated with folate from food or supplements have been reported. This does not mean that there is no potential for adverse effects resulting from high intakes. Because data on the adverse effects of folate are limited, caution may be warranted. The UL for folate applies to synthetic forms obtained from supplements and/or fortified foods.	In view of evidence linking folate intake with neural tube defects in the fetus, it is recommended that all women capable of becoming pregnant consume 400 µg from supplements or fortified foods in addition to intake of food folate from a varied diet. It is assumed that women will continue consuming 400 µg from supplements or fortified food until their pregnancy is confirmed and they enter prenatal care, which ordinarily occurs after the end of the periconceptional period—the critical time for formation of the neural tube.
		Children 1–3 y 4–8 y	150 200	300 400			
		Males 9–13 y 14–18 y 19–30 y 31–50 y 50–70 y >70 y	300 400 400 400 400 400	600 800 1,000 1,000 1,000 1,000			
		Females 9–13 y 14–18 y 19–30 y 31–50 y 50–70 y >70 y	300 400 400 400 400 400	600 800 1,000 1,000 1,000 1,000			
		Pregnancy ≤18 y 19–30y 31–50 y	600 600 600	800 1,000 1,000			
		Lactation ≤18 y 19–30y 31–50 y	500 500 500	800 1,000 1,000			

316

Niacin	Life Stage Group	(mg/d)	(mg/d)	Meat, fish, poultry, enriched and whole-grain breads and bread products, fortified ready-to-eat cereals	There is no evidence of adverse effects from the consumption of naturally occurring niacin in foods. Adverse effects from niacin containing supplements may include flushing and gastrointestinal distress. The UL for niacin applies to synthetic forms obtained from supplements, fortified foods, or a combination of the two.	Extra niacin may be required by persons treated with hemodialysis or peritoneal dialysis, or those with malabsorption syndrome.
Includes nicotinic acid amide, nicotinic acid (pyridine-3-carboxylic acid), and derivatives that exhibit the biological activity of nicotinamide. Note: Given as niacin equivalents (NE). 1 mg of niacin = 60 mg of tryptophan; 0–6 months = preformed niacin (not NE).	Infants					
Coenzyme or cosubstrate in many biological reduction and oxidation reactions—thus required for energy metabolism	0–6 mo	2*	ND			
	7–12 mo	4*	ND			
	Children					
	1–3 y	6	10			
	4–8 y	8	15			
	Males					
	9–13 y	12	20			
	14–18 y	16	30			
	19–30 y	16	35			
	31–50 y	16	35			
	50–70 y	16	35			
	>70 y	16	35			
	Females					
	9–13 y	12	20			
	14–18 y	14	30			
	19–30 y	14	35			
	31–50 y	14	35			
	50–70 y	14	35			
	>70 y	14	35			
	Pregnancy					
	≤18 y	18	30			
	19–30y	18	35			
	31–50 y	18	35			
	Lactation					
	≤18 y	17	30			
	19–30y	17	35			
	31–50 y	17	35			

NOTE: The table is adapted from the DRI reports, see www.nap.edu. It represents Recommended Dietary Allowances (RDAs) in **bold type**. Adequate Intakes (AIs) in ordinary type followed by an asterisk (*), and Tolerable Upper Intake Levels (ULs)[a]. RDAs and AIs may both be used as goals for individual intake. RDAs are set to meet the needs of almost all (97 to 98 percent) individuals in a group. For healthy breastfed infants, the AI is the mean intake. The AI for other life stage and gender groups is believed to cover the needs of all individuals in the group, but lack of data prevent being able to specify with confidence the percentage of individuals covered by this intake.

[a]UL = The maximum level of daily nutrient intake that is likely to pose no risk of adverse effects. Unless otherwise specified, the UL represents total intake from food, water, and supplements. Due to lack of suitable data, ULs could not be established for vitamin K, thiamin, riboflavin, vitamin B₁₂, pantothenic acid, biotin, or carotenoids. In the absence of ULs, extra caution may be warranted in consuming levels above recommended intakes.

[b]ND = Not determinable due to lack of data of adverse effects in this age group and concern with regard to lack of ability to handle excess amounts. Source of intake should be from food only to prevent high levels of intake.

SOURCES: *Dietary Reference Intakes for Calcium, Phosphorous, Magnesium, Vitamin D, and Fluoride* (1997); *Dietary Reference Intakes for Thiamin, Riboflavin, Niacin, Vitamin B₆, Folate, Vitamin B₁₂, Pantothenic Acid, Biotin, and Choline* (1998); *Dietary Reference Intakes for Vitamin C, Vitamin E, Selenium, and Carotenoids* (2000); and *Dietary Reference Intakes for Vitamin A, Vitamin K, Arsenic, Boron, Chromium, Copper, Iodine, Iron, Manganese, Molybdenum, Nickel, Silicon, Vanadium, and Zinc* (2001). These reports may be accessed via www.nap.edu.

Dietary Reference Intakes: Vitamins

Nutrient	Function	Life Stage Group	RDA/AI*	UL[a]	Selected Food Sources	Adverse effects of excessive consumption	Special Considerations
Pantothenic Acid	Coenzyme in fatty acid metabolism	Infants	(mg/d)	(mg/d)	Chicken, beef, potatoes, oats, cereals, tomato products, liver, kidney, yeast, egg yolk, broccoli, whole grains	No adverse effects associated with pantothenic acid from food or supplements have been reported. This does not mean that there is no potential for adverse effects resulting from high intakes. Because data on the adverse effects of pantothenic acid are limited, caution may be warranted.	None
		0–6 mo	1.7*	ND[b]			
		7–12 mo	1.8*	ND			
		Children					
		1–3 y	2*	ND			
		4–8 y	3*	ND			
		Males					
		9–13 y	4*	ND			
		14–18 y	5*	ND			
		19–30 y	5*	ND			
		31–50 y	5*	ND			
		50-70 y	5*	ND			
		> 70 y	5*	ND			
		Females					
		9–13 y	4*	ND			
		14–18 y	5*	ND			
		19–30 y	5*	ND			
		31–50 y	5*	ND			
		50-70 y	5*	ND			
		> 70 y	5*	ND			
		Pregnancy					
		≤ 18 y	6*	ND			
		19-30y	6*	ND			
		31-50 y	6*	ND			
		Lactation					
		≤ 18 y	7*	ND			
		19-30y	7*	ND			
		31–50 y	7*	ND			

Riboflavin

Also known as: Vitamin B₂

Function: Coenzyme in numerous redox reactions

Food sources: Organ meats, milk, bread products and fortified cereals

Adverse effects of excessive consumption: No adverse effects associated with riboflavin consumption from food or supplements have been reported. This does not mean that there is no potential for adverse effects resulting from high intakes. Because data on the adverse effects of riboflavin are limited, caution may be warranted.

Special considerations: None

Life Stage Group	RDA/AI (mg/d)	UL[b] (mg/d)
Infants		
0–6 mo	0.3*	ND
7–12 mo	0.4*	ND
Children		
1–3 y	0.5	ND
4–8 y	0.6	ND
Males		
9–13 y	0.9	ND
14–18 y	1.3	ND
19–30 y	1.3	ND
31–50 y	1.3	ND
50–70 y	1.3	ND
>70 y	1.3	ND
Females		
9–13 y	0.9	ND
14–18 y	1.0	ND
19–30 y	1.1	ND
31–50 y	1.1	ND
50–70 y	1.1	ND
>70 y	1.1	ND
Pregnancy		
≤18 y	1.4	ND
19–30y	1.4	ND
31–50 y	1.4	ND
Lactation		
≤18 y	1.6	ND
19–30y	1.6	ND
31–50 y	1.6	ND

NOTE: The table is adapted from the DRI reports, see www.nap.edu. It represents Recommended Dietary Allowances (RDAs) in **bold type**. Adequate Intakes (AIs) in ordinary type followed by an asterisk (*), and Tolerable Upper Intake Levels (ULs)[a]. RDAs and AIs may both be used as goals for individual intake. RDAs are set to meet the needs of almost all (97 to 98 percent) individuals in a group. For healthy breastfed infants, the AI is the mean intake. The AI for other life stage and gender groups is believed to cover the needs of all individuals in the group, but lack of data prevent being able to specify with confidence the percentage of individuals covered by this intake.

[a]UL = The maximum level of daily nutrient intake that is likely to pose no risk of adverse effects. Unless otherwise specified, the UL represents total intake from food, water, and supplements. Due to lack of suitable data, ULs could not be established for vitamin K, thiamin, riboflavin, vitamin B₁₂, pantothenic acid, biotin, or carotenoids. In the absence of ULs, extra caution may be warranted in consuming levels above recommended intakes.

[b]ND = Not determinable due to lack of data of adverse effects in this age group and concern with regard to lack of ability to handle excess amounts. Source of intake should be from food only to prevent high levels of intake.

SOURCES: *Dietary Reference Intakes for Calcium, Phosphorous, Magnesium, Vitamin D, and Fluoride* (1997); *Dietary Reference Intakes for Thiamin, Riboflavin, Niacin, Vitamin B₆, Folate, Vitamin B₁₂, Pantothenic Acid, Biotin, and Choline* (1998); *Dietary Reference Intakes for Vitamin C, Vitamin E, Selenium, and Carotenoids* (2000); and *Dietary Reference Intakes for Vitamin A, Vitamin K, Arsenic, Boron, Chromium, Copper, Iodine, Iron, Manganese, Molybdenum, Nickel, Silicon, Vanadium, and Zinc* (2001). These reports may be accessed via www.nap.edu.

Dietary Reference Intakes: Vitamins

Nutrient	Function	Life Stage Group	RDA/AI*	UL[a]	Selected Food Sources	Adverse effects of excessive consumption	Special Considerations
Thiamin Also known as: Vitamin B₁ Aneurin	Coenzyme in the metabolism of carbohydrates and branched-chain amino acids	Infants 0–6 mo 7–12 mo	(mg/d) 0.2* 0.3*	ND[b] ND	Enriched, fortified, or whole-grain products; bread and bread products, mixed foods whose main ingredient is grain, and ready-to-eat cereals	No adverse effects associated with thiamin from food or supplements have been reported. This does not mean that there is no potential for adverse effects resulting from high intakes. Because data on the adverse effects of thiamin are limited, caution may be warranted.	Persons who may have increased needs for thiamin include those being treated with hemodialysis or peritoneal dialysis, or individuals with malabsorption syndrome.
		Children 1–3 y 4–8 y	0.5 0.6	ND ND			
		Males 9–13 y 14–18 y 19–30 y 31-50 y 50-70 y > 70 y	0.9 1.2 1.2 1.2 1.2 1.2	ND ND ND ND ND ND			
		Females 9–13 y 14–18 y 19–30 y 31-50 y 50-70 y > 70 y	0.9 1.0 1.1 1.1 1.1 1.1	ND ND ND ND ND ND			
		Pregnancy ≤ 18 y 19-30y 31-50 y	1.4 1.4 1.4	ND ND ND			
		Lactation ≤ 18 y 19-30y 31–50 y	1.4 1.4 1.4	ND ND ND			

Vitamin A	Life Stage Group	(µg/d)	(µg/d)	Food sources	Adverse effects	Special considerations
Includes provitamin A carotenoids that are dietary precursors of retinol. Note: Given as retinol activity equivalents (RAEs). 1 RAE = 1 µg retinol, 12 µg β-carotene, 24 µg α-carotene, or 24 µg β-cryptoxanthin. To calculate RAEs from REs of provitamin A carotenoids in foods, divide the REs by 2. For preformed vitamin A in foods or supplements and for provitamin A carotenoids in supplements, 1 RE = 1 RAE. Required for normal vision, gene expression, reproduction, embryonic development and immune function	**Infants** 0–6 mo 7–12 mo	400* 500*	600 600	Liver, dairy products, fish, darkly colored fruits and leafy vegetables	Teratological effects, liver toxicity Note: From preformed Vitamin A only.	Individuals with high alcohol intake, pre-existing liver disease, hyperlipidemia or severe protein malnutrition may be distinctly susceptible to the adverse effects of excess preformed vitamin A intake. β-carotene supplements are advised only to serve as a provitamin A source for individuals at risk of vitamin A deficiency.
	Children 1–3 y 4–8 y	**300** **400**	600 900			
	Males 9–13 y 14–18 y 19–30 y 31–50 y 50–70 y >70 y	**600** **900** **900** **900** **900** **900**	1,700 2,800 3,000 3,000 3,000 3,000			
	Females 9–13 y 14–18 y 19–30 y 31–50 y 50–70 y >70 y	**600** **700** **700** **700** **700** **700**	1,700 2,800 3,000 3,000 3,000 3,000			
	Pregnancy ≤18 y 19–30y 31–50 y	**750** **770** **770**	2,800 3,000 3,000			
	Lactation ≤18 y 19–30y 31–50 y	**1,200** **1,300** **1,300**	2,800 3,000 3,000			

NOTE: The table is adapted from the DRI reports, see www.nap.edu. It represents Recommended Dietary Allowances (RDAs) in **bold type**. Adequate Intakes (AIs) in ordinary type followed by an asterisk (*), and Tolerable Upper Intake Levels (ULs)[a]. RDAs and AIs may both be used as goals for individual intake. RDAs are set to meet the needs of almost all (97 to 98 percent) individuals in a group. For healthy breastfed infants, the AI is the mean intake. The AI for other life stage and gender groups is believed to cover the needs of all individuals in the group, but lack of data prevent being able to specify with confidence the percentage of individuals covered by this intake.

[a]UL = The maximum level of daily nutrient intake that is likely to pose no risk of adverse effects. Unless otherwise specified, the UL represents total intake from food, water, and supplements. Due to lack of suitable data, ULs could not be established for vitamin K, thiamin, riboflavin, vitamin B$_{12}$, pantothenic acid, biotin, or carotenoids. In the absence of ULs, extra caution may be warranted in consuming levels above recommended intakes.

[b]ND = Not determinable due to lack of data of adverse effects in this age group and concern with regard to lack of ability to handle excess amounts. Source of intake should be from food only to prevent high levels of intake.

SOURCES: *Dietary Reference Intakes for Calcium, Phosphorous, Magnesium, Vitamin D, and Fluoride* (1997); *Dietary Reference Intakes for Thiamin, Riboflavin, Niacin, Vitamin B$_6$, Folate, Vitamin B$_{12}$, Pantothenic Acid, Biotin, and Choline* (1998); *Dietary Reference Intakes for Vitamin C, Vitamin E, Selenium, and Carotenoids* (2000); and *Dietary Reference Intakes for Vitamin A, Vitamin K, Arsenic, Boron, Chromium, Copper, Iodine, Iron, Manganese, Molybdenum, Nickel, Silicon, Vanadium, and Zinc* (2001). These reports may be accessed via www.nap.edu.

Dietary Reference Intakes: Vitamins

Nutrient	Function	Life Stage Group	RDA/AI* (mg/d)	UL[a] (mg/d)	Selected Food Sources	Adverse effects of excessive consumption	Special Considerations
Vitamin B6	Coenzyme in the metabolism of amino acids, glycogen and sphingoid bases	Infants			Fortified cereals, organ meats, fortified soy-based meat substitutes	No adverse effects associated with Vitamin B6 from food have been reported. This does not mean that there is no potential for adverse effects resulting from high intakes. Because data on the adverse effects of Vitamin B6 are limited, caution may be warranted.	None
		0–6 mo	0.1*	ND[b]			
		7–12 mo	0.3*	ND			
Vitamin B6 comprises a group of six related compounds: pyridoxal, pyridoxine, pyridoxamine, and 5'-phosphates (PLP, PNP, PMP)		Children					
		1–3 y	0.5	30			
		4–8 y	0.6	40			
		Males				Sensory neuropathy has occurred from high intakes of supplemental forms.	
		9–13 y	1.0	60			
		14–18 y	1.3	80			
		19–30 y	1.3	100			
		31-50 y	1.3	100			
		50-70 y	1.7	100			
		> 70 y	1.7	100			
		Females					
		9–13 y	1.0	60			
		14–18 y	1.2	80			
		19–30 y	1.3	100			
		31-50 y	1.3	100			
		50-70 y	1.5	100			
		> 70 y	1.5	100			
		Pregnancy					
		≤ 18 y	1.9	80			
		19-30y	1.9	100			
		31-50 y	1.9	100			
		Lactation					
		≤ 18 y	2.0	80			
		19-30y	2.0	100			
		31-50 y	2.0	100			

Vitamin B₁₂ Also known as: Cobalamin		(µg/d)	UL[a],[b]	Fortified cereals, meat, fish, poultry	No adverse effects have been associated with the consumption of the amounts of vitamin B₁₂ normally found in foods or supplements. This does not mean that there is no potential for adverse effects resulting from high intakes. Because data on the adverse effects of vitamin B₁₂ are limited, caution may be warranted.	Because 10 to 30 percent of older people may malabsorb food- bound vitamin B₁₂, it is advisable for those older than 50 years to meet their RDA mainly by consuming foods fortified with vitamin B₁₂ or a supplement containing vitamin B₁₂.
Coenzyme in nucleic acid metabolism; prevents megaloblastic anemia	Infants					
	0–6 mo	0.4*	ND			
	7–12 mo	0.5*	ND			
	Children					
	1–3 y	0.9	ND			
	4–8 y	1.2	ND			
	Males					
	9–13 y	1.8	ND			
	14–18 y	2.4	ND			
	19–30 y	2.4	ND			
	31–50 y	2.4	ND			
	50–70 y	2.4	ND			
	>70 y	2.4	ND			
	Females					
	9–13 y	1.8	ND			
	14–18 y	2.4	ND			
	19–30 y	2.4	ND			
	31–50 y	2.4	ND			
	50–70 y	2.4	ND			
	>70 y	2.4	ND			
	Pregnancy					
	≤18 y	2.6	ND			
	19–30y	2.6	ND			
	31–50 y	2.6	ND			
	Lactation					
	≤18 y	2.8	ND			
	19–30y	2.8	ND			
	31–50y	2.8	ND			

NOTE: The table is adapted from the DRI reports, see www.nap.edu. It represents Recommended Dietary Allowances (RDAs) in **bold type**. Adequate Intakes (AIs) in ordinary type followed by an asterisk (*), and Tolerable Upper Intake Levels (ULs)[a]. RDAs and AIs may both be used as goals for individual intake. RDAs are set to meet the needs of almost all (97 to 98 percent) individuals in a group. For healthy breastfed infants, the AI is the mean intake. The AI for other life stage and gender groups is believed to cover the needs of all individuals in the group, but lack of data prevent being able to specify with confidence the percentage of individuals covered by this intake.

[a]UL = The maximum level of daily nutrient intake that is likely to pose no risk of adverse effects. Unless otherwise specified, the UL represents total intake from food, water, and supplements. Due to lack of suitable data, ULs could not be established for vitamin K, thiamin, riboflavin, vitamin B₁₂, pantothenic acid, biotin, or carotenoids. In the absence of ULs, extra caution may be warranted in consuming levels above recommended intakes.

[b]ND = Not determinable due to lack of data of adverse effects in this age group and concern with regard to lack of ability to handle excess amounts. Source of intake should be from food only to prevent high levels of intake.

SOURCES: *Dietary Reference Intakes for Calcium, Phosphorous, Magnesium, Vitamin D, and Fluoride* (1997); *Dietary Reference Intakes for Thiamin, Riboflavin, Niacin, Vitamin B₆, Folate, Vitamin B₁₂, Pantothenic Acid, Biotin, and Choline* (1998); *Dietary Reference Intakes for Vitamin C, Vitamin E, Selenium, and Carotenoids* (2000); and *Dietary Reference Intakes for Vitamin A, Vitamin K, Arsenic, Boron, Chromium, Copper, Iodine, Iron, Manganese, Molybdenum, Nickel, Silicon, Vanadium, and Zinc* (2001). These reports may be accessed via www.nap.edu.

Dietary Reference Intakes: Vitamins

Nutrient	Function	Life Stage Group	RDA/AI*	UL[a]	Selected Food Sources	Adverse effects of excessive consumption	Special Considerations
Vitamin C Also known as: Ascorbic acid Dehydroascorbic acid (DHA)	Cofactor for reactions requiring reduced copper or iron metalloenzyme and as a protective antioxidant		(mg/d)	(mg/d)	Citrus fruits, tomatoes, tomato juice, potatoes, brussel sprouts, cauliflower, broccoli, strawberries, cabbage and spinach	Gastrointestinal disturbances, kidney stones, excess iron absorption	Individuals who smoke require an additional 35 mg/d of vitamin C over that needed by nonsmokers. Nonsmokers regularly exposed to tobacco smoke are encouraged to ensure they meet the RDA for vitamin C.
		Infants					
		0–6 mo	40*	ND[b]			
		7–12 mo	50*	ND			
		Children					
		1–3 y	15	400			
		4–8 y	25	650			
		Males					
		9–13 y	45	1,200			
		14–18 y	75	1,800			
		19–30 y	90	2,000			
		31–50 y	90	2,000			
		50–70 y	90	2,000			
		> 70 y	90	2,000			
		Females					
		9–13 y	45	1,200			
		14–18 y	65	1,800			
		19–30 y	75	2,000			
		31–50 y	75	2,000			
		50–70 y	75	2,000			
		> 70 y	75	2,000			
		Pregnancy					
		≤ 18 y	80	1,800			
		19–30y	85	2,000			
		31–50 y	85	2,000			
		Lactation					
		≤ 18 y	115	1,800			
		19–30y	120	2,000			
		31–50 y	120	2,000			

Vitamin D Also known as: Calciferol Note: 1 μg calciferol = 40 IU vitamin D The DRI values are based on the absence of adequate exposure to sunlight.	Maintain serum calcium and phosphorus concentrations.	Life stage group	(ug/d)	(ug/d)	Fish liver oils, flesh of fatty fish, liver and fat from seals and polar bears, eggs from hens that have been fed vitamin D, fortified milk products and fortified cereals	Elevated plasma 25 (OH) D concentration causing hypercalcemia	Patients on glucocorticoid therapy may require additional vitamin D.
		Infants					
		0–6 mo	5*	25			
		7–12 mo	5*	25			
		Children					
		1–3 y	5*	50			
		4–8 y	5*	50			
		Males					
		9–13 y	5*	50			
		14–18 y	5*	50			
		19–30 y	5*	50			
		31–50 y	5*	50			
		50-70 y	10*	50			
		> 70 y	15*	50			
		Females					
		9–13 y	5*	50			
		14–18 y	5*	50			
		19–30 y	5*	50			
		31–50 y	5*	50			
		50-70 y	10*	50			
		> 70 y	15*	50			
		Pregnancy					
		≤ 18 y	5*	50			
		19-30y	5*	50			
		31-50 y	5*	50			
		Lactation					
		≤ 18 y	5*	50			
		19-30y	5*	50			
		31-50 y	5*	50			

NOTE: The table is adapted from the DRI reports, see www.nap.edu. It represents Recommended Dietary Allowances (RDAs) in **bold type**. Adequate Intakes (AIs) in ordinary type followed by an asterisk (*), and Tolerable Upper Intake Levels (ULs)[a]. RDAs and AIs may both be used as goals for individual intake. RDAs are set to meet the needs of almost all (97 to 98 percent) individuals in a group. For healthy breastfed infants, the AI is the mean intake. The AI for other life stage and gender groups is believed to cover the needs of all individuals in the group, but lack of data prevent being able to specify with confidence the percentage of individuals covered by this intake.

[a]UL = The maximum level of daily nutrient intake that is likely to pose no risk of adverse effects. Unless otherwise specified, the UL represents total intake from food, water, and supplements. Due to lack of suitable data, ULs could not be established for vitamin K, thiamin, riboflavin, vitamin B₁₂, pantothenic acid, biotin, or carotenoids. In the absence of ULs, extra caution may be warranted in consuming levels above recommended intakes.

[b]ND = Not determinable due to lack of data of adverse effects in this age group and concern with regard to lack of ability to handle excess amounts. Source of intake should be from food only to prevent high levels of intake.

SOURCES: *Dietary Reference Intakes for Calcium, Phosphorous, Magnesium, Vitamin D, and Fluoride* (1997); *Dietary Reference Intakes for Thiamin, Riboflavin, Niacin, Vitamin B₆, Folate, Vitamin B₁₂, Pantothenic Acid, Biotin, and Choline* (1998); *Dietary Reference Intakes for Vitamin C, Vitamin E, Selenium, and Carotenoids* (2000); and *Dietary Reference Intakes for Vitamin A, Vitamin K, Arsenic, Boron, Chromium, Copper, Iodine, Iron, Manganese, Molybdenum, Nickel, Silicon, Vanadium, and Zinc* (2001). These reports may be accessed via www.nap.edu.

Dietary Reference Intakes: Vitamins

Nutrient	Function	Life Stage Group	RDA/AI* (mg/d)	UL^a (mg/d)	Selected Food Sources	Adverse effects of excessive consumption	Special Considerations
Vitamin E Also known as: α-tocopherol Note: As α-tocopherol. α-Tocopherol includes RRR-α-tocopherol, the only form of α-tocopherol that occurs naturally in foods, and the 2R-stereoisomeric forms of α-tocopherol (RRR-, RSR-, RRS-, and RSS-α-tocopherol) that occur in fortified foods and supplements. It does not include the 2S-stereoisomeric forms of α-tocopherol (SRR-, SSR-, SRS-, and SSS-α-tocopherol), also found in fortified foods and supplements.	A metabolic function has not yet been identified. Vitamin E's major function appears to be as a non-specific chain-breaking antioxidant.	**Infants** 0–6 mo 7–12 mo	4* 5*	ND^b ND	Vegetable oils, unprocessed cereal grains, nuts, fruits, vegetables, meats	There is no evidence of adverse effects from the consumption of vitamin E naturally occurring in foods. Adverse effects from vitamin E containing supplements may include hemorrhagic toxicity. The UL for vitamin E applies to any form of α-tocopherol obtained from supplements, fortified foods, or a combination of the two.	Patients on anticoagulant therapy should be monitored when taking vitamin E supplements.
		Children 1–3 y 4–8 y	6 7	200 300			
		Males 9–13 y 14–18 y 19–30 y 31–50 y 50–70 y > 70 y	11 15 15 15 15 15	600 800 1,000 1,000 1,000 1,000			
		Females 9–13 y 14–18 y 19–30 y 31–50 y 50–70 y > 70 y	11 15 15 15 15 15	600 800 1,000 1,000 1,000 1,000			
		Pregnancy ≤ 18 y 19-30y 31–50 y	15 15 15	800 1,000 1,000			
		Lactation ≤ 18 y 19-30y 31–50 y	19 19 19	800 1,000 1,000			

326

Vitamin K		(µg/d)		Green vegetables (collards, spinach, salad greens, broccoli), brussel sprouts, cabbage, plant oils and margarine	No adverse effects associated with vitamin K consumption from food or supplements have been reported in humans or animals. This does not mean that there is no potential for adverse effects resulting from high intakes. Because data on the adverse effects of vitamin K are limited, caution may be warranted.	Patients on anticoagulant therapy should monitor vitamin K intake.
Coenzyme during the synthesis of many proteins involved in blood clotting and bone metabolism	**Infants**					
	0–6 mo	2.0*	ND			
	7–12 mo	2.5*	ND			
	Children					
	1–3 y	30*	ND			
	4–8 y	55*	ND			
	Males					
	9–13 y	60*	ND			
	14–18 y	75*	ND			
	19–30 y	120*	ND			
	31–50 y	120*	ND			
	50–70 y	120*	ND			
	>70 y	120*	ND			
	Females					
	9–13 y	60*	ND			
	14–18 y	75*	ND			
	19–30 y	90*	ND			
	31–50 y	90*	ND			
	50–70 y	90*	ND			
	>70 y	90*	ND			
	Pregnancy					
	≤18 y	75*	ND			
	19–30y	90*	ND			
	31–50 y	90*	ND			
	Lactation					
	≤18 y	75*	ND			
	19–30y	90*	ND			
	31–50 y	90*	ND			

NOTE: The table is adapted from the DRI reports, see www.nap.edu. It represents Recommended Dietary Allowances (RDAs) in **bold type**. Adequate Intakes (AIs) in ordinary type followed by an asterisk (*), and Tolerable Upper Intake Levels (ULs)[a]. RDAs and AIs may both be used as goals for individual intake. RDAs are set to meet the needs of almost all (97 to 98 percent) individuals in a group. For healthy breastfed infants, the AI is the mean intake. The AI for other life stage and gender groups is believed to cover the needs of all individuals in the group, but lack of data prevent being able to specify with confidence the percentage of individuals covered by this intake.

[a]UL = The maximum level of daily nutrient intake that is likely to pose no risk of adverse effects. Unless otherwise specified, the UL represents total intake from food, water, and supplements. Due to lack of suitable data, ULs could not be established for vitamin K, thiamin, riboflavin, vitamin B₁₂, pantothenic acid, biotin, or carotenoids. In the absence of ULs, extra caution may be warranted in consuming levels above recommended intakes.

[b]ND = Not determinable due to lack of data of adverse effects in this age group and concern with regard to lack of ability to handle excess amounts. Source of intake should be from food only to prevent high levels of intake.

SOURCES: *Dietary Reference Intakes for Calcium, Phosphorous, Magnesium, Vitamin D, and Fluoride* (1997); *Dietary Reference Intakes for Thiamin, Riboflavin, Niacin, Vitamin B₆, Folate, Vitamin B₁₂, Pantothenic Acid, Biotin, and Choline* (1998); *Dietary Reference Intakes for Vitamin C, Vitamin E, Selenium, and Carotenoids* (2000); and *Dietary Reference Intakes for Vitamin A, Vitamin K, Arsenic, Boron, Chromium, Copper, Iodine, Iron, Manganese, Molybdenum, Nickel, Silicon, Vanadium, and Zinc* (2001). These reports may be accessed via www.nap.edu.

Dietary Reference Intakes: Elements

Nutrient	Function	Life Stage Group	RDA/AI*	UL[a]	Selected Food Sources	Adverse effects of excessive consumption	Special Considerations
Arsenic	No biological function in humans although animal data indicate a requirement	Infants 0–6 mo 7–12 mo	ND[b] ND	ND ND	Dairy products, meat, poultry, fish, grains and cereal	No data on the possible adverse effects of organic arsenic compounds in food were found. Inorganic arsenic is a known toxic substance. Although the UL was not determined for arsenic, there is no justification for adding arsenic to food or supplements.	None
		Children 1–3 y 4–8 y	ND ND	ND ND			
		Males 9–13 y 14–18 y 19–30 y 31–50 y 50–70 y > 70 y	ND ND ND ND ND ND	ND ND ND ND ND ND			
		Females 9–13 y 14–18 y 19–30 y 31–50 y 50–70 y > 70 y	ND ND ND ND ND ND	ND ND ND ND ND ND			
		Pregnancy ≤ 18 y 19–30y 31–50 y	ND ND ND	ND ND ND			
		Lactation ≤ 18 y 19–30y 31–50 y	ND ND ND	ND ND ND			

Boron	No clear biological function in humans although animal data indicate a functional role			(mg/d)	Fruit-based beverages and products, potatoes, legumes, milk, avocado, peanut butter, peanuts	Reproductive and developmental effects as observed in animal studies.	None
		Infants					
		0–6 mo	ND	ND			
		7–12 mo	ND	ND			
		Children					
		1–3 y	ND	3			
		4–8 y	ND	6			
		Males					
		9–13 y	ND	11			
		14–18 y	ND	17			
		19–30 y	ND	20			
		31–50 y	ND	20			
		50-70 y	ND	20			
		>70 y	ND	20			
		Females					
		9–13 y	ND	11			
		14–18 y	ND	17			
		19–30 y	ND	20			
		31–50 y	ND	20			
		50-70 y	ND	20			
		>70 y	ND	20			
		Pregnancy					
		≤18 y	ND	17			
		19-30y	ND	20			
		31–50 y	ND	20			
		Lactation					
		≤18 y	ND	17			
		19-30y	ND	20			
		31–50 y	ND	20			

NOTE: The table is adapted from the DRI reports, see www.nap.edu. It represents Recommended Dietary Allowances (RDAs) in **bold type**, Adequate Intakes (AIs) in ordinary type followed by an asterisk (*), and Tolerable Upper Intake Levels (ULs)[a] RDAs and AIs may both be used as goals for individual intake. RDAs are set to meet the needs of almost all (97 to 98 percent) individuals in a group. For healthy breastfed infants, the AI is the mean intake. The AI for other life stage and gender groups is believed to cover the needs of all individuals in the group, but lack of data prevent being able to specify with confidence the percentage of individuals covered by this intake.

[a]UL = The maximum level of daily nutrient intake that is likely to pose no risk of adverse effects. Unless otherwise specified, the UL represents total intake from food, water, and supplements. Due to lack of suitable data, ULs could not be established for vitamin K, thiamin, riboflavin, vitamin B_{12}, pantothenic acid, biotin, or carotenoids. In the absence of ULs, extra caution may be warranted in consuming levels above recommended intakes.

[b]ND = Not determinable due to lack of data of adverse effects in this age group and concern with regard to lack of ability to handle excess amounts. Source of intake should be from food only to prevent high levels of intake.

SOURCES: *Dietary Reference Intakes for Calcium, Phosphorous, Magnesium, Vitamin D, and Fluoride* (1997); *Dietary Reference Intakes for Thiamin, Riboflavin, Niacin, Vitamin B_6, Folate, Vitamin B_{12}, Pantothenic Acid, Biotin, and Choline* (1998); *Dietary Reference Intakes for Vitamin C, Vitamin E, Selenium, and Carotenoids* (2000); and *Dietary Reference Intakes for Vitamin A, Vitamin K, Arsenic, Boron, Chromium, Copper, Iodine, Iron, Manganese, Molybdenum, Nickel, Silicon, Vanadium, and Zinc* (2001). These reports may be accessed via www.nap.edu.

Dietary Reference Intakes: Elements

Nutrient	Function	Life Stage Group	RDA/AI*	UL[a]	Selected Food Sources	Adverse effects of excessive consumption	Special Considerations
Calcium	Essential role in blood clotting, muscle contraction, nerve transmission, and bone and tooth formation	Infants	(mg/d)	(mg/d)	Milk, cheese, yogurt, corn tortillas, calcium-set tofu, Chinese cabbage, kale, broccoli	Kidney stones, hypercalcemia, milk alkali syndrome, and renal insufficiency	Amenorrheic women (exercise- or anorexia nervosa-induced) have reduced net calcium absorption.
		0–6 mo	210*	ND[b]			
		7–12 mo	270*	ND			There is no consistent data to support that a high protein intake increases calcium requirement.
		Children					
		1–3 y	500*	2,500			
		4–8 y	800*	2,500			
		Males					
		9–13 y	1,300*	2,500			
		14–18 y	1,300*	2,500			
		19–30 y	1,000*	2,500			
		31-50 y	1,000*	2,500			
		50-70 y	1,200*	2,500			
		> 70 y	1,200*	2,500			
		Females					
		9–13 y	1,300*	2,500			
		14–18 y	1,300*	2,500			
		19–30 y	1,000*	2,500			
		31-50 y	1,000*	2,500			
		50-70 y	1,200*	2,500			
		> 70 y	1,200*	2,500			
		Pregnancy					
		≤ 18 y	1,300*	2,500			
		19-30y	1,000*	2,500			
		31-50 y	1,000*	2,500			
		Lactation					
		≤ 18 y	1,300*	2,500			
		19-30y	1,000*	2,500			
		31–50 y	1,000*	2,500			

330

Chromium	Helps to maintain normal blood glucose levels		(µg/d)		Some cereals, meats, poultry, fish, beer	Chronic renal failure	None
		Infants					
		0–6 mo	0.2*	ND			
		7–12 mo	5.5*	ND			
		Children					
		1–3 y	11*	ND			
		4–8 y	15*	ND			
		Males					
		9–13 y	25*	ND			
		14–18 y	35*	ND			
		19–30 y	35*	ND			
		31–50 y	35*	ND			
		50–70 y	30*	ND			
		>70 y	30*	ND			
		Females					
		9–13 y	21*	ND			
		14–18 y	24*	ND			
		19–30 y	25*	ND			
		31–50 y	25*	ND			
		50–70 y	20*	ND			
		>70 y	20*	ND			
		Pregnancy					
		≤18 y	29*	ND			
		19–30y	30*	ND			
		31–50 y	30*	ND			
		Lactation					
		≤18 y	44*	ND			
		19–30y	45*	ND			
		31–50 y	45*	ND			

NOTE: The table is adapted from the DRI reports, see www.nap.edu. It represents Recommended Dietary Allowances (RDAs) in **bold type**. Adequate Intakes (AIs) in ordinary type followed by an asterisk (*), and Tolerable Upper Intake Levels (ULs)[a]. RDAs and AIs may both be used as goals for individual intake. RDAs are set to meet the needs of almost all (97 to 98 percent) individuals in a group. For healthy breastfed infants, the AI is the mean intake. The AI for other life stage and gender groups is believed to cover the needs of all individuals in the group, but lack of data prevent being able to specify with confidence the percentage of individuals covered by this intake.

[a]UL = The maximum level of daily nutrient intake that is likely to pose no risk of adverse effects. Unless otherwise specified, the UL represents total intake from food, water, and supplements. Due to lack of suitable data, ULs could not be established for vitamin K, thiamin, riboflavin, vitamin B$_{12}$, pantothenic acid, biotin, or carotenoids. In the absence of ULs, extra caution may be warranted in consuming levels above recommended intakes.

[b]ND = Not determinable due to lack of data of adverse effects in this age group and concern with regard to lack of ability to handle excess amounts. Source of intake should be from food only to prevent high levels of intake.

SOURCES: *Dietary Reference Intakes for Calcium, Phosphorous, Magnesium, Vitamin D, and Fluoride* (1997); *Dietary Reference Intakes for Thiamin, Riboflavin, Niacin, Vitamin B$_6$, Folate, Vitamin B$_{12}$, Pantothenic Acid, Biotin, and Choline* (1998); *Dietary Reference Intakes for Vitamin C, Vitamin E, Selenium, and Carotenoids* (2000); and *Dietary Reference Intakes for Vitamin A, Vitamin K, Arsenic, Boron, Chromium, Copper, Iodine, Iron, Manganese, Molybdenum, Nickel, Silicon, Vanadium, and Zinc* (2001). These reports may be accessed via www.nap.edu.

331

Dietary Reference Intakes: Elements

Nutrient	Function	Life Stage Group	RDA/AI*	UL[a]	Selected Food Sources	Adverse effects of excessive consumption	Special Considerations
Copper	Component of enzymes in iron metabolism		(µg/d)	(µg/d)	Organ meats, seafood, nuts, seeds, wheat bran cereals, whole grain products, cocoa products	Gastrointestinal distress, liver damage	Individuals with Wilson's disease, Indian childhood cirrhosis and idiopathic copper toxicosis may be at increased risk of adverse effects from excess copper intake.
		Infants					
		0–6 mo	200*	ND[b]			
		7–12 mo	220*	ND			
		Children					
		1–3 y	340	1,000			
		4–8 y	440	3,000			
		Males					
		9–13 y	700	5,000			
		14–18 y	890	8,000			
		19–30 y	900	10,000			
		31–50 y	900	10,000			
		50–70 y	900	10,000			
		> 70 y	900	10,000			
		Females					
		9–13 y	700	5,000			
		14–18 y	890	8,000			
		19–30 y	900	10,000			
		31–50 y	900	10,000			
		50–70 y	900	10,000			
		> 70 y	900	10,000			
		Pregnancy					
		≤18 y	1000	8,000			
		19–30y	1000	10,000			
		31–50 y	1000	10,000			
		Lactation					
		≤18 y	1300	8,000			
		19–30y	1300	10,000			
		31–50 y	1300	10,000			

332

Fluoride	Inhibits the initiation and progression of dental caries and stimulates new bone formation	Life stage group	(mg/d)	(mg/d)	Fluoridated water, teas, marine fish, fluoridated dental products	Enamel and skeletal fluorosis	None
		Infants					
		0–6 mo	0.01*	0.7			
		7–12 mo	0.5*	0.9			
		Children					
		1–3 y	0.7*	1.3			
		4–8 y	1*	2.2			
		Males					
		9–13 y	2*	10			
		14–18 y	3*	10			
		19–30 y	4*	10			
		31–50 y	4*	10			
		50–70 y	4*	10			
		>70 y	4*	10			
		Females					
		9–13 y	2*	10			
		14–18 y	3*	10			
		19–30 y	3*	10			
		31–50 y	3*	10			
		50–70 y	3*	10			
		>70 y	3*	10			
		Pregnancy					
		≤ 18 y	3*	10			
		19–30y	3*	10			
		31–50 y	3*	10			
		Lactation					
		≤ 18 y	3*	10			
		19–30y	3*	10			
		31–50y	3*	10			

NOTE: The table is adapted from the DRI reports, see www.nap.edu. It represents Recommended Dietary Allowances (RDAs) in **bold type.** Adequate Intakes (AIs) in ordinary type followed by an asterisk (*), and Tolerable Upper Intake Levels (ULs)[a]. RDAs and AIs may both be used as goals for individual intake. RDAs are set to meet the needs of almost all (97 to 98 percent) individuals in a group. For healthy breastfed infants, the AI is the mean intake. The AI for other life stage and gender groups is believed to cover the needs of all individuals in the group, but lack of data prevent being able to specify with confidence the percentage of individuals covered by this intake.

[a]UL = The maximum level of daily nutrient intake that is likely to pose no risk of adverse effects. Unless otherwise specified, the UL represents total intake from food, water, and supplements. Due to lack of suitable data, ULs could not be established for vitamin K, thiamin, riboflavin, vitamin B₁₂, pantothenic acid, biotin, or carotenoids. In the absence of ULs, extra caution may be warranted in consuming levels above recommended intakes.

[b]ND = Not determinable due to lack of data of adverse effects in this age group and concern with regard to lack of ability to handle excess amounts. Source of intake should be from food only to prevent high levels of intake.

SOURCES: *Dietary Reference Intakes for Calcium, Phosphorous, Magnesium, Vitamin D, and Fluoride* (1997); *Dietary Reference Intakes for Thiamin, Riboflavin, Niacin, Vitamin B₆, Folate, Vitamin B₁₂, Pantothenic Acid, Biotin, and Choline* (1998); *Dietary Reference Intakes for Vitamin C, Vitamin E, Selenium, and Carotenoids* (2000); and *Dietary Reference Intakes for Vitamin A, Vitamin K, Arsenic, Boron, Chromium, Copper, Iodine, Iron, Manganese, Molybdenum, Nickel, Silicon, Vanadium, and Zinc* (2001). These reports may be accessed via www.nap.edu.

333

Dietary Reference Intakes: Elements

Nutrient	Function	Life Stage Group	RDA/AI* (µg/d)	UL^a (µg/d)	Selected Food Sources	Adverse effects of excessive consumption	Special Considerations
Iodine	Component of the thyroid hormones; and prevents goiter and cretinism	Infants			Marine origin, processed foods, iodized salt	Elevated thyroid stimulating hormone (TSH) concentration	Individuals with autoimmune thyroid disease, previous iodine deficiency, or nodular goiter are distinctly susceptible to the adverse effect of excess iodine intake. Therefore, individuals with these conditions may not be protected by the UL for iodine intake for the general population.
		0–6 mo	110*	ND^b			
		7–12 mo	130*	ND			
		Children					
		1–3 y	90	200			
		4–8 y	90	300			
		Males					
		9–13 y	120	600			
		14–18 y	150	900			
		19–30 y	150	1,100			
		31–50 y	150	1,100			
		50–70 y	150	1,100			
		> 70 y	150	1,100			
		Females					
		9–13 y	120	600			
		14–18 y	150	900			
		19–30 y	150	1,100			
		31–50 y	150	1,100			
		50–70 y	150	1,100			
		> 70 y	150	1,100			
		Pregnancy					
		≤ 18 y	220	900			
		19–30y	220	1,100			
		31–50 y	220	1,100			
		Lactation					
		≤ 18 y	290	900			
		19–30y	290	1,100			
		31–50 y	290	1,100			

Iron (mg/d)	Component of hemoglobin and numerous enzymes; prevents microcytic hypochromic anemia		(mg/d)[a]	(mg/d)	Fruits, vegetables and fortified bread and grain products such as cereal (non-heme iron sources), meat and poultry (heme iron sources)	Gastrointestinal distress	Non-heme iron absorption is lower for those consuming vegetarian diets than for those eating nonvegetarian diets. Therefore, it has been suggested that the iron requirement for those consuming a vegetarian diet is approximately 2-fold greater than for those consuming a nonvegetarian diet. Recommended intake assumes 75% of iron is from heme iron sources.
		Infants					
		0–6 mo	0.27*	40			
		7–12 mo	**11**	40			
		Children					
		1–3 y	7	40			
		4–8 y	**10**	40			
		Males					
		9–13 y	**8**	40			
		14–18 y	**11**	45			
		19–30 y	**8**	45			
		31–50 y	**8**	45			
		50–70 y	**8**	45			
		>70 y	**8**	45			
		Females					
		9–13 y	**8**	40			
		14–18 y	**15**	45			
		19–30 y	**18**	45			
		31–50 y	**18**	45			
		50–70 y	**8**	45			
		>70 y	**8**	45			
		Pregnancy					
		≤18 y	**27**	45			
		19–30y	**27**	45			
		31–50 y	**27**	45			
		Lactation					
		≤18 y	**10**	45			
		19–30y	**9**	45			
		31–50 y	**9**	45			

NOTE: The table is adapted from the DRI reports, see www.nap.edu. It represents Recommended Dietary Allowances (RDAs) in **bold type**. Adequate Intakes (AIs) in ordinary type followed by an asterisk (*), and Tolerable Upper Intake Levels (ULs)[a]. RDAs and AIs may both be used as goals for individual intake. RDAs are set to meet the needs of almost all (97 to 98 percent) individuals in a group. For healthy breastfed infants, the AI is the mean intake. The AI for other life stage and gender groups is believed to cover the needs of all individuals in the group, but lack of data prevent being able to specify with confidence the percentage of individuals covered by this intake.

[a]UL = The maximum level of daily nutrient intake that is likely to pose no risk of adverse effects. Unless otherwise specified, the UL represents total intake from food, water, and supplements. Due to lack of suitable data, ULs could not be established for vitamin K, thiamin, riboflavin, vitamin B12, pantothenic acid, biotin, or carotenoids. In the absence of ULs, extra caution may be warranted in consuming levels above recommended intakes.

[b]ND = Not determinable due to lack of data of adverse effects in this age group and concern with regard to lack of ability to handle excess amounts. Source of intake should be from food only to prevent high levels of intake.

SOURCES: *Dietary Reference Intakes for Calcium, Phosphorous, Magnesium, Vitamin D, and Fluoride* (1997); *Dietary Reference Intakes for Thiamin, Riboflavin, Niacin, Vitamin B6, Folate, Vitamin B12, Pantothenic Acid, Biotin, and Choline* (1998); *Dietary Reference Intakes for Vitamin C, Vitamin E, Selenium, and Carotenoids* (2000); and *Dietary Reference Intakes for Vitamin A, Vitamin K, Arsenic, Boron, Chromium, Copper, Iodine, Iron, Manganese, Molybdenum, Nickel, Silicon, Vanadium, and Zinc* (2001). These reports may be accessed via www.nap.edu.

Dietary Reference Intakes: Elements

Nutrient	Function	Life Stage Group	RDA/AI*	UL[a]	Selected Food Sources	Adverse effects of excessive consumption	Special Considerations
Magnesium	Cofactor for enzyme systems		(mg/d)	(mg/d)	Green leafy vegetables, unpolished grains, nuts, meat, starches, milk	There is no evidence of adverse effects from the consumption of naturally occurring magnesium in foods.	None
		Infants					
		0–6 mo	30*	ND[b]			
		7–12 mo	75*	ND			
		Children				Adverse effects from magnesium containing supplements may include osmotic diarrhea.	
		1–3 y	80	65			
		4–8 y	130	110			
		Males				The UL for magnesium represents intake from a pharmacological agent only and does not include intake from food and water.	
		9–13 y	240	350			
		14–18 y	410	350			
		19–30 y	400	350			
		31–50 y	420	350			
		50–70 y	420	350			
		> 70 y	420	350			
		Females					
		9–13 y	240	350			
		14–18 y	360	350			
		19–30 y	310	350			
		31–50 y	320	350			
		50–70 y	320	350			
		> 70 y	320	350			
		Pregnancy					
		≤ 18 y	400	350			
		19–30y	350	350			
		31–50 y	360	350			
		Lactation					
		≤ 18 y	360	350			
		19–30y	310	350			
		31–50 y	320	350			

Manganese		(mg/d)	(mg/d)	Nuts, legumes, tea, and whole grains	Elevated blood concentration and neurotoxicity	Because manganese in drinking water and supplements may be more bioavailable than manganese from food, caution should be taken when using manganese supplements especially among those persons already consuming large amounts of manganese from diets high in plant products. In addition, individuals with liver disease may be distinctly susceptible to the adverse effects of excess manganese intake.
Involved in the formation of bone, as well as in enzymes involved in amino acid, cholesterol, and carbohydrate metabolism	**Infants**					
	0–6 mo	0.003*	ND			
	7–12 mo	0.6*	ND			
	Children					
	1–3 y	1.2*	2			
	4–8 y	1.5*	3			
	Males					
	9–13 y	1.9*	6			
	14–18 y	2.2*	9			
	19–30 y	2.3*	11			
	31–50 y	2.3*	11			
	50–70 y	2.3*	11			
	>70 y	2.3*	11			
	Females					
	9–13 y	1.6*	6			
	14–18 y	1.6*	9			
	19–30 y	1.8*	11			
	31–50 y	1.8*	11			
	50–70 y	1.8*	11			
	>70 y	1.8*	11			
	Pregnancy					
	≤18 y	2.0*	9			
	19–30y	2.0*	11			
	31–50 y	2.0*	11			
	Lactation					
	≤18 y	2.6*	9			
	19–30y	2.6*	11			
	31–50 y	2.6*	11			

NOTE: The table is adapted from the DRI reports, see www.nap.edu. It represents Recommended Dietary Allowances (RDAs) in **bold type**. Adequate Intakes (AIs) in ordinary type followed by an asterisk (*), and Tolerable Upper Intake Levels (ULs)[a]. RDAs and AIs may both be used as goals for individual intake. RDAs are set to meet the needs of almost all (97 to 98 percent) individuals in a group. For healthy breastfed infants, the AI is the mean intake. The AI for other life stage and gender groups is believed to cover the needs of all individuals in the group, but lack of data prevent being able to specify with confidence the percentage of individuals covered by this intake.

[a]UL = The maximum level of daily nutrient intake that is likely to pose no risk of adverse effects. Unless otherwise specified, the UL represents total intake from food, water, and supplements. Due to lack of suitable data, ULs could not be established for vitamin K, thiamin, riboflavin, vitamin B₁₂, pantothenic acid, biotin, or carotenoids. In the absence of ULs, extra caution may be warranted in consuming levels above recommended intakes.

[b]ND = Not determinable due to lack of data of adverse effects in this age group and concern with regard to lack of ability to handle excess amounts. Source of intake should be from food only to prevent high levels of intake.

SOURCES: *Dietary Reference Intakes for Calcium, Phosphorous, Magnesium, Vitamin D, and Fluoride* (1997); *Dietary Reference Intakes for Thiamin, Riboflavin, Niacin, Vitamin B₆, Folate, Vitamin B₁₂, Pantothenic Acid, Biotin, and Choline* (1998); *Dietary Reference Intakes for Vitamin C, Vitamin E, Selenium, and Carotenoids* (2000); and *Dietary Reference Intakes for Vitamin A, Vitamin K, Arsenic, Boron, Chromium, Copper, Iodine, Iron, Manganese, Molybdenum, Nickel, Silicon, Vanadium, and Zinc* (2001). These reports may be accessed via www.nap.edu.

Dietary Reference Intakes: Elements

Nutrient	Function	Life Stage Group	RDA/AI*	UL[a]	Selected Food Sources	Adverse effects of excessive consumption	Special Considerations
Molybdenum	Cofactor for enzymes involved in catabolism of sulfur amino acids, purines and pyridines.		(µg/d)	(µg/d)	Legumes, grain products and nuts	Reproductive effects as observed in animal studies.	Individuals who are deficient in dietary copper intake or have some dysfunction in copper metabolism that makes them copper-deficient could be at increased risk of molybdenum toxicity.
		Infants					
		0–6 mo	2*	ND[b]			
		7–12 mo	3*	ND			
		Children					
		1–3 y	17	300			
		4–8 y	22	600			
		Males					
		9–13 y	34	1,100			
		14–18 y	43	1,700			
		19–30 y	45	2,000			
		31–50 y	45	2,000			
		50–70 y	45	2,000			
		> 70 y	45	2,000			
		Females					
		9–13 y	34	1,100			
		14–18 y	43	1,700			
		19–30 y	45	2,000			
		31–50 y	45	2,000			
		50–70 y	45	2,000			
		> 70 y	45	2,000			
		Pregnancy					
		≤ 18 y	50	1,700			
		19-30y	50	2,000			
		31-50 y	50	2,000			
		Lactation					
		≤ 18 y	50	1,700			
		19-30y	50	2,000			
		31–50 y	50	2,000			

Nickel	No clear biological function in humans has been identified. May serve as a cofactor of metalloenzymes and facilitate iron absorption or metabolism in microorganisms.	Life Stage Group		(mg/d)	Nuts, legumes, cereals, sweeteners, chocolate milk powder, chocolate candy	Decreased body weight gain Note: As observed in animal studies	Individuals with preexisting nickel hypersensitivity (from previous dermal exposure) and kidney dysfunction are distinctly susceptible to the adverse effects of excess nickel intake
		Infants					
		0–6 mo	ND	ND			
		7–12 mo	ND	ND			
		Children					
		1–3 y	ND	0.2			
		4–8 y	ND	0.3			
		Males					
		9–13 y	ND	0.6			
		14–18 y	ND	1.0			
		19–30 y	ND	1.0			
		31–50 y	ND	1.0			
		50–70 y	ND	1.0			
		>70 y	ND	1.0			
		Females					
		9–13 y	ND	0.6			
		14–18 y	ND	1.0			
		19–30 y	ND	1.0			
		31–50 y	ND	1.0			
		50–70 y	ND	1.0			
		>70 y	ND	1.0			
		Pregnancy					
		≤18 y	ND	1.0			
		19–30y	ND	1.0			
		31–50 y	ND	1.0			
		Lactation					
		≤18 y	ND	1.0			
		19–30y	ND	1.0			
		31–50 y	ND	1.0			

NOTE: The table is adapted from the DRI reports, see www.nap.edu. It represents Recommended Dietary Allowances (RDAs) in **bold type**. Adequate Intakes (AIs) in ordinary type followed by an asterisk (*), and Tolerable Upper Intake Levels (ULs)[a]. RDAs and AIs may both be used as goals for individual intake. RDAs are set to meet the needs of almost all (97 to 98 percent) individuals in a group. For healthy breastfed infants, the AI is the mean intake. The AI for other life stage and gender groups is believed to cover the needs of all individuals in the group, but lack of data prevent being able to specify with confidence the percentage of individuals covered by this intake.

[a]UL = The maximum level of daily nutrient intake that is likely to pose no risk of adverse effects. Unless otherwise specified, the UL represents total intake from food, water, and supplements. Due to lack of suitable data, ULs could not be established for vitamin K, thiamin, riboflavin, vitamin B_{12}, pantothenic acid, biotin, or carotenoids. In the absence of ULs, extra caution may be warranted in consuming levels above recommended intakes.

[b]ND = Not determinable due to lack of data of adverse effects in this age group and concern with regard to lack of ability to handle excess amounts. Source of intake should be from food only to prevent high levels of intake.

SOURCES: *Dietary Reference Intakes for Calcium, Phosphorous, Magnesium, Vitamin D, and Fluoride* (1997); *Dietary Reference Intakes for Thiamin, Riboflavin, Niacin, Vitamin B_6, Folate, Vitamin B_{12}, Pantothenic Acid, Biotin, and Choline* (1998); *Dietary Reference Intakes for Vitamin C, Vitamin E, Selenium, and Carotenoids* (2000); and *Dietary Reference Intakes for Vitamin A, Vitamin K, Arsenic, Boron, Chromium, Copper, Iodine, Iron, Manganese, Molybdenum, Nickel, Silicon, Vanadium, and Zinc* (2001). These reports may be accessed via www.nap.edu.

Dietary Reference Intakes: Elements

Nutrient	Function	Life Stage Group	RDA/AI*	UL[a]	Selected Food Sources	Adverse effects of excessive consumption	Special Considerations
Molybdenum	Cofactor for enzymes involved in catabolism of sulfur amino acids, purines and pyridines.	Infants	(µg/d)	(µg/d)	Legumes, grain products and nuts	Reproductive effects as observed in animal studies.	Individuals who are deficient in dietary copper intake or have some dysfunction in copper metabolism that makes them copper-deficient could be at increased risk of molybdenum toxicity.
		0–6 mo	2*	ND[b]			
		7–12 mo	3*	ND			
		Children					
		1–3 y	17	300			
		4–8 y	22	600			
		Males					
		9–13 y	34	1,100			
		14–18 y	43	1,700			
		19–30 y	45	2,000			
		31–50 y	45	2,000			
		50–70 y	45	2,000			
		> 70 y	45	2,000			
		Females					
		9–13 y	34	1,100			
		14–18 y	43	1,700			
		19–30 y	45	2,000			
		31–50 y	45	2,000			
		50–70 y	45	2,000			
		> 70 y	45	2,000			
		Pregnancy					
		≤ 18 y	50	1,700			
		19–30 y	50	2,000			
		31–50 y	50	2,000			
		Lactation					
		≤ 18 y	50	1,700			
		19–30 y	50	2,000			
		31–50 y	50	2,000			

Selenium	Defense against oxidative stress and regulation of thyroid hormone action, and the reduction and oxidation status of vitamin C and other molecules		(µg/d)	(µg/d)	Organ meats, seafood, plants (depending on soil selenium content)	Hair and nail brittleness and loss	None
		Infants					
		0–6 mo	15*	45			
		7–12 mo	20*	60			
		Children					
		1–3 y	**20**	90			
		4–8 y	**30**	150			
		Males					
		9–13 y	**40**	280			
		14–18 y	**55**	400			
		19–30 y	**55**	400			
		31–50 y	**55**	400			
		50–70 y	**55**	400			
		>70 y	**55**	400			
		Females					
		9–13 y	**40**	280			
		14–18 y	**55**	400			
		19–30 y	**55**	400			
		31–50 y	**55**	400			
		50–70 y	**55**	400			
		>70 y	**55**	400			
		Pregnancy					
		≤18 y	**60**	400			
		19–30y	**60**	400			
		31–50 y	**60**	400			
		Lactation					
		≤18 y	**70**	400			
		19–30y	**70**	400			
		31–50 y	**70**	400			

NOTE: The table is adapted from the DRI reports, see www.nap.edu. It represents Recommended Dietary Allowances (RDAs) in **bold type**. Adequate Intakes (AIs) in ordinary type followed by an asterisk (*), and Tolerable Upper Intake Levels (ULs)[a]. RDAs and AIs may both be used as goals for individual intake. RDAs are set to meet the needs of almost all (97 to 98 percent) individuals in a group. For healthy breastfed infants, the AI is the mean intake. The AI for other life stage and gender groups is believed to cover the needs of all individuals in the group, but lack of data prevent being able to specify with confidence the percentage of individuals covered by this intake.

[a]UL = The maximum level of daily nutrient intake that is likely to pose no risk of adverse effects. Unless otherwise specified, the UL represents total intake from food, water, and supplements. Due to lack of suitable data, ULs could not be established for vitamin K, thiamin, riboflavin, vitamin B12, pantothenic acid, biotin, or carotenoids. In the absence of ULs, extra caution may be warranted in consuming levels above recommended intakes.

[b]ND = Not determinable due to lack of data of adverse effects in this age group and concern with regard to lack of ability to handle excess amounts. Source of intake should be from food only to prevent high levels of intake.

SOURCES: *Dietary Reference Intakes for Calcium, Phosphorous, Magnesium, Vitamin D, and Fluoride* (1997); *Dietary Reference Intakes for Thiamin, Riboflavin, Niacin, Vitamin B6, Folate, Vitamin B12, Pantothenic Acid, Biotin, and Choline* (1998); *Dietary Reference Intakes for Vitamin C, Vitamin E, Selenium, and Carotenoids* (2000); and *Dietary Reference Intakes for Vitamin A, Vitamin K, Arsenic, Boron, Chromium, Copper, Iodine, Iron, Manganese, Molybdenum, Nickel, Silicon, Vanadium, and Zinc* (2001). These reports may be accessed via www.nap.edu.

Dietary Reference Intakes: Elements

Nutrient	Function	Life Stage Group	RDA/AI*	ULa	Selected Food Sources	Adverse effects of excessive consumption	Special Considerations
Silicon	No biological function in humans has been identified. Involved in bone function in animal studies.	Infants 0–6 mo 7–12 mo	NDb ND	ND ND	Plant-based foods	There is no evidence that silicon that occurs naturally in food and water produces adverse health effects.	None
		Children 1–3 y 4–8 y	ND ND	ND ND			
		Males 9–13 y 14–18 y 19–30 y 31-50 y 50-70 y > 70 y	ND ND ND ND ND ND	ND ND ND ND ND ND			
		Females 9–13 y 14–18 y 19–30 y 31-50 y 50-70 y > 70 y	ND ND ND ND ND ND	ND ND ND ND ND ND			
		Pregnancy ≤ 18 y 19-30y 31-50 y	ND ND ND	ND ND ND			
		Lactation ≤ 18 y 19-30y 31–50 y	ND ND ND	ND ND ND			

Vanadium	No biological function in humans has been identified.				(mg/d)	Mushrooms, shellfish, black pepper, parsley, and dill seed.	Renal lesions as observed in animal studies.	None
		Infants						
		0–6 mo	ND	ND	ND			
		7–12 mo	ND	ND	ND			
		Children						
		1–3 y	ND	ND	ND			
		4–8 y	ND	ND	ND			
		Males						
		9–13 y	ND	ND	ND			
		14–18 y	ND	ND	ND			
		19–30 y	ND	ND	1.8			
		31–50 y	ND	ND	1.8			
		50–70 y	ND	ND	1.8			
		>70 y	ND	ND	1.8			
		Females						
		9–13 y	ND	ND	ND			
		14–18 y	ND	ND	ND			
		19–30 y	ND	ND	1.8			
		31–50 y	ND	ND	1.8			
		50–70 y	ND	ND	1.8			
		>70 y	ND	ND	1.8			
		Pregnancy						
		≤18 y	ND	ND	ND			
		19–30y	ND	ND	ND			
		31–50 y	ND	ND	ND			
		Lactation						
		≤18 y	ND	ND	ND			
		19–30y	ND	ND	ND			
		31–50 y	ND	ND	ND			

NOTE: The table is adapted from the DRI reports, see www.nap.edu. It represents Recommended Dietary Allowances (RDAs) in **bold type**. Adequate Intakes (AIs) in ordinary type followed by an asterisk (*), and Tolerable Upper Intake Levels (ULs). RDAs and AIs may both be used as goals for individual intake. RDAs are set to meet the needs of almost all (97 to 98 percent) individuals in a group. For healthy breastfed infants, the AI is the mean intake. The AI for other life stage and gender groups is believed to cover the needs of all individuals in the group, but lack of data prevent being able to specify with confidence the percentage of individuals covered by this intake.

[a]UL = The maximum level of daily nutrient intake that is likely to pose no risk of adverse effects. Unless otherwise specified, the UL represents total intake from food, water, and supplements. Due to lack of suitable data, ULs could not be established for vitamin K, thiamin, riboflavin, vitamin B12, pantothenic acid, biotin, or carotenoids. In the absence of ULs, extra caution may be warranted in consuming levels above recommended intakes.

[b]ND = Not determinable due to lack of data of adverse effects in this age group and concern with regard to lack of ability to handle excess amounts. Source of intake should be from food only to prevent high levels of intake.

SOURCES: *Dietary Reference Intakes for Calcium, Phosphorous, Magnesium, Vitamin D, and Fluoride* (1997); *Dietary Reference Intakes for Thiamin, Riboflavin, Niacin, Vitamin B6, Folate, Vitamin B12, Pantothenic Acid, Biotin, and Choline* (1998); *Dietary Reference Intakes for Vitamin C, Vitamin E, Selenium, and Carotenoids* (2000); and *Dietary Reference Intakes for Vitamin A, Vitamin K, Arsenic, Boron, Chromium, Copper, Iodine, Iron, Manganese, Molybdenum, Nickel, Silicon, Vanadium, and Zinc* (2001). These reports may be accessed via www.nap.edu.

Dietary Reference Intakes: Elements

Nutrient	Function	Life Stage Group	RDA/AI*	UL[a]	Selected Food Sources	Adverse effects of excessive consumption	Special Considerations
Zinc	Component of multiple enzymes and proteins; involved in the regulation of gene expression.	Infants	(mg/d)	(mg/d)	Fortified cereals, red meats, certain seafood	Reduced copper status	Zinc absorption is lower for those consuming vegetarian diets than for those eating nonvegetarian diets. Therefore, it has been suggested that the zinc requirement for those consuming a vegetarian diet is approximately 2-fold greater than for those consuming a nonvegetarian diet.
		0–6 mo	2*	4			
		7–12 mo	3	5			
		Children					
		1–3 y	3	7			
		4–8 y	5	12			
		Males					
		9–13 y	8	23			
		14–18 y	11	34			
		19–30 y	11	40			
		31–50 y	11	40			
		50–70 y	11	40			
		> 70 y	11	40			
		Females					
		9–13 y	8	23			
		14–18 y	9	34			
		19–30 y	8	40			
		31–50 y	8	40			
		50–70 y	8	40			
		> 70 y	8	40			
		Pregnancy					
		≤ 18 y	12	34			
		19–30y	11	40			
		31–50 y	11	40			
		Lactation					
		≤ 18 y	13	34			
		19–30y	12	40			
		31–50 y	12	40			

NOTE: The table is adapted from the DRI reports, see www.nap.edu. It represents Recommended Dietary Allowances (RDAs) in **bold type**. Adequate Intakes (AIs) in ordinary type followed by an asterisk (*), and Tolerable Upper Intake Levels (ULs)[a]. RDAs and AIs may both be used as goals for individual intake. RDAs are set to meet the needs of almost all (97 to 98 percent) individuals in a group. For healthy breastfed infants, the AI is the mean intake. The AI for other life stage and gender groups is believed to cover the needs of all individuals in the group, but lack of data prevent being able to specify with confidence the percentage of individuals covered by this intake.

[a]UL = The maximum level of daily nutrient intake that is likely to pose no risk of adverse effects. Unless otherwise specified, the UL represents total intake from food, water, and supplements. Due to lack of suitable data, ULs could not be established for vitamin K, thiamin, riboflavin, vitamin B₁₂, pantothenic acid, biotin, or carotenoids. In the absence of ULs, extra caution may be warranted in consuming levels above recommended intakes.

[b]ND = Not determinable due to lack of data of adverse effects in this age group and concern with regard to lack of ability to handle excess amounts. Source of intake should be from food only to prevent high levels of intake.

SOURCES: *Dietary Reference Intakes for Calcium, Phosphorous, Magnesium, Vitamin D, and Fluoride* (1997); *Dietary Reference Intakes for Thiamin, Riboflavin, Niacin, Vitamin B₆, Folate, Vitamin B₁₂, Pantothenic Acid, Biotin, and Choline* (1998); *Dietary Reference Intakes for Vitamin C, Vitamin E, Selenium, and Carotenoids* (2000); and *Dietary Reference Intakes for Vitamin A, Vitamin K, Arsenic, Boron, Chromium, Copper, Iodine, Iron, Manganese, Molybdenum, Nickel, Silicon, Vanadium, and Zinc* (2001). These reports may be accessed via www.nap.edu.

Dietary Reference Intakes: Macronutrients

Nutrient	Function	Life Stage Group	RDA/AI* g/d	AMDR	Selected Food Sources	Adverse effects of excessive consumption
Carbohydrate— Total digestible	RDA based on its role as the primary energy source for the brain; AMDR based on its role as a source of kilocalories to maintain body weight	Infants			Starch and sugar are the major types of carbohydrates. Grains and vegetables (corn, pasta, rice, potatoes, breads) are sources of starch. Natural sugars are found in fruits and juices. Sources of added sugars are soft drinks, candy, fruit drinks, and desserts.	While no defined intake level at which potential adverse effects of total digestible carbohydrate was identified, the upper end of the adequate macronutrient distribution range (AMDR) was based on decreasing risk of chronic disease and providing adequate intake of other nutrients. It is suggested that the maximal intake of added sugars be limited to providing no more than 25 percent of energy.
		0–6 mo	60*	ND[b]		
		7–12 mo	95*	ND		
		Children				
		1–3 y	130	45-65		
		4–8 y	130	45-65		
		Males				
		9–13 y	130	45-65		
		14–18 y	130	45-65		
		19–30 y	130	45-65		
		31-50 y	130	45-65		
		50-70 y	130	45-65		
		> 70 y	130	45-65		
		Females				
		9–13 y	130	45-65		
		14–18 y	130	45-65		
		19–30 y	130	45-65		
		31-50 y	130	45-65		
		50-70 y	130	45-65		
		> 70 y	130	45-65		
		Pregnancy				
		≤ 18 y	175	45-65		
		19-30y	175	45-65		
		31-50 y	175	45-65		
		Lactation				
		≤ 18 y	210	45-65		
		19-30y	210	45-65		
		31–50 y	210	45-65		

Continued on next page

Total Fiber	Improves laxation, reduces risk of coronary heart disease, assists in maintaining normal blood glucose levels.		Includes dietary fiber naturally present in grains (such as found in oats, wheat, or unmilled rice) and functional fiber synthesized or isolated from plants or animals and shown to be of benefit to health	Dietary fiber can have variable compositions and therefore it is difficult to link a specific source of fiber with a particular adverse effect, especially when phytate is also present in the natural fiber source. It is concluded that as part of an overall healthy diet, a high intake of dietary fiber will not produce deleterious effects in healthy individuals. While occasional adverse gastrointestinal symptoms are observed when consuming some isolated or synthetic fibers, serious chronic adverse effects have not been observed. Due to the bulky nature of fibers, excess consumption is likely to be self-limiting. Therefore, a UL was not set for individual functional fibers.
	Infants			
	0–6 mo	ND		
	7–12 mo	ND		
	Children			
	1–3 y	19*		
	4–8 y	25*		
	Males			
	9–13 y	31*		
	14–18 y	38*		
	19–30 y	38*		
	31–50 y	38*		
	50–70 y	30*		
	>70 y	30*		
	Females			
	9–13 y	26*		
	14–18 y	26*		
	19–30 y	25*		
	31–50 y	25*		
	50–70 y	21*		
	>70 y	21*		
	Pregnancy			
	≤ 18 y	28*		
	19–30 y	28*		
	31–50 y	28*		
	Lactation			
	≤ 18 y	29*		
	19–30 y	29*		
	31–50 y	29*		

NOTE: The table is adapted from the DRI reports, see www.nap.edu. It represents Recommended Dietary Allowances (RDAs) in **bold type**. Adequate Intakes (AIs) in ordinary type followed by an asterisk (*). RDAs and AIs may both be used as goals for individual intake. RDAs are set to meet the needs of almost all (97 to 98 percent) individuals in a group. For healthy breastfed infants, the AI is the mean intake. The AI for other life stage and gender groups is believed to cover the needs of all individuals in the group, but lack of data prevent being able to specify with confidence the percentage of individuals covered by this intake.

a Acceptable Macronutrient Distribution Range (AMDR)ᵃ is the range of intake for a particular energy source that is associated with reduced risk of chronic disease while providing intakes of essential nutrients. If an individual consumes in excess of the AMDR, there is a potential of increasing the risk of chronic diseases and/or insufficient intakes of essential nutrients.

bND = Not determinable due to lack of data of adverse effects in this age group and concern with regard to lack of ability to handle excess amounts. Source of intake should be from food only to prevent high levels of intake.

SOURCES: *Dietary Reference Intakes for Energy, Carbohydrate. Fiber, Fat, Fatty Acids, Cholesterol, Protein, and Amino Acids (2002).* This report may be accessed via www.nap.edu

346

Dietary Reference Intakes: Macronutrients

Nutrient	Function	Life Stage Group	RDA/AI* g/d	AMDR[a]	Selected Food Sources	Adverse effects of excessive consumption
Total Fat	Energy source and when found in foods, is a source of n-6 and n-3 polyunsaturated fatty acids. Its presence in the diet increases absorption of fat soluble vitamins and precursors such as vitamin A and pro-vitamin A carotenoids.	Infants			Butter, margarine, vegetable oils, whole milk, visible fat on meat and poultry products, invisible fat in fish, shellfish, some plant products such as seeds and nuts, and bakery products.	While no defined intake level at which potential adverse effects of total fat was identified, the upper end of AMDR is based on decreasing risk of chronic disease and providing adequate intake of other nutrients. The lower end of the AMDR is based on concerns related to the increase in plasma triacylglycerol concentrations and decreased HDL cheolesterol concentrations seen with very low fat (and thus high carbohydrate) diets.
		0–6 mo	31*			
		7–12 mo	30*			
		Children				
		1–3 y		30-40		
		4–8 y		25-35		
		Males				
		9–13 y		25-35		
		14–18 y		25-35		
		19–30 y		20-35		
		31–50 y		20-35		
		50–70 y		20-35		
		> 70 y		20-35		
		Females				
		9–13 y		25-35		
		14–18 y		25-35		
		19–30 y		20-35		
		31–50 y		20-35		
		50–70 y		20-35		
		> 70 y		20-35		
		Pregnancy				
		≤ 18 y		20-35		
		19–30y		20-35		
		31–50 y		20-35		
		Lactation				
		≤ 18 y		20-35		
		19–30y		20-35		
		31–50 y		20-35		

Continued on next page

347

n-6 polyunsaturated fatty acids (linoleic acid)	Essential component of structural membrane lipids, involved with cell signaling, and precursor of eicosanoids. Required for normal skin function.		ND[b]	Nuts, seeds, and vegetable oils such as soybean, safflower, and corn oil.	While no defined intake level at which potential adverse effects of n-6 polyunsaturated fatty acids was identified, the upper end of the AMDR is based on the lack of evidence that demonstrates long-term safety and human in vitro studies which show increased free-radical formation and lipid peroxidation with higher amounts of n-6 fatty acids. Lipid peroxidation is thought to be a component of in the development of atherosclerotic plaques.
	Infants				
	0–6 mo	4.4*	ND		
	7–12 mo	4.6*	ND		
	Children				
	1–3 y	7*	5-10		
	4–8 y	10*	5-10		
	Males				
	9–13 y	12*	5-10		
	14–18 y	16*	5-10		
	19–30 y	17*	5-10		
	31–50 y	17*	5-10		
	50–70 y	14*	5-10		
	>70 y	14*	5-10		
	Females				
	9–13 y	10*	5-10		
	14–18 y	11*	5-10		
	19–30 y	12*	5-10		
	31–50 y	12*	5-10		
	50–70 y	11*	5-10		
	>70 y	11*	5-10		
	Pregnancy				
	≤ 18 y	13*	5-10		
	19-30y	13*	5-10		
	31-50y	13*	5-10		
	Lactation				
	≤ 18 y	13*	5-10		
	19-30y	13*	5-10		
	31–50 y	13*	5-10		

NOTE: The table is adapted from the DRI reports, see www.nap.edu. It represents Recommended Dietary Allowances (RDAs) in **bold type**. Adequate Intakes (AIs) in ordinary type followed by an asterisk (*). RDAs and AIs may both be used as goals for individual intake. RDAs are set to meet the needs of almost all (97 to 98 percent) individuals in a group. For healthy breastfed infants, the AI is the mean intake. The AI for other life stage and gender groups is believed to cover the needs of all individuals in the group, but lack of data prevent being able to specify with confidence the percentage of individuals covered by this intake.

[a] Acceptable Macronutrient Distribution Range (AMDR)[a] is the range of intake for a particular energy source that is associated with reduced risk of chronic disease while providing intakes of essential nutrients. If an individuals consumed in excess of the AMDR, there is a potential of increasing the risk of chronic diseases and insufficient intakes of essential nutrients.

[b] ND = Not determinable due to lack of data of adverse effects in this age group and concern with regard to lack of ability to handle excess amounts. Source of intake should be from food only to prevent high levels of intake.

SOURCES: *Dietary Reference Intakes for Energy, Carbohydrate. Fiber, Fat, Fatty Acids, Cholesterol, Protein, and Amino Acids (2002).* This report may be accessed via www.nap.edu

348

Dietary Reference Intakes: Macronutrients

Nutrient	Function	Life Stage Group	RDA/AI* g/d	AMDR[a]	Selected Food Sources	Adverse effects of excessive consumption
n-3 polyunsaturated fatty acids (α-linolenic acid)	Involved with neurological development and growth. Precursor of eicosanoids.	Infants			Vegetable oils such as soybean, canola, and flax seed oil, fish oils, fatty fish, with smaller amounts in meats and eggs.	While no defined intake level at which potential adverse effects of n-3 polyunsaturated fatty acids was identified, the upper end of AMDR is based on maintaining the appropriate balance with n-6 fatty acids and on the lack of evidence that demonstrates long-term safety, along with human in vitro studies which show increased free-radical formation and lipid peroxidation with higher amounts of polyunsaturated fatty acids. Lipid peroxidation is thought to be a component of in the development of atherosclerotic plaques.
		0–6 mo	0.5*	ND[b]		
		7–12 mo	0.5*	ND		
		Children				
		1–3 y	0.7*	0.6-1.2		
		4–8 y	0.9*	0.6-1.2		
		Males				
		9–13 y	1.2*	0.6-1.2		
		14–18 y	1.6*	0.6-1.2		
		19–30 y	1.6*	0.6-1.2		
		31-50 y	1.6*	0.6-1.2		
		50-70 y	1.6*	0.6-1.2		
		>70 y	1.6*	0.6-1.2		
		Females				
		9–13 y	1.0*	0.6-1.2		
		14–18 y	1.1*	0.6-1.2		
		19–30 y	1.1*	0.6-1.2		
		31-50 y	1.1*	0.6-1.2		
		50-70 y	1.1*	0.6-1.2		
		>70 y	1.1*	0.6-1.2		
		Pregnancy				
		≤ 18 y	1.4*	0.6-1.2		
		19-30y	1.4*	0.6-1.2		
		31-50 y	1.4*	0.6-1.2		
		Lactation				
		≤ 18 y	1.3*	0.6-1.2		
		19-30y	1.3*	0.6-1.2		
		31–50 y	1.3*	0.6-1.2		

Continued on next page

Nutrient	Function	Life Stage Group		Selected Food Sources	Adverse Effects of Overconsumption
Saturated and *trans* fatty acids, and cholesterol	No required role for these nutrients other than as energy sources was identified; the body can synthesize its needs for saturated fatty acids and cholesterol from other sources.	Infants 0–6 mo 7–12 mo Children 1–3 y 4–8 y Males 9–13 y 14–18 y 19–30 y 31–50 y 50–70 y >70 y Females 9–13 y 14–18 y 19–30 y 31–50 y 50–70 y >70 y Pregnancy ≤18 y 19–30y 31–50 y Lactation ≤18 y 19–30y 31–50 y	ND ND	Saturated fatty acids are present in animal fats (meat fats and butter fat), and coconut and palm kernel oils. Sources of cholesterol include liver, eggs, and foods that contain eggs such as cheesecake and custard pies. Sources of *trans* fatty acids include stick margarines and foods containing hydrogenated or partially-hydrogenated vegetable shortenings.	There is an incremental increase in plasma total and low-density lipoprotein cholesterol concentrations with increased intake of saturated or *trans* fatty acids or with cholesterol at even very low levels in the diet. Therefore, the intakes of each should be minimized while consuming a nutritionally adequate diet.

NOTE: The table is adapted from the DRI reports, see www.nap.edu. It represents Recommended Dietary Allowances (RDAs) in **bold type**. Adequate Intakes (AIs) in ordinary type followed by an asterisk (*). RDAs and AIs may both be used as goals for individual intake. RDAs are set to meet the needs of almost all (97 to 98 percent) individuals in a group. For healthy breastfed infants, the AI is the mean intake. The AI for other life stage and gender groups is believed to cover the needs of all individuals in the group, but lack of data prevent being able to specify with confidence the percentage of individuals covered by this intake.

a Acceptable Macronutrient Distribution Range (AMDR)[a] is the range of intake for a particular energy source that is associated with reduced risk of chronic disease while providing intakes of essential nutrients. If an individuals consumed in excess of the AMDR, there is a potential of increasing the risk of chronic diseases and insufficient intakes of essential nutrients.

b ND = Not determinable due to lack of data of adverse effects in this age group and concern with regard to lack of ability to handle excess amounts. Source of intake should be from food only to prevent high levels of intake.

SOURCES: *Dietary Reference Intakes for Energy, Carbohydrate. Fiber, Fat, Fatty Acids, Cholesterol, Protein, and Amino Acids (2002).* This report may be accessed via www.nap.edu

Dietary Reference Intakes: Macronutrients

Nutrient	Function	Life Stage Group	RDA/AI* g/d[a]	AMDR[b]	Selected Food Sources	Adverse effects of excessive consumption
Protein and amino acids	Serves as the major structural component of all cells in the body, and functions as enzymes, in membranes, as transport carriers, and as some hormones. During digestion and absorption dietary proteins are broken down to amino acids, which become the building blocks of these structural and functional compounds. Nine of the amino acids must be provided in the diet; these are termed indispensable amino acids. The body can make the other amino acids needed to synthesize specific structures from other amino acids.	**Infants** 0–6 mo	9.1*	ND[c]	Proteins from animal sources, such as meat, poultry, fish, eggs, milk, cheese, and yogurt, provide all nine indispensable amino acids in adequate amounts, and for this reason are considered "complete proteins". Proteins from plants, legumes, grains, nuts, seeds, and vegetables tend to be deficient in one or more of the indispensable amino acids and are called 'incomplete proteins'. Vegan diets adequate in total protein content can be "complete" by combining sources of incomplete proteins which lack different indispensable amino acids.	While no defined intake level at which potential adverse effects of protein was identified, the upper end of AMDR based on complementing the AMDR for carbohydrate and fat for the various age groups. The lower end of the AMDR is set at approximately the RDA..
		7–12 mo	**13.5**	ND		
		Children 1–3 y	**13**	**5-20**		
		4–8 y	**19**	10-30		
		Males 9–13 y	**34**	10-30		
		14–18 y	**52**	10-30		
		19–30 y	**56**	10-35		
		31-50 y	**56**	10-35		
		50-70 y	**56**	10-35		
		> 70 y	**56**	10-35		
		Females 9–13 y	**34**	10-30		
		14–18 y	**46**	10-30		
		19–30 y	**46**	10-35		
		31-50 y	**46**	10-35		
		50-70 y	**46**	10-35		
		> 70 y	**46**	10-35		
		Pregnancy ≤ 18 y	**71**	10-35		
		19-30y	**71**	10-35		
		31-50y	**71**	10-35		
		Lactation ≤ 18 y	**71**	10-35		
		19-30y	**71**	10-35		
		31-50 y	**71**	10-35		

NOTE: The table is adapted from the DRI reports, see www.nap.edu. It represents Recommended Dietary Allowances (RDAs) in **bold type.** Adequate Intakes (AIs) in ordinary type followed by an asterisk (*). RDAs and AIs may both be used as goals for individual intake. RDAs are set to meet the needs of almost all (97 to 98 percent) individuals in a group. For healthy breastfed infants, the AI is the mean intake. The AI for other life stage and gender groups is believed to cover the needs of all individuals in the group, but lack of data prevent being able to specify with confidence the percentage of individuals covered by this intake.

[a] Based on 1.5 g/kg/day for infants, 1.1 g/kg/day for 1-3 y, 0.95 g/kg/day for 4-13 y, 0.85 g/kg/day for 14-18 y, 0.8 g /kg/day for adults, and 1.1 g/kg/day for pregnant (using pre-pregnancy weight) and lactating women.

[b] Acceptable Macronutrient Distribution Range (AMDR)[a] is the range of intake for a particular energy source that is associated with reduced risk of chronic disease while providing intakes of essential nutrients. If an individuals consumed in excess of the AMDR, there is a potential of increasing the risk of chronic diseases and insufficient intakes of essential nutrients.

[c]ND = Not determinable due to lack of data of adverse effects in this age group and concern with regard to lack of ability to handle excess amounts. Source of intake should be from food only to prevent high levels of intake.

SOURCES: *Dietary Reference Intakes for Energy, Carbohydrate, Fiber, Fat, Fatty Acids, Cholesterol, Protein, and Amino Acids (2002).* This report may be accessed via www.nap.edu

351

Dietary Reference Intakes: Macronutrients

Nutrient	Function	IOM/FNB 2002 Scoring Pattern[a]	Mg /g protein	Adverse effects of excessive consumption
Indispensable amino acids:	The building blocks of all proteins in the body and some hormones. These nine amino acids must be provided in the diet and thus are termed indispensable amino acids. The body can make the other amino acids needed to synthesize specific structures from other amino acids and carbohydrate precursors.			Since there is no evidence that amino acids found in usual or even high intakes of protein from food present any risk, attention was focused on intakes of the L-form of these and other amino acid found in dietary protein and amino acid supplements. Even from well-studied amino acids, adequate dose-response data from human or animal studies on which to base a UL were not available. While no defined intake level at which potential adverse effects of protein was identified for any amino acid, this does not mean that there is no potential for adverse effects resulting from high intakes of amino acids from dietary supplements. Since data on the adverse effects of high levels of amino acid intakes from dietary supplements are limited, caution may be warranted.
Histidine		Histidine	18	
Isoleucine		Isoleucine	25	
Lysine		Lysine	55	
Leucine		Leucine	51	
Methionine & Cysteine		Methionine & Cysteine	25	
Phenylalanine & Tyrosine		Phenylalanine & Tyrosine	47	
Threonine		Threonine	27	
Tryptophan		Tryptophan	7	
Valine		Valine	32	

NOTE: The table is adapted from the DRI reports, see www.nap.edu.

[a] Based on the amino acid requirements derived for Preschool Children (1-3 y): (EAR for amino acid ÷ EAR for protein); for 1-3 y group where EAR for protein = 0.88 g/kg/d.

SOURCES: *Dietary Reference Intakes for Energy, Carbohydrate. Fiber, Fat, Fatty Acids, Cholesterol, Protein, and Amino Acids (2002)*. This report may be accessed via www.nap.edu

352

Appendix D

Cranial Nerve Assessment

Cranial Nerve Assessment

Cranial Nerve	Function	Examination	Presentation
I. Olfactory	*S* Sensation to nasal mucosa. Smell.	*S* Test presence and ability to distinguish scents using fragrant foods, flavor extracts, or spices.	*S* Limitation in ability to smell.
II. Optic	*S* Visual acuity. Visual field. Convey visual information from the retina.	*S* Stand behind patient with arms extended outward. Bring arms together and have patient identify when they can see your hands.	*S* Limitation in ability to see.
III. Oculomotor	*M* Motor function to eye, pupillary constriction to light.	*M* Test movement of eye with "H" or "box" test. Test pupillary light reaction with penlight. Test III, IV, VI together.	*M* Limitation in ability to move eye downward, upward or toward nose (adduction), unable to adapt to light and dark. Ptosis (drooping eyelid).
IV. Trochlear	*M* Motor function to superior oblique muscle.	Test III, IV, VI together.	*M* Limitation in ability to move eye downward and inward. Double vision.
V. Trigeminal [a]	*S* Sensation to dura, skin of forehead, scalp, roof of nasal cavity, nose, skin around the eye, cheek, lip, teeth, hard palate, ear, chin, lining of cheek and gums. *M* Mastication. Motor function to temporalis, masseter, medial and lateral pterygoid, mylohyoid.	*S* Test face along the mandible, maxilla, and forehead with sharp (pinprick), dull (tongue depressor), and light touch (cotton swab). *M* Have patient open and close the jaw. Then have patient resist attempts of examiner to close jaw.	*S* Decreased facial or oral sensation. • Drooling • Pocketing of food *M* Weak jaw closing, asymmetric opening, muscle atrophy. • Easily fatigues • Food leakage
VI. Abducens	*M* Motor function to lateral rectus muscle (for precise movement of the eye for visual tracking or fixation on an object).	Test III, IV, VI together.	*M* Limitation in ability to follow object with eye, or move away from nose (abduction).

Cranial Nerve	Function	Assessment	Abnormal Findings

VII. Facial [a]	S Taste anterior 2/3 of tongue, palate.
	M Facial expressions, muscles of lips and cheeks.
	A Secretion of lacrimal, sublingual, and submandibular glands.
		S Test taste sensation of sweet, salt, and sour.
		M Have patient smile to show teeth, raise eyebrows, close eyelids tightly.
			S Altered taste.
			M Facial asymmetry, unequal nasolabial folds, poor lip seal.
			  • Drooling
			  • Pocketing of food
			A Decreased saliva.
			  • Increased oral preparatory stage.

VIII. Vestibulocochlear (Acoustic)	S Sensation from cochlea for hearing and from semicircular canals and vestibule for equilibrium.	S Rub hair or fingers near patient's ears.	S Deafness, vertigo.

IX. Glossopharyngeal [a]	S Taste posterior 1/3 of tongue; sensation to pharynx, tonsils, soft palate.
	M Elevation of soft palate; swallowing.
	A Secretion of parotid gland.
		S Test taste sensation of bitter. Gag reflex: Touch posterior pharynx with a cotton swab. Look for pharyngeal elevation and tongue retraction.
		M Have patient say "AH." Look for bilateral soft palate elevation and midline uvula.
			S Altered taste. No pharyngeal elevation.
			  • Increased risk of aspiration.
			M Limited palate elevation.
			  • Pocketing
			  • Prolonged eating time
			A Decreased saliva.

X. Vagus [a]	S Taste base of tongue and epiglottis. Sensation to soft palate, upper larynx. M Movement of soft palate, pharynx, and larynx.	Test IX and X together. (See above.)	(See above.)
XI. Spinal Accessory	M Motor function to vagus, sternomastoid, and trapezius muscles.	M Test neck range of motion. Have patient lift shoulders with and without pressure. Have patient turn head with and without pressure.	M Limitation in ability to raise shoulders or turn head, muscle atrophy and weakness.
XII. Hypoglossal [a]	M Movement of tongue.	M Protrude tongue. Should be midline. Test tongue strength with tongue blade.	M Limitation in tongue movement or deviation.

S Sensor response; M motor response; A autonomic response; [a] CN involved in dysphagia screening.
From Norman, W. Cranial Nerves. Website: (http://mywebpages.comcast.net/wnor/cranialnerves.htm). Accessed October 24, 2003.

Appendix E
Diet Education Tools

The authors share the following diet education materials that may be reproduced for patient education purposes only without permission. However, we ask that the appropriate references citation to the originators of the materials be listed. These materials may not be reproduced to be sold or used in any publication without written permission.

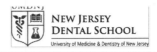

NEW JERSEY
DENTAL SCHOOL
University of Medicine & Dentistry of New Jersey

Department of Diagnostic Sciences
Division of Nutrition

Dealing with Dry Mouth (Xerostomia)

➢ Suck on sugar-free hard candy, ice chips, frozen grapes, sugar-free gum or sugar-free ice pops

➢ Use xylitol gums and mints, such as Smints ®, to help prevent caries

➢ Eat soft foods that may be easier to swallow, such as custards, soups, ice cream, puddings or sorbets

➢ Use yogurt, cottage cheese, or bean soups as protein sources

➢ Dunk or soak foods in liquids to make them softer and easier to swallow

➢ Use lip balm to keep lips moist

➢ Cut food into small pieces and mix with sauces and gravies to make them moist and easy to swallow

➢ Have a sip of water every few minutes during meals to help you swallow

➢ Try mashed potatoes and rice instead of dry crackers and bread

➢ Try applesauce, fruit cocktail and other fruits canned in their own juices instead of raw or citrus fruits

➢ Try herbs in place of spices, citrus juices and salt for seasonings

➢ Eating papaya may help break up thick "ropy" saliva

➢ Carry a bottle of water with a fresh-squeezed lemon with you for easy access

Calcium

❖ Calcium is essential for body functions including regulation of the heartbeat, conduction of nerve impulses, stimulation of hormone secretions, clotting of blood, and for the building and maintaining of healthy bones.

❖ Calcium is a mineral found in many foods, higher in dairy products such as milk, yogurt, cheese, and ice cream. Calcium is important in the diet because the human body can not produce adequate amounts of calcium alone.

❖ Calcium supplements may be indicated in individuals who are unable to get enough calcium in their regular diet or may have a higher need for calcium. For example, pregnancy, nursing, osteoporosis, hypocalcemia, and at times of growth.

Normal Daily Recommended Intakes for Calcium	
Infants & Children: Birth to 3 years	400-800 mg
4 to 6 years of age	800 mg
7 to 10 years of age	800 mg
Adolescent and adult males	800-1200 mg
Adolescent and adult females	800-1200 mg
Pregnant females	1200 mg
Breast-feeding females	1200 mg

Calcium Supplements May Come in Several Different Compounds

Amount of Elemental Calcium of Select Compounds	
Calcium Supplement	Amount of elemental calcium per tablet (mg)
Calcium carbonate	260
	600
Calcium citrate	200
Calcium gluconate	45
	90
Calcium lactate	84
Calcium phosphate, dibasic	115
Calcium phosphate, tribasic	304

• Calcium is best absorbed from the citrate malate form, or the type of calcium found in some juices, calcium carbonate is recommended for the overall amount of calcium it offers and its affordability.

• Calcium carbonate is relatively insoluble, and is best absorbed when taken with meals. Food slows down the time it takes substances to travel through the GI tract, giving the calcium more time to be absorbed. Antactids. like Tums, contain calcium carbonate and may be an acceptable source of calcium

Continued on next page

- Calcium citrate, although only containing half as much as calcium by weight as calcium carbonate, is a more soluble form and does not require gastric acid for absorption. It is best taken between meals. Calcium citrate is useful for patients with limited gastric acid production.
- Calcium citrate, calcium lactate, and calcium gluconate are well absorbed at any time.
- Look for calcium supplements with vitamin D, magnesium, or phosphorous, which are essential for quick absorption.
- Intestinal absorption is limited to 500 mg of elemental calcium at one time, and should be taken with adequate water.
- Name brand supplements may be more bioavailable than generic products because of better manufacturing processes. Look for USP (United States Pharmacopeia) or NSF seal of quality.

Calcium/Drug Interactions:

- **Calcium-containing medicines**: Taking too much calcium may cause excess levels of calcium in the blood or urine, leading to additional medical problems. The current recommended upper limit of intake for calcium is 2500 mg/day.
- **Cellulose sodium phosphate (Calcibind):** If used with calcium supplements, they may decrease the effects of cellulose sodium phosphate.
- **Digitalis glycosides (heart medicine):** Used with calcium supplements by injection may increase the regular heartbeat.
- **Etidronate (Didronel):** Effects of etidronate may be decreased if calcium supplements are taken within two hours of medication.
- **Gallium nitrate (Ganite):** May not work properly if calcium supplements are being taken.
- **Magnesium sulfate (injections):** If calcium supplements are also taken, either medication may become less effective.
- **Phenytoin (Dilantin):** Calcium supplements should not be taken within 1-3 hours of phenytoin, may decrease the effects of either medication.
- **Tetracyclines (for infections) by mouth:** Tetracycline effects may be decreased if calcium supplements are taken 1-3 hours of medication.

Information was obtained from the following resources:
Kapes, Beth. Gale Encyclopedia of Alternative Medicine.
Medline Plus Drug Information: Calcium Supplements (Systemic)
Clarke, Mary. Timely Topic: Calcium Supplements. Dairy Council Digest 66(1), January/February 1995.

Calcium Requirements
Calcium Supplements and Food Sources

Recommended daily values by age:

Birth to 3 years	4-10 years	11-24 years	Women 25-50 years	Post-menopausal women on estrogen	Post-menopausal women not on estrogen	Pregnant/ Lactating women	Men 25-50 years	Men and women 65 years and older
400-800 mg	800 mg	1200-1500 mg	1000 mg	1000 mg	1500 mg	1200 mg	1000 mg	1500 mg

*Different calcium supplements vary in calcium content, the following table includes the different dosages of oral calcium supplements available and it also explains how many tablets of each type of supplement will provide 1000 milligrams of elemental calcium. When looking for a calcium supplement, it is important to look at the number of milligrams on the label since this refers to the amount of elemental calcium, and not to the strength of each tablet.

Calcium supplement	Amount of elemental calcium per tablet (in milligrams)	Number of tablets to provide 1000 milligrams of calcium
Calcium carbonate	250	4
	260	4
	300	4
	334	3
	500	2
	600	2
Calcium citrate	200	5
Calcium gluconate	45	22
	58	17
	90	11
Calcium lactate	42	24
	84	12

Food Sources of Calcium:

*The following table includes some foods that are rich in calcium along with the amount of calcium in each of the servings indicated.

Food (amount)	Milligrams of calcium
Nonfat dry milk, reconstituted (1 cup)	375
Lowfat, skim, or whole milk (1 cup)	290 to 300
Yogurt (1 cup)	275 to 400
Sardines with bones (3 ounces)	370
Ricotta cheese, part skim (1/2 cup)	340
Salmon, canned, with bones (3 ounces)	285
Cheese, Swiss (1 ounce)	272
Cheese, cheddar (1 ounce)	204
Cheese, American (1 ounce)	174
Cottage cheese, lowfat (1 cup)	154
Tofu (4 ounces)	154
Shrimp (1 cup)	147
Ice milk (3/4 cup)	132

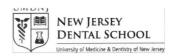

NEW JERSEY
DENTAL SCHOOL
University of Medicine & Dentistry of New Jersey

Department of Diagnostic Sciences
Division of Nutrition

Diabetes and Dentures
A guide to successful diet management

Use the tips below to advise your patients on what foods to consume to maintain a healthy diabetic diet and proper denture care. It is important that Diabetics do not have an excessive amount of carbohydrates at one time, but rather to balance them throughout the day. Listed below are some food choices along with the amount of carbohydrates they contain that you can recommend your patients have with their new dentures.

First meal after placement of dentures:
1 cup cream based soup (1 CHO exchange)

1 cup sugar-free pudding (2 CHO exchange)
1 cup sugar-free jello (free food)
8 oz Oral supplement (Glucerna, Choice) (2 CHO exchange)
8 oz vanilla milkshake prepared with sugar-free ice cream (2 CHO exchanges)

Suggestions for soft-solid meal:
1 cup cooked plain oatmeal (2 CHO exchanges)
8 oz light, fat-free yogurt (1.5 CHO exchanges)
$3/4$ cup non-sugar sweetened cereal (1 CHO exchange)
soaked in 8 oz milk (additional 1 CHO exchange)
1 cup cooked pasta (2 CHO exchanges)

* CHO=Carbohydrate

Helpful Hints When Treating a Patient With Diabetes

Questions to Ask When Assessing a Patient With Diabetes:

1. Do you have Type 1 or Type 2 diabetes?

2. When were you diagnosed with diabetes?

3. How do you control your blood sugar? (Diet, Oral Hypoglycemic Agents, Insulin)

4. How well is your diabetes controlled?

5. What is your medication regimen? (Dose and Frequency)

6. When did you take your medication today?

7. When was the last time you ate today? What did you eat?

8. How often do you monitor your glucose?

9. When was your last fingerstick? What was the number?

10. What is your Hgb A1c?

11. How often have you experienced a hypoglycemic reaction?

12. Have you ever been hospitalized due to diabetes?

13. When was your last visit to your physician?

Remember:

> ➤ Before starting a procedure, make sure the patient has taken his medications and has eaten
> ➤ Have juice readily available in case the procedure takes longer than anticipated
> ➤ Provide a time estimate on the length of the next dental visit so patient can prepare accordingly

References

www.ada.org/prof/resources/pubs/jada/reports/diabetes.asp
Journal articles related to diabetes and oral health.
www.diabetes.org
Evidence-Based nutrition principles and recommendations for the treatment and prevention of diabetes and related complications
www.drymouth.info
Provides explanations, treatments, and causes of dry mouth.

Continued on next page

Hypoglycemic Agents

Drug	Mechanisms of action
Sulfonylureas o Glipizide o Amaryl o Prandin o Starlix	Increases insulin production.
Biguanides o Glucophage o Glucovance	Anti-hyperglycemic/ Insulin Sensitizers decreases hepatic glucose production and improves insulin sensitivity.
Thiazolidediones o Avandia o Actos	Insulin Sensitizers improves insulin sensitivity
Alpha-glucosidase inhibitors o Precose o Glyset	Starch Blockers Inhibits alpha-glucosidase enzymes to delay glucose absorption.

Actions of insulin

Insulin	Onset (hours)	Peak Action (hours)	Duration (hours)
Short acting o Human Regular	1/2 to 1	2 to 3	4 to 6
o Human Lispro	Within 15 minutes	1 to 1.5	4 to 5
Intermediate acting o NPH	2 to 4	4 to 10	10 to 16
o Human Lente	3 to 4	4 to 12	12 to 18
Long acting o Human Ultralente	6 to 10	14 to 24	18 to 20

Blood Glucose measures of whole blood	Normal values	Goal values
Preprandial glucose (mg/dl)	< 110	80-120
Postprandial glucose (mg/dl)	< 140	No more than 50mg/dl higher than Preprandial
Bedtime glucose (mg/dl)	< 110	100 to 140
Hgb A1c (%)	< 6%	< 7%

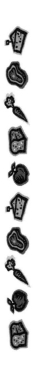

Tips for Successful Diet Management for Denture Wearers

Provided to you by:

_____
Your Student Dentist

&

_____
Registered Dietitian

Dear Patient,

This has been prepared for you to help you through the adjustment to your new immediate dentures. The gums will swell after the extraction of the teeth and the new denture will act like a big oral Band Aid. Since the mouth will be tender at first, it may make it difficult to eat your usual diet.

In order to maintain proper nutrition during the adjustment phase, the following menu suggestions are provided. Remember to drink at least 8 cups of fluid daily especially water.

If you have any questions, please feel free to call us at (973)-972-4160.

Sincerely,

_____
Your Dentist & Your Dietitian

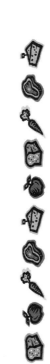

Continued on next page

First meal immediately after dentures:

(choose one or two)

1 cup cream soup

8 oz vanilla milkshake

8 oz apple or grape juice

8 oz Carnation Instant Breakfast or other oral
    supplement like: Ensure, Sustacal
        (these are lactose-free)

Progress to soft-solid meal:

2 scrambled eggs	1 cup applesauce
or	or
1 cup yogurt	1 cup canned fruit
1 cup hot cereal	1 cup mashed potatoes
or	or
1 cup cold cereal	1 cup cooked pasta
soaked with milk	

First Night Denture Care Instructions:

Do not remove the denture the first night.
Rinse mouth with bland mouthwash
with denture in mouth. Your dentist
will remove the denture at the 24
hour post-insertion appointment.

Sample menu for 2nd day after denture insertion:

Breakfast:

8 oz glass low fat milk

4 oz grape juice

1 cup oatmeal

8 oz Carnation Instant Breakfast or other oral
    supplement like: Ensure, Sustacal
        (these are lactose-free)

Morning Snack:

1 cup applesauce

Lunch:

1 cup lentil soup
w/ soaked crackers

1 cup fruit yogurt

1 cup warm tea

Afternoon Snack:

$^1/_2$ cup peaches

1 cup vanilla ice cream

Dinner:

1$^1/_2$ cups steamed
    rice/pasta

1 cup refried beans

1 cup well-cooked string beans

8 oz low fat milk

Evening Snack:

1 cup bran flakes cereal
    soaked with cold milk

Continued on next page

366

Second Day Home Care Instructions:

If you can remove and insert the denture without difficulty, do so. If it should be too painful, repeat the first night program. You can brush the denture while it is in your mouth. *The denture must be cleaned after every meal.* If you can remove the denture, take it out and scrub it with a denture toothbrush and denture toothpaste (Dent-u-Cr me). Rinse and place in a denture cup with Polident or Efferdent cleanser. Leave in cup overnight.

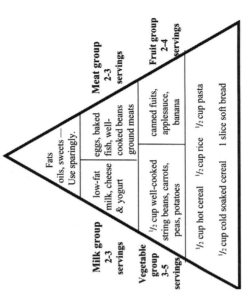

In morning, again brush denture with denture toothpaste, rinse and carefully put it into your mouth. Close together slowly to make sure denture is well seated. Always fill sink with some water and brush denture slightly above water. The denture will get slippery when wet and the water will cushion the blow if dropped.

Third day after denture insertion:

You may begin to eat foods as usual.

Let your comfort be your guide.

Refer to the following Food Guide Pyramid which

Has examples of foods that may be better tolerated as

you get used to your new dentures

Fats
oils, sweets —
Use sparingly.

Milk group 2-3 servings	low-fat milk, cheese & yogurt	eggs, baked fish, well-cooked beans ground meats	Meat group 2-3 servings
		canned fuits, applesauce, banana	Fruit group 2-4 servings
Vegetable group 3-5 servings	½ cup well-cooked string beans, carrots, peas, potatoes		
	½ cup hot cereal ½ cup rice ½ cup pasta		
	½ cup cold soaked cereal 1 slice soft bread		

Bread group 6 — 11 servings

Continued on next page

367

Other easy to bite/ chew foods ideas you can try:

❖ pudding, Jello, ice cream, sherbet
❖ sandwiches — grill cheese, egg salad, tuna fish
❖ macaroni & cheese, chili with rice
❖ pasta salads with chopped steamed vegetables
❖ soft breads (those that are chewy may be difficult at first)
❖ bite size crackers, tortilla chips, rice cakes
❖ fruit smoothies (see recipe below)

Peaches and Cream Sipper

1, 16 oz package of frozen unsweetened peaches
1, 6 oz can frozen apple juice concentrate
1, 8 oz carton vanilla nonfat yogurt
1/3 cup instant nonfat dry milk powder
1/4 cup water
1/8 tsp vanilla extract
ice cubes

1) Combine first 6 ingredients in electric blender cover and process until smooth
2) Gradually add enough ice to measure 4 cups in blender cover and process until smooth
3) Pour into glasses makes 4 (1 cup servings)

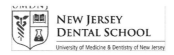

Department of Diagnostic Sciences
Division of Nutrition

People with Diabetes Need Special Attention: Don't Forget About Your Teeth!

If you have diabetes (high blood sugar) you need to take extra special care of your mouth to prevent gum disease & tooth decay.

If your blood sugar stays high, your teeth and gums may be at greater risk for dental diseases.

High blood sugar can cause dry mouth. This leaves you with less saliva to rinse your mouth and protect your teeth from germs.

Dry mouth leads to cut, dry and cracked lips, and sores of the mouth, making eating painful. It can also cause a burning feeling in your mouth or on your tongue.

When your blood sugar is high, there is more sugar in your saliva, which can change your taste, and may cause cavities.

When you have high blood sugar, your body cannot fight off the bacteria, increasing risk of gum disease and tooth decay and loss.

Continued on next page

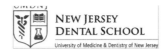

<u>What You Can Do To Protect Your Teeth:</u>

- Maintain the right blood sugar level.
- Get a dental checkup & cleaning every 3-6 months.
- Brush your teeth at least twice a day (preferably after each meal.)
- Rinse with water after meals or chew sugar-free gum if you can't brush.
- Ask your dentist to show you how to brush the right way.
- Floss daily
- If you have dry mouth, drink water, and suck on sugar-free candy or sugar-free gum.

Limit	*Choose*
<u>*Foods that are harmful to teeth*</u>	<u>*Foods that are friendly for teeth*</u>
Cookies, cakes	Cheese
Candy	Low fat milk
Chips	Sugar-free yogurt
Snack crackers	Fresh vegetables
Pretzels, cereals	Nuts

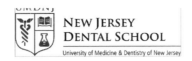

NEW JERSEY
DENTAL SCHOOL
University of Medicine & Dentistry of New Jersey

Department of Diagnostic Sciences
Division of Nutrition

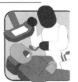

Do You Have a Hard Time Eating?

If you have missing teeth or have a hard time chewing then you may
want to try these types of foods. If you are also diabetic it is
important to remember to eat about the same amount of food at the
same time each day and try not to skip meals or snacks.

Foods To Choose To Keep You Healthy

Food Group	# Of Servings/Day	Serving Size Examples	Modified Consistency
Starches	6-11	1 slice bread 1 small potato 1/2 cup cooked cereal or pasta 3/4 cup cold cereal	Cut bread into small pieces and dunk into milk or coffee, mash potatoes, soak cold cereal in milk until very soft
Fruits	3-4	1 small fresh fruit 1/2 cup fruit juice 1/2 cup canned fruit	Use canned fruits (in juice, not syrup), chop, mash, or puree fresh fruits such as 1/2 banana, small ripe pear
Vegetables	3-5	1 cup raw vegetables 1/2 cup cooked	Cook or steam, used canned foods, chop, mash, or puree
Meats & Other Protein	2-3	1 oz egg = 1 egg 4 ounces tofu 2 to 3 oz cheese 2 to 3 oz lean meat, chicken or fish 1/2 cup to 3/4 cup tuna or cottage cheese	Boil or stew, chop into small pieces, slice thinly, grind in food processor, puree, grate or melt cheeses,
Milk	2-3	1 cup milk 1 cup yogurt (sugar free)	Puree sugar free fruited yogurts

Continued on next page

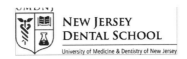

NEW JERSEY
DENTAL SCHOOL
University of Medicine & Dentistry of New Jersey

Helpful Hints

- To puree foods, first cut foods into medium size pieces. Place desired amount in food processor or blender. Add hot broth or gravy to meats and hot starches. Add juice or milk to fruits and cold starches. Blend until smooth.
- Dry items such as meat, biscuits, cereal, and crackers can be moistened with milk, gravy or soup.
- Remember to always clean blending equipment and other utensils properly in hot soapy water after each use to keep foods safe from bacteria. Do not put uncooked meat in the blender with foods that will be eaten raw such as vegetables. Blend these items separately and wash equipment after each use. Wash and scrub all fruits and vegetables in running water before blending them to get rid of dirt and bacteria.

Sample Menu

Breakfast

¾ cup Cheerios soaked in ½ cup skim milk
½ banana mashed
1 egg scrambled
1 slice cinnamon swirl bread dipped in ½ cup skim milk
4 oz orange juice
Coffee or tea

Lunch

3 oz thinly sliced turkey breast w/gravy
1 slice rye bread dipped in gravy
½ cup cooked green beans (pureed)
½ cup mashed potato
½ cup canned peaches in juice
1 cup skim milk

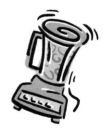

Dinner

4 oz apple juice
¾ cup tuna salad w/mayo
1 cup lentil soup w/soaked crackers
1 cup steamed carrots (mashed if desired)
1 cup sugar free yogurt (As a Snack)

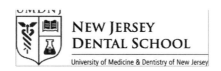

NEW JERSEY
DENTAL SCHOOL
University of Medicine & Dentistry of New Jersey

Department of Diagnostic Sciences
Division of Nutrition

Post Surgical Nutrition Recommendations

This information has been prepared to help you identify foods that are more easily tolerated after your dental extractions. After an extraction you may feel oral discomfort. In order to maintain good nutrition, the following food tips are provided.

First meal after extractions

❖ Carbohydrate sources: hot cereal or cream soups
❖ Protein sources: pureed meats or cottage cheese
❖ Vegetable sources: mashed potatoes or pureed/mashed vegetables such squash, carrots, sweet potatoes.
❖ Fruit sources: applesauce or pureed/mashed fruits
❖ Dairy sources: milk, yogurt, pudding, ice-cream, sherbet, milkshakes, or fruit smoothies
❖ Fluids: tea, juices and water
❖ Supplements: Carnation Instant breakfast or other oral supplement like: Ensure or Boost
❖ Do not use straws to sip liquids. Follow guidelines provided by your dentist

Progress to soft-solid foods

❖ Carbohydrate sources: cold cereal soaked with milk, lentil soup with soaked crackers, cooked pasta, soft bread
❖ Protein sources: scramble eggs, mashed beans, egg salad, tuna salad
❖ Fruit sources canned fruit
❖ Vegetables sources: boiled or steamed vegetables
❖ Dairy sources: cream or soft cheeses

Sample menu

Breakfast:
4 oz juice
8oz cup Carnation Instant Breakfast
1 cup cottage cheese or scramble eggs

Morning Snack:
1 cup yogurt or canned fruit / applesauce
Oatmeal

Lunch:
1 cup cream or lentil soup
1 scoop tuna salad w/ diced tomatoes
1 cup of ice-cream
8 oz water

Afternoon Snack:
½ cup pudding or milkshake

Dinner:
1 cup of mashed potatoes or cooked pasta
1 cup of mashed beans or pureed meat
1 cup mashed or pureed vegetable
1 cup of tea

Evening Snack:
1 cup of cereal soaked in milk

As mouth begins to feel better, you may want to try soft-solid foods. Advance your diet as tolerated!

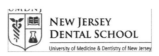

NEW JERSEY
DENTAL SCHOOL
University of Medicine & Dentistry of New Jersey

Department of Diagnostic Sciences
Division of Nutrition

Dealing With A Sore Mouth

Mouth sores, tender gums, and sore throats are often side effects of radiation therapy. Some foods can irritate an already tender mouth and make chewing and swallowing difficult. Proper food selection and good oral hygiene can make eating easier. Here are some suggestions that may help:

- **Include soft foods that are easy to chew and swallow such as:**
  - bananas, applesauce, peach, pear, and apricot (fresh or canned)
  - milkshakes, cottage cheese, yogurt
  - mashed potatoes, noodles, macaroni and cheese
  - custards, puddings, and gelatin
  - oatmeal or other cooked cereals, soaked cereals
  - scrambled eggs and pureed meats and vegetables
  - Carnation instant breakfast

- **Avoid Foods that can cause irritation such as:**
  - oranges, grapefruits, lemons, or other citrus fruit or juice
  - tomato sauces, spicy or salty foods
  - raw vegetables, granola, toast, crackers
  - commercial mouthwashes that contain alcohol

- **Food Preparation:**
  - Cook foods until they are soft and tender.
  - Cut foods into small pieces.
  - Puree food with a blender or food processor
  - Mix food with butter, margarine, thin gravy, or sauce to make it easier to swallow.

- **Tips on consuming food:**
  - Try foods cold or at room temperature. Hot foods can irritate a tender mouth and throat.
  - Try sucking on ice chips and rinsing your mouth often with water to remove food and bacteria
  - Try drinking through a straw

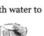

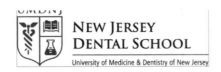

NEW JERSEY
DENTAL SCHOOL
University of Medicine & Dentistry of New Jersey

Department of Diagnostic Sciences
Division of Nutrition

WHEN THINGS DON'T TASTE THE SAME

Chemotherapy, radiation, cancer itself, diabetes, or other diseases and medications may cause some food to taste different than what you are used to. If this occurs, follow the tips below to modify your diet and continue to eat healthy balanced meals.

To enhance the flavor of food
1. Marinate meat in a variety of sauces such as:
    Soy sauce
    Barbeque sauce
    Sweet-n-sour sauce
    Salad dressing
2. Use a variety of seasonings on vegetables such as:
    Garlic powder
    Lemon juice/ lemon pepper
    Basil
3. Use fresh fruit or vanilla extract to enhance the flavor of milkshakes, ice cream and pudding.

To minimize the metallic taste of food
1. Use plastic utensils and dishes
2. Tart foods will overcome a metallic taste such as:
    Citrus juices
    Pickles, relish
    Fruit (ex: grapefruit, cranberry, Granny Smith apple)

Food Substitutions
1. If red meat tastes unusual, use other protein sources such as:
    Chicken, Turkey, Fish
    Dairy Products
2. Adding sugar can improve the flavor of salty foods
3. Adding salt can decrease the sweetness of sugary foods.
    * Caution- some diets require a restriction of salt and sugar

Other Suggestions:
1. Serve food cold or at room temperature to decrease strong odors (Remember to use food safety precautions with room temperature foods)
2. Use a variety of foods to complement your taste preferences
3. Serve food attractively and in a pleasant atmosphere to enhance acceptance.

Eating Guidelines for Times When Biting and Chewing are Compromised Due to Dental Procedures / Temporary Conditions

Hints:
1. Turn fruits and vegetables into chopped salads —
    Fruit salad in bite size pieces made from fresh cut up fruit
    Chopped greens, tomatoes, cucumbers
    Corn salsa (take fresh corn off the cob and mix with salsa)

2. Choose either very soft breads, crackers or very crisp ones
    (limit those that are chewy such as bagels, soft rolls, bread crusts)

3. If raw vegetables are tough to chew even chopped; steam or stir fry for 5
    minutes and then chop and chill for a salad

4. Pasta salads — pasta mixed with chopped vegetables or beans and chilled

Snacks Foods That Are Easy to Eat
1. Bite size tortilla chips broken in half

2. Bite size rice cakes

3. Fruit smoothies — frozen fresh fruit + yogurt or milk in the blender (high in
    calcium also)

4. Frozen berries or grapes — great to suck on

5. Flour tortilla pizza strips (flour tortillas with a layer of salsa and cheese,
    microwave for 1 minute then cut in strips

Drinking
Remember to drink at least 8 cups of liquid (= amount of water) daily

Adequate Fiber
When eating ability is compromised dietary fiber intake may drop; using these tips for eating chopped and cut food will help maintain fiber intake.
However if needed or desired, try $^1/_2$ to 1 cup of bran cereal daily (FIBER ONE or ALL BRAN) and emphasize high fiber foods such as corn, blueberries, dried beans.

c2001RTD-UMDNJ

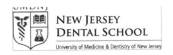

Department of Diagnostic Sciences
Division of Nutrition

<u>Smart Snacks For Healthy Teeth!</u>

- **Apples and Cheese**
- **Fruit Slices with Yogurt**
- **Baby Carrots**
- **Popcorn**
- **Tortilla Chips and Salsa topped with shredded cheese**
- **Animal Crackers with Milk**
- **Fruit Shakes**

✓ **Always brush your teeth after eating to prevent cavities, especially after eating candy, cookies, cake, chips, soft drinks, cereals, and sticky foods.**

Remember!!

❖ **Choose sugary foods less often**
❖ **Avoid sweets between meals**
❖ **Brush with toothpaste that has fluoride between meals and snacks**

Index

ABOUT THE EDITORS

Dr. Touger-Decker is an Associate Professor, Director of the Graduate Programs in Clinical Nutrition in the UMDNJ School of Health Related Professions (SHRP) and Director of the Nutrition Division at the New Jersey Dental School (NJDS). She completed her BS at New York State University College at Buffalo and her MA and PhD degrees in Clinical Nutrition from New York University.

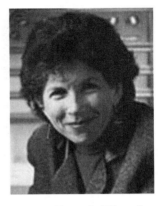

Dr. Touger-Decker's academic and research interests include nutrition and oral diseases, oral manifestations of systemic disease, and nutrition education of dietetics, dental and medical students, and practitioners. Her research experience includes nutrition education of dental students, technology-based approaches to graduate education, and nutrition and oral diseases.

She is recognized as a speaker internationally and has published in refereed journals and texts. Dr. Touger-Decker has received numerous awards including the American Dietetic Association Medallion Award and Excellence in Education awards from the American Dietetic Association Foundation and the American Society for Clinical Nutrition.

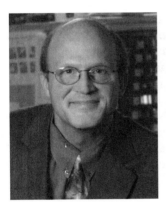

Dr. Sirois received his DMD degree from the University of Pennsylvania where he is also completed the PhD in neuroscience and clinical specialty in oral medicine. Presently, he is Chairman of Oral Medicine and Head, Division of Reconstructive and Comprehensive Care at NYU College of Dentistry. Dr. Sirois is a Diplomat of the American Board of Oral Medicine. He is a nationally recognized expert in oral medicine and lectures widely on topics related to oral mucosal disease, salivary gland disorders, chronic pain, and nutrition in dentistry. In addition to his academic and research responsibilities at NYU, Dr. Sirois also provides patient care in a private, faculty practice setting at NYU Hospital-Tisch Medical Center, where he is also a member of the Departments of Neurology and Surgery. He has published widely in the clinical and basic sciences, focusing on oral mucosal disease, medicine and dentistry, and trigeminal sensory physiology and pain.

Dr. Mobley is a Professor of Nutrition at The University of Nevada Las Vegas School of Dental Medicine and was previously at The University of Texas Health Science Center in San Antonio. She completed nutrition/dietetic degrees and clinical internships at The University of Southwestern Louisiana, Florida International University, Texas A&M University, and the University of Oklahoma Medical Center. She is a funded investigator in several hallmark multicenter National Institutes of Health dietary intervention studies examining the prevention and management of obesity and diabetes in children and adults. Her contributions as an investigator and clinical instructor include infant and child dental nutrition, aging and oral health, and nutrition education in dental schools. She has been an invited speaker at international meetings. She has numerous publications in books, monographs, and refereed journals and serves on local, state, and national public health committees. She has received awards from public broadcasting radio for her work in women's health, the American Cancer Society, and was selected as Distinguished Scientist by the Texas Dietetic Association.

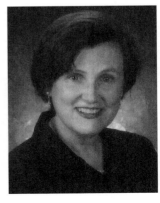

ABOUT THE SERIES EDITOR

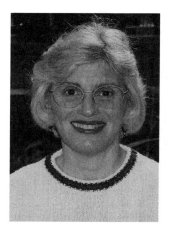

Dr. Adrianne Bendich is Clinical Director of Calcium Research at GlaxoSmithKline Consumer Healthcare, where she is responsible for leading the innovation and medical programs in support of TUMS and Os-Cal. Dr. Bendich has primary responsibility for the direction of GSK's support for the Women's Health Initiative intervention study. Prior to joining GlaxoSmithKline, Dr. Bendich was at Roche Vitamins Inc., and was involved with the groundbreaking clinical studies proving that folic acid-containing multivitamins significantly reduce major classes of birth defects. Dr. Bendich has co-authored more than 100 major clinical research studies in the area of preventive nutrition. Dr. Bendich is recognized as a leading authority on antioxidants, nutrition, immunity, and pregnancy outcomes, vitamin safety, and the cost-effectiveness of vitamin/mineral supplementation.

In addition to serving as Series Editor for Humana Press and initiating the development of the 15 currently published books in the *Nutrition and Health*™ series, Dr. Bendich is the editor of nine books, including *Preventive Nutrition: The Comprehensive Guide for Health Professionals.* She also serves as Associate Editor for *Nutrition: The International Journal of Applied and Basic Nutritional Sciences,* and Dr. Bendich is on the Editorial Board of the *Journal of Women's Health and Gender-Based Medicine,* as well as a past member of the Board of Directors of the American College of Nutrition.

Dr. Bendich was the recipient of the Roche Research Award, a *Tribute to Women and Industry* Awardee, and a recipient of the Burroughs Wellcome Visiting Professorship in Basic Medical Sciences, 2000–2001. Dr. Bendich holds academic appointments as Adjunct Professor in the Department of Preventive Medicine and Community Health at UMDNJ, Institute of Nutrition, Columbia University P&S, and Adjunct Research Professor, Rutgers University, Newark Campus. She is listed in *Who's Who in American Women.*